WOMEN'S FITNESS PROGRAM DEVELOPMENT

Ann F. Cowlin, MA
Yale University

Human Kinetics

Library of Congress Cataloging-in-Publication Data

Cowlin, Ann F., 1946-
   Women's fitness program development / Ann F. Cowlin.
      p. cm.
Includes bibliographical references and index.
   ISBN 0-088011-937-3
   1. Physical fitness for women. I. Title.
   GV482 .C69 2002
   613.7'045--dc21

                                    2002002997

ISBN: 0-088011-937-3

Acquisitions Editor: Michael S. Bahrke, PhD; **Developmental Editor:** Christine M. Drews; **Managing Editor:** Sandra Merz Bott; **Copyeditor:** Joyce Sexton; **Proofreader:** Jim Burns; **Indexer:** Marie Rizzo; **Permission Manager:** Dalene Reeder; **Graphic Designer:** Fred Starbird; **Graphic Artist:** Dawn Sills; **Photo Manager:** Leslie A. Woodrum; **Cover Designer:** Keith Blomberg; **Photographer (cover):** Carl D. Johnson; **Photographer (interior):** Ann F. Cowlin; **Art Managers:** Carl D. Johnson and Kelly Hendren; **Illustrators:** Mic Greenberg and Tom Roberts; **Printer:** Versa Press

Printed in the United States of America   10 9 8 7 6 5 4 3 2 1

Human Kinetics
Web site: www.HumanKinetics.com

United States: Human Kinetics
P.O. Box 5076
Champaign, IL 61825-5076
800-747-4457
e-mail: humank@hkusa.com

Canada: Human Kinetics
475 Devonshire Road Unit 100
Windsor, ON N8Y 2L5
800-465-7301 (in Canada only)
e-mail: orders@hkcanada.com

Europe: Human Kinetics
107 Bradford Road, Stanningley
Leeds LS28 6AT, United Kingdom
+44 (0)113 255 5665
e-mail: hk@hkeurope.com

Australia: Human Kinetics
57A Price Avenue
Lower Mitcham, South Australia 5062
08 8277 1555
e-mail: liahka@senet.com.au

New Zealand: Human Kinetics
P.O. Box 105-231, Auckland Central
09-523-3462
e-mail: hkp@ihug.co.nz

CONTENTS

PREFACE

Women are different from men in fundamental ways. Physically, mentally, emotionally, and socially they differ from men, and they go through a very different life cycle than men. Why are these differences important to the fitness field? Most current models of fitness programs are based on male paradigms. Even where women are involved, they are participating in activities originally based on male-centered values and philosophies. Although some women have adapted to this male-based system, some more easily than others, most have not.

We need to step back and view women as a whole population, not just the women currently operating within the sport and fitness world. In so doing, we may find that we can design fitness programs that reach and benefit many more women than are currently participating, and we may find new ways of presenting fitness programs that better meet women's needs.

Bringing more women into a lifestyle that includes fitness is important. Public health experts agree that adequate physical activity contributes to health at all stages of life and for both sexes. To bring more women into this arena, we need models that are attractive and understandable to women. Adolescence, childbearing, and menopause are experiences within the female life cycle that provide platforms for the development of meaningful models. Whether or not a woman reproduces, her reproductive physiology and the psychosocial milieu in which it is played out profoundly affect her participation in what we consider physical fitness.

This text deals with the process of evolving effective gender-based fitness models for women. It comprises an introductory chapter followed by four major parts: Adolescence, Pregnancy, Postpartum Period, and Menopause. Each of the four parts opens with background information relevant to understanding the given period in the female life cycle and its relationship to physical activity. Subsequent discussion concerns the setting of goals and priorities based on this understanding. Each part of the book concludes with suggestions for program design to meet the goals and priorities for that particular period in women's lives.

ACKNOWLEDGMENTS

Preparing a manuscript starts well before the first words are put on paper. In the case of this book, it began many years ago. A life-long mentor to me has been E. Noel McIntosh, physician, researcher, educator, and currently the president of the Johns Hopkins Program for International Education in Reproductive Health (JHPIEGO). Under Noel's auspices doors have opened for me in the world and in my mind. He has helped me turn research into practice and to do work that is meaningful and that makes a significant, positive contribution to women's health. Two other physician/researchers have been truly generous, making it possible for me to learn first-hand how women benefit from becoming mentally and physically empowered: John C. Hobbins and James F. Clapp, III.

I have also been fortunate to have as mentors a number of nursing professionals, including Helen Varney Burst, professor, Yale University School of Nursing, past director of the nurse-midwifery program at the school, and past president of the American College of Nurse-Midwives; and, Lois S. Sadler, associate professor, Yale University School of Nursing, and director of the pediatric nurse practitioner program at the school. Ann Dacey, perinatal nurse educator at the West Virginia University Medical Center, is a valued friend. It is she who first asked me to begin a movement program for pregnant women and provided me with a supportive environment in which to do so. Peggy DeZinno, coordinator of the Women's Education, Life Learning (WELL) program at Yale-New Haven Hospital; Judy Maddeux, associate director of the Yale Health Plan; and, Marilyn Hirsch, ob/gyn care coordinator at Yale-New Haven Hospital, are great compatriots in learning, teaching, and facilitating.

During my dance career and academic pursuits in movement and exercise, I have had the good fortune to learn from or work with many notable professionals. Iris Merrick (my first ballet teacher), Evelyn LeMone, Alma M. Hawkins, Mia Slavenska, Alwin Nikolais, Jose Limon, Beth Lessard, Phyllis Haskell, Florence Davich, Bill Evans, Douglas Dunn, Barbara Feldman, and June Kennedy are present with me in every movement. Valerie Hunt, my first kinesiology professor, brought the analysis of human movement alive for me in terms I was burning to hear. Pam Matt and Andre Bernard—with whom I studied ideokinesis—opened the world of mindful movement and helped me find a methodology for moving and teaching in a centered way. Two exercise scientists—Christine Wells and Loretta DiPietro—have been generous friends, listening and providing feedback for many of my maverick concepts. Many colleagues at Yale have allowed me to sit in on lectures, audit courses (thank you, Tom Brown, for the graduate seminar in systems of the brain), and participate in conversations outside my field.

When I started Dancing Thru Pregnancy® in 1979, I knew it would grow, but had no idea how much. Deborah DeLap Palmer, Virginia W. Eicher, Dana Zygmont, Barbara Perry, Gina Donato, Sue McHenry, Kathy LaMountain, Wendy Meyer-Goodwin, Monique Nemarich, Rena V. O'Connor, Betsy B. Wasiniak, Pamela Hutchinson, and Jamie Levine are among the faculty members and advisors involved at various stages with the company's development. Feedback from the thousands of pre/postnatal and menopause instructors and trainers we have put into the field through our educational seminars, and from the hundreds of thousands of women who have participated in our programs, has been invaluable in preparing this text. The adolescent mothers with whom I work are a constant source of inspiration.

I have also had great good fortune in my editors at Human Kinetics. Scott Wikgren—with whom I first spoke about this project—was so *sympatico* that I knew I was in the right place. Mike Bahrke has been a most patient acquisition editor. Managing editor Sandra Merz Bott has, in very calm and reassuring ways, provided the relentless attention to detail required by this tangled subject. The copyeditor, Joyce Sexton, and the graphic artist who provided the layout, Dawn Sills, have both contributed greatly to the cogency of the work. A special note of gratitude is due to Chris Drews, the development editor, who did the surgery! Chris handed me the literary tools to take an overgrown garden, in which it was sometimes difficult to tell the treasures from the weeds, and turn it into an organized and sensible whole.

Finally, I express gratitude to my family—each and every one. You have been constant and more than generous throughout the process. I am sure you are as much relieved as pleased to see this in print. To my husband: I never could have done it without you and the singing fish.

CHAPTER 1

FOCUSING ON FEMALES

This introductory chapter starts by identifying how it is that one0"ccomes a *female*, then looks at women's anatomy and physiology, life cycle issues, and social preferences. Next it briefly reviews current models of exercise for indications of why they do or don't appeal to women. The chapter closes with a discussion of how this knowledge aids the derivation of new fitness models focusing on women's needs and desires.

DEVELOPMENT OF SEX, GENDER, AND BODY IMAGE

The genes of most women include two X chromosomes, while most men have one X and one Y chromosome. This genetic material is responsible for generating many of the characteristics we refer to as *female* or *male*. Occasionally there are three chromosomes, which can confuse matters. There are also factors beyond genes that contribute to gender identities and social roles. Despite having genes of one sex, a person may develop physical, mental, emotional, or social characteristics of the other sex as a consequence of biological or cultural influences. For most of the 20th century, the question whether an individual became female or male, and to what extent, was considered a nature versus nurture issue.

In 1985, sex researcher John Money of Johns Hopkins University suggested expanding our concept of the development of gender from the simple dualism of nature versus nurture to the more complex model of nature-critical period-nurture [1]. Studying determinants of gender identity/role, including genetics and psychosexual development [2], prenatal hormone exposures [3], sex assignment at birth [4], and abnormal genetic syndromes [5-8],

Money concluded that the only irreducible sex differences are that females menstruate, gestate, and lactate and that males impregnate. Although his practical experiments have become controversial, Money is credited with bringing about a breakthrough in our understanding of how sexuality develops: the programming of sexual dimorphism into the brain under the influence of prenatal hormones appears to be sex-shared and threshold-dimorphic (i.e., the components of femininity and masculinity that will shape brain structure and activity can be influenced by a variety of sequential hormonal events at critical periods in utero) [1]. From conception through adolescent development and with decreasing plasticity through adulthood, aspects of gender can be influenced by genetics, hormonal expression, and behavior.

For purposes of this text, two important observations accompany this information. First, the majority of those who identify themselves as girls and women develop the capacity for irreducible female sex characteristics (menstruation, gestation, and lactation); and second, it is the underlying biological causes of these same characteristics that so greatly affect the life experience of girls and women. Menstruation, gestation, lactation, and the biological events that cause them are a large part of the genetic, environmental, and hormonal flux in which females exist and accrue their body image, which serves as a foundation for self-image.

When we examine brain function, it is easy to see why body image is literally the basis of self-image: the *homunculus* (see figure 1.1), or "little person," within the cerebral cortex is an ephemeral entity whose existence derives from actual experience. Sensation and movement activate brain cells within the sensory and motor cortex regions that correspond to the participating body parts, literally turning on awareness of the body parts and plugging them into our sense of self within our experiences. When we think *I,* the foundation is the homunculus.

If the images and messages about ourselves that we receive from the culture reinforce this inner experience, there is consonance. If the images and messages run counter to experience, there is dissonance. Girls and women experience the body as a menstruating, gestating, and lactating form—in a cycle during which several circulating female hormones plug into receptors in the brain, organs, heart, bones, and glands. The body offers up a variety of sensations during the month, and the mood shifts. At some life stages (i.e., puberty, pregnancy, and menopause), the body changes dramatically, and thoughts and feelings diverge from previous norms. At the same time, girls and women are exposed to the static, androgynous images of women that dominate Western culture. The ultrathin model's body and boylike superstar athletic build are everywhere present in advertising: *Buy this thing so you can look like this.* When pregnancy is portrayed in the media, it is the Hollywood version—gleaming and ripe, a desirable state of being. But when adolescent girls become pregnant, they are somehow bad, representing one of society's ills. The media serves up idealized midlife and older women who deny age. Being female in today's world is no simple task. Where are girls and women to look in order to see themselves pictured in an authentic way?

EMPHASIZING FEMALE ANATOMY

The starting point may be rewriting the books on anatomy, beginning with the skeleton. In that venerable grandfather of anatomy textbooks, *Gray's Anatomy,* the description of the skeleton begins with the spine; continues with rib cage, shoulder girdle, and head; then proceeds to the *extremities* (arms, legs, and pelvis). Both the 1977 and 1993 editions of the *Anatomy Coloring Book* identify the axial skeleton as the "skull, vertebrae, sternum, ribs, hyoid bone" and the remainder as "the appendicular skeleton." These descriptions were written by men—as were similar descriptions in a number of other standard anatomy texts—and that they are never challenged holds a clue to how deeply embedded in Western culture the male perspective of the body is.

For women, the axial skeleton is the spine, head, and pelvis. Reimaging the skeleton is central to teaching girls to know who they are and how their bodies work. The male image of the core body, with its emphasis on the upper torso and its deletion of the pelvis, devalues the physics and the experience of the female form.

During and after adolescence, the male's upper-body muscle mass becomes larger than the female's. The adult male upper body is actually and proportionally larger and the pelvis proportionally more narrow, resulting in a cen-

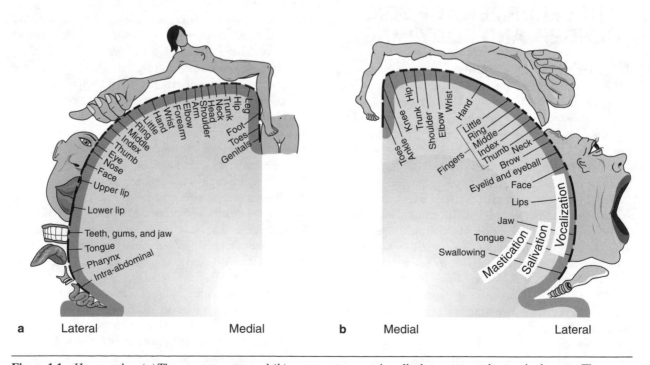

| a | Lateral | Medial | b | Medial | Lateral |

Figure 1.1   Homunculus. *(a)* The sensory cortex and *(b)* motor cortex contain cells that correspond to our body parts. They are activated when we have sensations or move, and form the physiological basis of our sense of self.

ter of gravity that is above the pelvis and less stable. But the male physique also has the ability to manipulate the environment through powerful arms. Women, with a lower center of gravity that is within the pelvis, are more stable; women move more three-dimensionally in the lower extremities because of a greater rotation in the iliofemoral (hip) joint during weight-bearing functional motion.

For women there are a greater number and variety of pelvis-based experiences than for men. Women center their body weight, menstruate, experience sex, and reproduce all within the pelvis. Research has focused on quantitative issues, such as how much high intensity exercise will affect fertility, whether women and men vary in muscle damage in response to power lifting, or how much training produces an increased risk for anterior cruciate ligament (ACL) injury in women. In the design of programs for girls and women, the importance of an accurate description of female anatomy and of female-based principles of biomechanical function remains unappreciated.

Research Shows Damage

There are, however, indications for study. There is an incongruity between how females are taught to image their bodies and how their bodies prefer to move; and this discrepancy does, in fact, lead to damage. Consider the following findings, which taken together suggest the need to design fitness experiences around women's anatomy.

The first piece of the puzzle is a finding from the Minnesota Heart Health Program study, showing that the approach of using multiple intervention components can produce lasting improvement in adolescent females' physical activity levels [9]. For girls, it is critical to approach the material from a variety of angles, to set up multiple tasks around an issue. The second piece is the Child and Adolescent Trial for Cardiovascular Health study, a multisite (California, Louisiana, Minnesota, and Texas) prospective school-based study of 6000 students, looking at health behaviors in an intervention group versus control group, which showed that girls reported significantly greater perceived reinforcement for healthy eating than did boys [10]. The third piece is from the Adolescent Injury Control Study, a large, population-based prospective study of adolescent injuries conducted in western Pennsylvania. In a cohort of 641 males and 604 females ages 12 to 16, of the reported 1076 injuries, 55% of injuries to males occurred in unsupervised settings [11]—an important, but not surprising, finding. What is not directly reported, but can be inferred from information about the percentage of female injuries oc-

curring in physical education classes (16%) and the percentage of female injuries occurring in interscholastic sports (48%), is that *64% of female injuries occurred in supervised settings*. The fourth piece of the puzzle is establishment of the fact that one of the most devastating athletic injuries—ACL damage—occurs more frequently in collegiate and elite female soccer and basketball players than in similar males [12-14]. The fifth and last piece of the puzzle is the finding that women's ACL injuries occur more frequently during ovulation when levels of estrogen, and particularly relaxin (the hormone responsible for softening female connective tissue), are increased [15].

These seemingly unrelated bits of information point toward a theory proposing that during the maturing process, when girls are developing lifestyle habits, they are more readily influenced by reinforcement from carefully structured social settings than boys—and that this influence may not always be in their best interest. If their injuries frequently occur in supervised activities, might they be receiving information that predisposes them to danger? When we see this taken to the extreme, as in the case of highly motivated amateur and professional athletes, are we seeing the result of long-term training methods that are inappropriate for female bodies?

Female-Based Biomechanics

The point of departure for biomechanics appropriate to the female form is the pelvis. There are four basic types of pelvises: gynecoid, android, anthropoid, and platypelloid—based largely on proportions of bony structures that affect giving birth [16]. As with ectomorphic, mesomorphic, and endomorphic body types, most persons are a mixture of pelvic types. However, women and men tend toward differing pelvic types, and this is evident as early as three or four months of gestation. A starting point in protecting girls' bodies might be to replace the standard image of the pelvis as the typically male, or android type, with images of the more typically female gynecoid and anthropoid types, and to create more activities in which movements are based on resulting female biomechanics. One specific, concrete feature of a more female pelvis that affects biomechanics is the placement of the acetabulum, the pelvic half of the iliofemoral joint that is often referred to as a socket. In the female pelvis the acetabulum is at a slightly more lateral, downward angle than in the male pelvis (see figure 1.2). This phenomenon affects all motion involving the legs.

The principle of the pie is at work here. Through small, but significant, alterations in the way a female moves at the level of the pelvis, the effect at the distal ends of the anatomy may be quite large—much as a slight change in

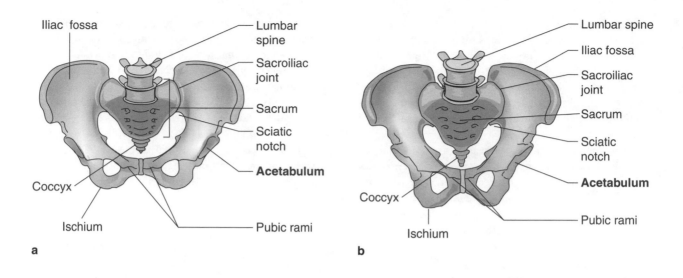

Figure 1.2   Pelvis (anterior views). Note the difference in the placement of the acetabulum for *(a)* the female pelvis which is at a slightly more lateral, downward angle than in *(b)* the male pelvis which is more frontal and has a less downward pitch than the female.

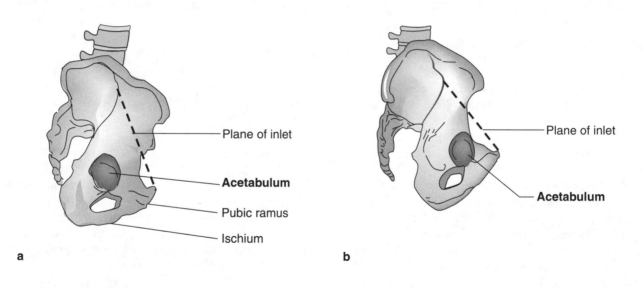

Figure 1.3   Pelvis (right lateral views). Note the longer distance from the pubis to the sacral table in *(a)* the female pelvis compared to that of *(b)* the male. Also note the relative placement of the coccyx in relation to the pubis in each figure.

the angle of a piece of pie at the center drastically changes the length of the arc at the outer rim. Consequently, the entire volume of a motion is affected, as is distribution of weights, forces, and stresses.

For example, there is a strength exercise that is done in the lunge position, with one leg forward and one behind the pelvis. The muscles of the forward thigh are strengthened through the lowering and raising of the torso as the person flexes and extends the forward leg. As traditionally taught, the motion at the hip (iliofemoral joint) of the forward leg consists purely of flexion and extension, which is consistent with the placement of the ac-

etabulum in the more typically male pelvis. This placement also explains why running is often a more efficient movement for the male than for the female. However, in female biomechanics, inward rotation accompanies the flexion and outward rotation accompanies the extension in the hip of the forward leg to accommodate the placement of the acetabulum in the more typically female pelvis. This results in spiraling of the entire torso toward the front thigh as the weight is lowered and spiraling away from the front leg as it is raised. If the hands are placed on the hips, with elbows bent, the arc of the elbows through space is quite large. Iliofemoral rotation also alters the adjustments made in the legs. If the hip of the back leg remains fixed, there is a small arc of the back knee through space and a pivot action on the ball of the back foot. On the front leg, supination and pronation in the forward ankle are needed, as well as small adjustments in the front knee. As we teach this exercise to women, it is important to teach them to do these actions in their individual bodies to the degree that most reduces stressful sensations in the forward knee associated with the traditional way of executing the action.

A second significant, concrete feature of the female pelvis that affects biomechanics is the vertical distance between the sacral table and pubis symphysis. In women, the vertical distance tends to be greater than in men so that the inlet is larger, making more space for a baby to enter the birth canal (see figure 1.3). It is partly because of this difference in arrangement that the center of gravity falls lower in relation to the sacrum in women than in men, contributing to the stability of the female. This difference also brings the acetabula closer together in the male than in the female, so that the carriage of weight from the top of the male body—where the width of the shoulder mass is much greater than the width of the pelvis—via the iliofemoral joints to the ground resembles an inverted triangle, which is highly unstable. This greatly affects the choice of a stable stance for the male as one in which the feet are far enough apart to form a base at least as wide as the shoulders. With the feet pointed forward, this sets up the body as two opposing, immobile second-class levers. This wide parallel stance for stability is frequently employed in fitness programs as a starting position.

A helpful change to make with females is to alter the stance used as a starting point, especially in preparation for movement. Because the axial skeleton in women is head, spine, and pelvis, the carriage of weight in the upper body conforms to the plumb line in the torso, then flows outward from the sacrum (functioning as the keystone of an arch) through the right and left iliacus bones to the acetabula and straight down the plumb lines of each leg. Placing the ankles directly under the acetabula permits the carriage of weight to resemble a tall, thin upright triangle. Thus, for women, a stance with the feet about 6 or 8 inches apart is helpful for balance and alignment and as a preparation for movement. In this narrower stance, the principle of balance is equipoise, or use of the body as a first-class lever. In the female model, this stance reduces stress at the knee as weight is lowered and raised to warm up muscles of the legs. It also makes it possible to move in any direction without a preparation. With a wider stance, it is necessary for a female to shift weight to one leg prior to moving in a direction in space.

Figure 1.4 shows an often practiced male model of a preparatory stance. With feet at least shoulder-width apart so that stability provides balance, the male's legs are slightly abducted. In executing a squat, the male's knees flex safely over the feet as the iliofemoral joint flexes in parallel posture, as shown in figure 1.5. However, in the female, the action of inward rotation often accompanies iliofemoral flexion in this position as shown in figure 1.6, placing the knees in a vulnerable position. Placing the ankles in line vertically below the acetabula improves this position considerably, as shown in figure 1.7.

For safely aligning the knees in a wider stance, the alternative is to allow females to use their six outward deep rotator muscles: piriformis, gemellus superior, gemellus inferior, obturator externus, obturator internus, and quadratus femoris (see figure 1.8). These muscles, which work in synchrony, attach proximally at the lateral aspect of the lower sacrum and posterior portions of the ischium, and attach distally at the greater trochanter. Contracting these muscles to aim the knees safely over the feet prompts the outward rotation of the entire leg as a natural response, shown in figure 1.9. It can also be helpful to prompt women to supinate the feet slightly ("Lift the arches" or "Cup your feet") to assist rotation.

Mechanical advantages derive from outward rotation of the leg, including an extended range of motion in abduction because the greater trochanter is no longer limited by the iliacus. In flexion and extension of the iliofemoral joint, the adductors and pelvic floor muscles are also brought into play as synergists and antagonists, thus enabling control of rotary action. The interplay of internal and external rotators during locomotion guides rotation at the center of the iliofemoral joint, reducing stress at the knee.

While women are warming up the legs for locomotion or developing strength in the muscles that control hip action, it is important to caution them not to generate outward rotation by forcing the toes out from the distal end. Rather they should initiate rotation with the deep rotators from the proximal end (iliofemoral joint) by bringing the greater trochanter (side of the upper thigh) toward the ischial tuberosities (sitsbones). Inward rotation is initiated with the gracilis and/or medial hamstrings through slight adduction of the knee. Stabilizing is accomplished with the pelvic floor muscles, allowing the leg to rotate in the acetabulum (socket) to a comfortable degree. An example of application of this principle in practice is learning to execute a step that appears in almost every culture's dance vocabulary and is also a popular aerobic dance step known as the grapevine. In this step, the participant makes an open step to the right side with the right leg, followed by a step on the left foot that crosses over in front of the right foot, then another open right step, and a step with the left leg that crosses behind the right foot. Often, people are taught only to put the feet in the correct place in the correct order. But it is also

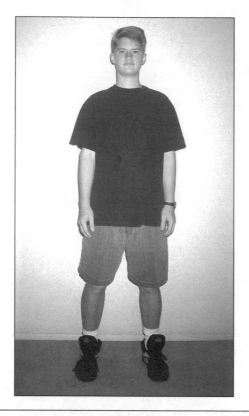

Figure 1.4 A typical preparatory stance when an adolescent male is asked to prepare for movement is wider than the hip sockets.

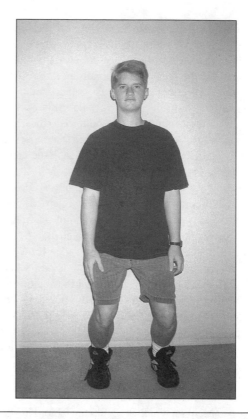

Figure 1.5 When the adolescent male is asked to squat, his knees go over his feet.

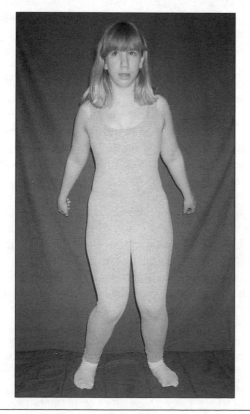

Figure 1.6 When an adolescent female takes the typical stance and squats, her femurs rotate inwardly.

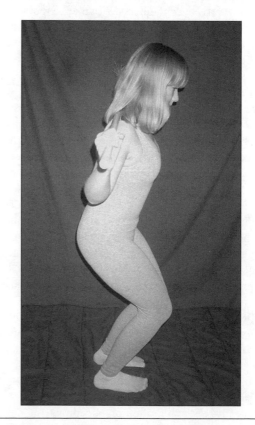

Figure 1.7 By bringing her legs closer together so her feet are directly below her iliofemoral joints, the adolescent female's biomechanics are in line with gravity when she bends.

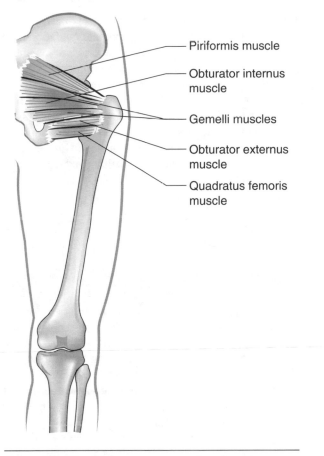

Piriformis muscle

Obturator internus muscle

Gemelli muscles

Obturator externus muscle

Quadratus femoris muscle

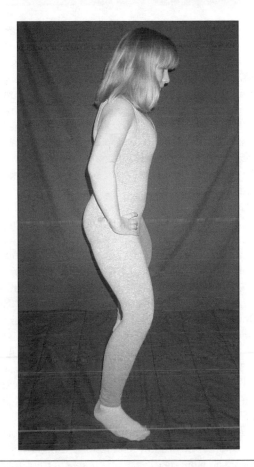

Figure 1.8 The six deep rotators seen here from the posterior aspect of the right hip joint, rotate the femur in the acetabulum in an outward circle. In a wide stance, the deep rotators guide the knees safely over the feet in the typical female anatomy.

Figure 1.9 Female squat, or plie, in the open position. Using the deep rotators as she squats, the female open position resembles a ballet plie.

important to teach how to generate the appropriate size and direction of each step based on the strength and range of the outward rotators during the open steps and the inward rotators during the crossing steps. This produces the most biomechanically sound execution of the movement in the female model.

EMPHASIZING FEMALE PHYSIOLOGY

While these anatomical revisions produce substantial alterations in motion in the female, it is equally important to note physiological differences between females and males that contribute to other alterations. Some of the changes are physical, but others are mental or emotional. Endocrine function is a realm in which the sexes diverge, and one that has an impact on the appetite for motion. Prior to puberty, the primary hormone promoting growth is pituitary growth hormone. The pituitary is active in

several regulatory functions in the endocrine system, as well as maintaining a relationship with the thyroid system. This contributes—in both sexes—to the ability of a number of organs to utilize oxygen. In the prepubescent period, improvements in strength as well as coordination, balance, and the development of individual motor skills are a result of neurological function and are similar in girls and boys [17]. However, with the onset of puberty, gonadal hormones (testosterone in males, estrogen and progesterone in females) become the primary factors in growth, and sex differences emerge.

Testosterone and androgens (anabolic steroids) from the adrenal cortex promote fusion of the epiphyses and the cessation of vertical growth (hence early maturers tend to be shorter than later maturers). In addition, estrogen, which girls secrete in much greater proportion than boys, also hastens sealing of the epiphyseal plates, contributing to the generally shorter stature of girls and women. This affects movement size and proportion. The presence of greater levels of testosterone in boys also implies that they can develop greater strength, which research would seem to bear out [17]. However, authors such as Kathleen Haywood have raised questions about the effect of cultural factors in our evaluation of this situation, pointing out that differences in absolute strength may actually be limited to the more massive male upper body [18]. Cross-sectional fiber strength in women and men is, in fact, equal. Strength factors in movement preferences may largely manifest themselves in the female's need to recruit more of her lower-body power in manipulating her environment.

What other factors related to these hormonal changes might affect movement? Differences in body composition become pronounced during puberty and adolescence. Male muscle mass continues to increase until about age 17, but female muscle mass is added only until about age 13, contributing to a lower percentage of lean body mass in women [19]. Differences in adipose (fat) tissue development and distribution during adolescence are also sex dependent. Until the age of 6 or 7, fatness varies greatly from individual to individual, with internal fat (i.e., the fat surrounding organs) growing more rapidly than subcutaneous fat. Around age 6, both sexes experience a growth spurt, with subcutaneous fat increasing until about age 12 or 13. At this point, girls' subcutaneous fat deposition shows increases for both trunk and limbs, whereas boys show decreases in limb fat and hold steady or show late-adolescent increases in trunk fat [18].

While the evolutionary imperative that led to these differences can only be guessed at, it is possibly related to the survival advantage of the female's capacity to store energy for gestation and nursing and to give birth to offspring. Is this related in some way to girls' and women's appetite for motion? Is there an association between these bodily changes and changes in interest or meaning? During adolescence, girls begin drifting away from physical activity as a satisfying experience, just as their bodies make these shifts in shape and composition. As adults, there is little to entice them back. Are we missing cues in this shift that could help us create more relevant and satisfying forms of movement?

Women also have higher levels of relaxin and elastin, two hormones that regulate the molecular structure and elasticity of collagen as well as other components of connective tissue. These hormones contribute to joint flexibility and to connective tissue's ability to stretch. They could, in part, account for women's proclivity for activities involving a large range of motion. During pregnancy, these hormones increase dramatically, allowing the abdomen to stretch to contain the growing uterus and the pelvic joints to soften to permit greater mobility within the birth canal.

Female hormones also affect the nervous system. Estrogen dominates the first portion of the menstrual cycle; follicle stimulating hormone and luteinizing hormone affect the brief midportion and generate ovulation; and progesterone dominates the last portion. Each of these has an impact on the brain. The most pronounced impact may be estrogen's effect of proliferating dendrites—the communication strands of neurons in the brain—during the first half of the cycle. This phenomenon permits enhanced communication among sections of the brain. In the latter portion of the cycle, under the influence of progesterone (when the dendrites wilt), many women feel irritable and more vulnerable to stress. Oxytocin, another female hormone, is responsible for uterine contractions in labor and is also present in the female brain during orgasm and breast-feeding, providing clues to possible differences in how women and men process pain and pleasure.

Cardiovasculature also diverges. The female heart exhibits dramatic differences from the male heart, especially from puberty on. Size, cardiac rhythm, disease etiology, and other factors all seem to be affected by sex. Estrogen appears to protect the heart during the fertile years. There is evidence that following menopause, exercise-trained women who take supplementary estrogen demonstrate higher cardiac output and lower peripheral resistance than exercise-trained women who do not take supplementary estrogen [20].

Rowland has pointed out that prior to puberty the response to endurance training appears to be blunted and that puberty probably represents a period when the body becomes more capable of an aerobic training effect [17]. The ability of the body to increase the maximum amount of oxygen it can consume during exertion before becoming anaerobic (its $\dot{V}O_2max$) is most likely due to the cardiotropic effect of testosterone and growth hormone at that time [17]. Krahenbuhl's cross-sectional meta-analysis of $\dot{V}O_2max$ for healthy, untrained children demonstrated that the mean value for boys exceeded the mean value for girls at all ages, although prior to 12 the difference was small and the rate of rise similar, while by age 16 the gender difference grew to 50% [21]. In addition, analysis demonstrated that while boys' $\dot{V}O_2max$ per kilogram remains stable through the age span of 6 to 16, girls show a progressive decline across the same age span [21]. Some of this variance may be attributable to differences in body composition; but even with correction for that factor, gender differences persist [22-24] and continue through adulthood.

Physiological differences between women and men raise questions about the applicability of aspects of many current fitness activities. Their purpose, movement shapes, intensity, or rhythm may not be optimal for many women. Might some women have better cardiovascular enhancement if they learned to keep the tennis ball in play by cooperating with other players, instead of trying to beat them? Might some of the military-style choreography in aerobics classes be replaced by motions derived from real life—loading the dryer, getting in and out of the car, brushing your hair while putting your feet into your clogs, or changing the ink cartridge in the computer printer? Might we avoid some of the incontinence problems of our female athletes by teaching them how to integrate their pelvic floor into many movements? Might we look closely at the naturally occurring patterns of aerobic intensity in the life of a young mother before telling her what her target heart rate should be when she exercises?

THE FEMALE LIFE CYCLE

We know that being a female only begins with genes. Prenatally, the female is exposed to a variety of sex hormones—and how much of which ones will profoundly affect her development. The critical period of prenatal androgen exposure will affect her physical appearance, brain development, and the way she chooses to identify herself. As a child, she will receive socialization. Some of it will be appropriate; some may not be. Her appearance as female (or male) will affect how she is treated. Observant parents, teachers, and others will take their cues from the child. But unobservant, unskilled, or abusive parents, teachers, and others may provide inappropriate feedback and contribute to identity problems. A girl may be assertive or subtly able to prevail in her quest to survive psychologically, but she may not.

During her maturation process, a girl undergoes major changes. Cognitive function as well as physical development alters drastically. She becomes subject to the rhythmic patterns of her menstrual cycle. Again, her hormone exposure dramatically affects her being, this time influencing not only her identity, but also her health. The habits she forms during this time will play a critical role in her long-term well-being, and social influences will profoundly affect her identity and sense of self-worth. If she is athletic and develops difficulties maintaining a balance of energy intake and expenditure, she may incur major health problems.

She may choose to bear children early; she may choose to postpone or eliminate childbearing; or a choice may be thrust on her. In any case, her choices or situation will follow her throughout her life. If she has children, she will forever carry aspects of the process within her body structure, all the way down to her cells. Her biomechanics, muscle balance, metabolic processes, immune system, risk of diseases, and identity are altered in powerful ways by gestation, birth, and parenting. During pregnancy, her physical balance shifts, stressing the skeleton and requiring muscles to work in new ways. Her immune system is suppressed while the baby—foreign genetic material—develops within her; later, this may translate into autoimmune disorders. Pregnancy can affect her thyroid, either increasing or decreasing its function. Birth is a major event; parenting is long and trying. Women's health is also affected by a lack of childbearing. If she is never pregnant, never carries a child to term, and never breast-feeds, a woman's mammary glands never fully mature, leaving her at increased risk of breast cancer.

When childbearing is over, and perhaps also when it is still in progress, there are again changes in a woman's hormonal cycle. As early as her mid-30s, she may begin to experience menstrual irregularities that foreshadow changes in fertility. With so much cultural focus on the attractiveness of fertile women, her self-worth may undergo much consideration as she enters the period that signals loss of fertility. As she proceeds through midlife, she loses the cardiovascular protection of high estrogen levels. This time may also signal another major change in her caretaking role, as her children prepare to leave home and her parents become more dependent. She may also be a financial provider. All of these combined stresses come at a time when she begins to lose some of her natural defenses against disease, and she is faced with decisions about how to proceed through midlife: Does she take hormones to prolong heart and bone protection or not take them to reduce her risk of cancer? Does she prolong her youth? Whatever her decisions, her lifestyle habits will play a crucial role in her well-being.

Once she is past the fertile years, a woman's lifestyle continues to play a crucial role. Forging a new identity as manager, advisor, or mentor or as a provider of care for grandchildren, she again shifts gears, recycling herself and learning new demands. Her body bears the marks. Often in Western culture, aging women have lost their value. But with the aging of the post-World War II babies, as with every stage of life through which this group of women has passed, new definitions of what it means to be a woman are emerging.

Each of these life cycle landmarks represents a challenging and meaningful experience in women's lives. If we view these landmarks as potential content around which physical activity can occur, they represent a means for creating and sustaining women's interest in being fit.

THE SOCIAL NATURE OF GIRLS AND WOMEN

In 1989, Spiegel and colleagues published a groundbreaking study showing that female breast cancer patients who participated in a supportive weekly group therapy program lived significantly longer than those who did not attend the support sessions [25]. Women with female labor support have shorter and less complicated births (see chapter 6). Research tells us that social support has a positive effect on health in relation to cardiovascular diseases (and that lack of support has a negative influence) [26]. Mounting evidence points toward the realization that social networking is a feature that appears throughout the female life cycle and is a key component in women's health.

This feature extends into physical activity. One of the differences between female and male participation in physical activities has to do with social experience. Research has shown that 10- to 11-year-old girls are motivated to participate in exercise programs as much for the social networking as for the game, while boys are motivated largely by the opportunity to practice competition and dominance [27]. Projects like a buddy system, icebreaker exercises, or the use of peer leaders to demonstrate activities encourage camaraderie and teamwork among girls and women at all stages of life. Women in prenatal and postpartum group exercise programs form profound and often lifelong friendships.

What is it about the nature of women that makes them such social creatures, dependent on contacts for meaning, motivation, and health? It could be that the particular events women undergo in their lives require assistance, or that women perceive themselves as having identity in relation to others in a way men do not. Whatever generates this phenomenon, it is another feature that must be kept in mind when it comes to designing and implementing women-centered fitness programs.

CURRENT EXERCISE MODELS

Do existing models adequately benefit girls and women? It is useful to start this inquiry with a large overview. By examining models of exercise—settings where physical activity occurs within long-standing structured regimens—we can peer into history, finding the major threads and their underlying assumptions, and ask how these models affect girls and women. Looking at history, we can easily identify three major threads that contribute to what we today call *exercise* or *physical activity:* first, competitive games and sports; second, ceremonies, festivals, and movement arts; and third, military culture and warfare.

Games and Sports

We have only to look at the Olympics to see the connection between past and present with respect to physical competition. But the ancient Greek and current modern Olympics are just one example. Many cultures have games with balls, spears, weights, and a variety of other accoutrements that teach mastery of the environment and forces of nature and that have developed into structured competitions such as soccer, javelin throwing, weightlifting, or ice skating. One of the fundamental features of games and sports is the assumption that there will be a winner and a loser, based on objective measures such as distance, speed, or the number of times something is accomplished. Does this match women-centered thinking? Some girls and women enjoy this type of competition, but many do not. Fortunately there are other assumptions underlying games and sports.

An assumption that one hopes motivates physical educators is that socialization and learning processes are taking place on the field or court or in the dance studio that extend far beyond these settings. Not only do people develop self-awareness, strength, endurance, range of motion, and other physical skills; they also develop cooperation, sharing, discipline, a sense of accomplishment, and even knowledge of basic science (gravity, force, momentum) and math (two on the right and two on the left makes four altogether) and perceptual skills (if I bend my body this way, I can squeak through that space) [28]. In well-run sport programs, girls gain self-confidence [29]. The significance of girls' participation in games and sports is so strong that one major athletic shoe manufacturer aimed an entire advertising campaign at girls based on the concept "let me play sports," illustrating the positive effect on girls' lives of participating in these activities.

Historically speaking, it has been only recently that many games requiring intense physical exertion have included women. For example, it was in 1984 that the first women's marathon was run in the modern Olympics. In press interviews following her win in the event, Joan Benoit Samuelson often remarked on her focus of running her own race, of staying within herself. While it remains clear that objectively defined winning is the chief goal of games and sports, the concept of *playing within oneself* is often cited by both winners and nonwinners as the method or primary focus in achieving the best of which one is capable. Feminizing forces in recreation and physical activity have contributed to this enlargement of the concept of winning in ritualized games and sports. In a female model, features of socialization and learning, skill building, and self-awareness form valuable aspects of games and sports, especially for girls.

Ceremonies, Festivals, and Movement Arts

Another area in which physical activity has been ritualized is the extension of the human response to recurring events in nature and human discourse—building shelter, harvesting food, giving birth, observing the equinox or the force of gravity or other stimuli—to produce ceremonies, festivals, or the ritualized movement arts we generally call dance. Every culture, on every continent, has ritual physical activities that involve expressive movement. These are preverbal expressions—movement rituals that have evolved over time. Dance clubs, parties, theater, martial arts, the circus, rodeos, arts festivals, and other settings and occasions provide contemporary opportunities to experience this preverbal activity. An assumption underlying these events is that important phenomena or occasions such as sexual attraction, marriage, birth, death, a plentiful harvest, or victory in battle—or subjective values such as beauty, truth, joy, or authenticity—can be shared experiences that give us moments of ecstasy or a glimpse of the divine.

At some point, celebration emerges from this preverbal, expressive, and transformational human behavior, and movement becomes dance. At its core, dance arises from pulse and breath, from the rhythm of work and sex, from feelings of joy and pain, from the physical condition of being human. "Before man can do anything, he must draw breath, he must move. Movement is the source and condition of life" [30]. As a result, this celebratory movement we call dance underlies all the expressive arts. Without it, one cannot paint or sculpt, play an instrument, or sing. As ethnomusicologist and dance historian Curt Sachs noted,

> The dance is the mother of the arts. . . . The creator and the thing created, the artist and the work are still one and the same thing. Rhythmical patterns of movement, the plastic sense of space, the vivid representation of a world seen and imagined—these things man creates in his own body in the dance before he uses substance and stone and word to give expression to his inner experiences. [31]

Egyptian murals, pre-Columbian artifacts, African and Native American dolls, and myriad other sources tell us that both sexes participate in ceremonies and rituals. At various times and places, one sex or the other may have dominated a particular art or ritual (Elizabethan men, for example, acting all the roles in a Shakespeare play; or the focus on women in the era of the Romantic ballet); but within the larger framework, all community members participate in such events. To the Ubakala in Nigeria, for example, ceremonies have political as well as social meaning, and these community physical activities provide the primary method of educating all adolescents in how to behave as adults [32].

The transformational properties of expressive movement provide a clue to why and how women might find these celebratory events meaningful and therefore become motivated to participate in a physical activity. Moving with others in a joyful way explains some of the ongoing popularity of well-designed and well-led aerobic dance, step aerobics, water aerobics, and similar activities whose participants are primarily women. In school, envisioning and creating an art project around a theme or event involves physical activity—large motor movements as girls show each other where an object might be placed in space or on a wall, and fine motor skills if they are drawing, cutting paper, or gluing things together. There is a sense of belonging, of intimate contact, in the ritual of bringing the vision into physical reality. Ceremony, festivity, and creativity—these are beneficial but underused conduits for bringing girls and women into the fitness realm.

Military and Warfare Culture

The recorded history of military culture and warfare is extensive. Extant literature and present-day armies provide proof of the long-standing existence of fighting mechanisms within human cultures. An underlying assumption of war is that people will fight and die and that it is therefore advantageous for warriors to be obedient, aggressive (even hypermasculine), and physically fit—that these qualities are tools of survival. Opponents of women in the military in the United States note that it is the nature of fighting in war that argues against bringing women into military culture. Discussing this issue in the *New York Times Magazine,* Fred C. Ikle, Undersecretary of Defense for Policy during the Reagan presidency, noted, "You can't cultivate the necessary commitment to physical violence and fully protect against the risk of harassment. Military life may *correctly* foster the attitudes that tend toward rape, such as aggression and single-minded assertion" [33].

Although much of the discussion regarding women in the military is not of concern here, the impact of military culture on the culture of sport and fitness is a major issue in this text. One of the first observations one makes when looking at a fitness class, a contemporary gym (or health club or wellness center), a team meeting, or any of a number of other sport or fitness activities, is the arrangement of authority. Military calisthenics, basic training, and maneuvers are the primary models for fitness training sessions. As a result, we often see what amounts to the sergeant leading the troops and a hierarchical chain of command. This may be the best method to guarantee a fighting force willing to lay down its life, but is it the best training model for girls and women?

The question is complicated by the fact that some females wish to join military culture as it has evolved, understanding all that this implies. This raises questions about the nature of sexuality. What is female? What is male? Why are some girls and women more aggressive and competitive than others? Why do some girls and women seek experiences in which they can be dominated? And, of course, how will answers affect the design of appropriate activity models for girls?

We know that the answer has something to do with the hormone exposure referred to at the beginning of the chapter. But how does hormone exposure affect motivation? Research on rats and other small mammals sheds some light on the question; rats are particularly useful in research because of their genetic and neuroendocrinological similarities to humans. Both the genetic (nature) and environmental (nurture) bases of behavior are affected by hormonal expression [1]. Increased endogenous testosterone levels (nature) can cause an increase in fighting behaviors, but so can environmental events (nurture). Victory raises the testosterone level and increases the likelihood of repeated aggressive behavior, while defeat lowers testosterone and reduces the risk of aggression in both sexes [34].

Military behavior, by necessity, relies on these phenomena. With this in mind, it may be useful to broaden the concept of sexuality into a continuum. At one end are females whose genetic material, hormone history, and consequential brain structure, genitalia, and socialization are all female. At the other end of the continuum are the corresponding males. In between there are numerous variations—a person, for example, with 46,XX congenital virilizing adrenal hyperplasia syndrome. While clearly female genetically, a woman with this syndrome has received prenatal brain androgenization (unusual doses of testosterone) and often prefers socialization as a "tomboy." This person may identify herself as female but appear less feminine than many other people. Will this person have a greater capacity for exercise than a more feminine person? Not necessarily. Will this person have different preferences for activity modes than a more feminine person? Very likely. Can this person's behavior be made more or less aggressive depending on environmental factors? Certainly.

The question whether the male military model of physical activity is beneficial for girls and women has more than one answer. There will likely always be a percentage of women for whom this model of activity is fulfilling. There will be women for whom this model now and then offers satisfaction. However, for many girls and women, this model represents the greatest potential for incongruity between an inner sense of self and outer experience, despite its prevalence. Whether the future will bring more feminizing changes to military culture and fitness culture, and whether more women will adopt a masculinizing gender identity, remain to be seen.

FEMALE-BASED EXERCISE MODELS

Having reviewed women's physical and social distinctions as well as current models of exercise, we can use this knowledge to build women-centered models. To start this process, we look at the two general areas that are most affected—movement alterations and psychosocial design factors. What alterations in movement would we expect to see in programs that are guided by female-based anatomy and physiology? What psychosocial elements would need to be present in order for us to create, implement, and evaluate programs that are meaningful and effective for girls and women? To finish this chapter, we review general concepts of what female-based exercise models could look like. Subsequent chapters will expand these concepts and look at them in detail.

Movement Alterations

In female-based exercise models, girls and women are taught to adjust their stance and posture, utilize their lower center of gravity, and work with more three-dimensional lower-body motion. Regarding stance and posture, this might mean adjusting the conventional wisdom of sport stances: teaching a narrower stance or a more outward rotation in a wide stance for playing an outfield position in softball, using a narrower stance in calisthenics and dance moves, and teaching centering to women of all ages. Sensorimotor skills that are easier for females are preferable for developing self-efficacy [35]. School physical education classes as well as community offerings for adults might encourage using balance boards and exercise balls—drawing on women's balance ability—prior to working on strength or endurance activities.

Women's three-dimensional lower-body motion leads safety-conscious instructors to teach different calisthenic and sport moves and to teach them differently to girls and women than to boys and men. For instance, when teaching girls how to find and strengthen leg rotator muscles, instructors might have girls sit to eliminate weight-bearing and then use imagery; as one example, girls could sit on the ground with their legs straight in front of them and roll their legs in and out like logs. Once they can do this easily, a buddy could offer resistance by holding the leg just above the knee. Midlife women might like to learn to draw or paint with their feet to develop lower-body motion and power. Rising from a chair in a biomechanically sound way develops leg strength and functionality for older women. For young mothers, learning to use rotation while squatting to pick up household items or children—or weighted objects that represent children—will do the same. Manufacturers might want to rethink resistance equipment design. For instance, with leg press machines it is presently not possible to generate rotation in the iliofemoral joint as the resistance plate is moved.

Specific areas of the female body are emphasized in women-centered programs. Lower-body strength is needed to support movement and lifting with the arms. Because there is less muscle mass in the upper body of females, pressure against the floor or ground with the feet provides some of the thrust that men's arms and shoulders provide. Integrated movements of the arms and legs involving resistance against the floor can be emphasized (e.g., have the participant extend the whole body by reaching up with the arms as she rises onto the balls of her feet by pushing down through the balls of her feet; the movement can be sequenced to arrive at maximum extension simultaneously in the legs, torso, and arms). Once the participant learns the technique, she can add weight to the hands, moving the weight up and overhead close to the central axis of the body.

Also, the abdomen and pelvic floor are more vulnerable in women than in men and therefore need specialized exercises. Strengthening exercises for the transverse abdominal muscle and Kegel exercises for the pelvic floor should be done by all women, at all stages of life, from adolescence forward. During pregnancy and the postpartum period, abdominal exercises become problematic, and many modifications are needed (see later chapters). Stretching the pelvic floor and learning the mechanisms involved in pushing a baby out are special activities that must be added to the Kegel exercises in pregnancy.

Psychosocial Design Factors

In designing women-centered programs, it may be necessary to reconsider what we mean by fitness as well as how it is achieved. If we are building programs for the public health sector of women, as opposed to the competitive or professional female athlete, we have to ask what the health goals at various stages of a woman's life are and how physical activity can best help achieve them. Because reproductive function plays such a critical role in making women who they are, we need to look for clues to the answers in three key periods in women's lives: adolescence, childbearing, and menopause. The concept of fitness, and also the goals and the methods for achieving goals, are different for a girl developing self-awareness as a fertile creature, a pregnant or postpartum woman, and a woman seeking relief from hot flashes or recovering from breast cancer surgery.

Traditionally, physical fitness refers to the measurable ability to perform tasks of muscle strength and endurance, cardiorespiratory endurance, flexibility, balance, and coordination, in addition to body composition. The natural ability to perform many of these tasks is seen as peaking during adolescence. Through progressive training, most people can continue to increase their fitness quotient in a steady upward direction until midlife or beyond, when the effects of aging appear to cause a decline. But women's bodies, minds, and feelings are subject to flux. Is it reasonable to expect that a single rise and then a fall will be the form of progress in women's fitness? A spiral might be more appropriate. During some periods of life, achieving a high level of fitness makes sense; when one is looking for a mate, for example, it is helpful to appear strong and desirable as a fertile creature. But at other times, just being healthy, feeling positive, moving for satisfaction, or learning about one's body is desirable. With adolescent girls, using fitness as a means to teach cognitive information may be more appropriate than making fitness the goal. For example, learning about circulation by trying activities that provide a variety of challenges to the cardiovascular system can introduce girls to how exertion alters their body. From this experience they become familiar with different types of exertion—low- or high-intensity activity, sprinting or sustained movement, gross motor activity or fine motor skill—and have a chance to register their preferences. They spend time in fitness activities but are responsible for the cognitive piece that concerns circulatory responses, rather than for changing their measurable performance of a certain event. Even with traditional strength training for young women, designing peaks and valleys within each month, quarter, or year may be more effective than a linear approach for keeping women involved in the long run.

Another aspect of designing women-centered programs relates to how results are assessed. The benchmark for success is participant response rather than quantitative analysis of performance. Of course, measurement and analysis may be needed for research purposes; but even here, we are starting to ask questions about what we should measure. Do we need to know the $\dot{V}O_2$max of a pregnant woman? Can we use Likert scales to assess how a woman feels about her motor skills in pregnancy? Can we look at her maternal adaptation after birth to assess the success of her physical activity pattern?

Integrating a variety of health-inducing activities into new models and finding new markers for health are more important in women-centered programs than determining the dose effect of individual factors. For example, a large quantity of high-intensity exercise is needed to prevent obesity and cardiovascular disorders related to detrimental body composition. However, this quantity-oriented method does not work well with many girls and women. It requires a great deal of high-intensity exercise in a population that is not favorably inclined in this direction. It may prove more useful to ask what activity pattern improves markers for type 2 diabetes than to ask how much activity reduces body fat. Sugar metabolism serves as a marker for a complex of disease factors, including stress, diet, hormone history, and immune function, as well as lifestyle. While there is much work to be done in this arena, we have good reason to believe that new models of active women and new ways of assessing health will go hand in hand.

Exercises that gradually increase range of movement are used in helping girls and women see progress. For many, this is more agreeable than measuring how much they can lift or how many times they can do something. Most women have a larger range of motion than men, which provides a starting point. If taught to develop balanced alignment, as well as strong abdominals, hip rotators, and pelvic floor muscles, they can generate greater and greater power in a larger and larger range of motion with more and more variation of movements. This result is achieved with predictability in disciplines like ballet and tai chi. One popular exercise form, aerobic dancing, aims at something similar, but runs into problems for all but the most physically talented or persevering participants. It relies on laterally symmetrical movements in sets of fours or eights, adding more and more of these phrases together in a linear fashion. This focuses attention on quantity and uniformity, thus removing awareness of the bodily sensations associated with projecting one's energy into space. In women-centered programs, it is these very sensations of manipulating energy that are tapped to help participants delineate progress. This is a concept that goes beyond kinesthesia into the perceptual realm of space beyond one's body and assessing the quality of effort.

When we peek in on a successful women-centered program, one of the key features we see is socialization: working in circles, partnering, enabling, playing follow-the-leader, or breaking into groups to improvise movements. We also see expressive, joyful, and transformational experiences, as well as choices and multitasking. We don't necessarily see a detachment from everyday life. Many successful programs take place in churches, at playgrounds, during off-hours at gyms, or even in people's homes. A successful postpartum women's exercise class might look like this:

- Periods of endurance activities in which some women are jogging, others are dancing behind strollers, some are carrying small infants, and all are chatting

- All women doing abdominal and pelvic floor exercises, but not necessarily at the same time

- Women sometimes interrupting their activities to address their infants' needs or help each other

- A point at which everyone is doing something together, laughing, and feeling exhilarated

- A chance to get centered and another chance to relax

- A seemingly disorganized group of women who are actually accomplishing many things at the same time—just as in real life

LOOKING AHEAD

This is an exciting time for girls and women, as both sexes are gaining better understanding of the female view of life. As a result, information in many fields—including fitness—is expanding. Developing new models that are gender based is a necessary step as knowledge grows. This introduction has identified central concepts for this step within the fitness field: increasing education about what distinguishes females from males, understanding how existing fitness regimens do and don't support being female, and examining what physical and psychosocial adjustments make fitness programs more women centered. The following chapters further explore these ideas, their roots, and their consequences, for adolescence, pregnancy, the postpartum period, and menopause.

REFERENCES

1. Money, J. 1985. Pediatric sexology and hermaphroditism. *Journal of Sex and Marital Therapy* 11(3):139-156.
2. Money, J. 1972. Phyletic and idiosyncratic determinants of gender identity. *Danish Medical Bulletin* 19(8):259-264.
3. Money, J. 1973. Effects of prenatal androgenization and deandrogenization on behavior in human beings. *Frontiers in Neuroendocrinology* 0(0):249-266.
4. Money, J. 1975. Ablatio penis: Normal male infant sex-reassigned as a girl. *Archives of Sexual Behavior* 41(1):65-71.
5. Watson, M.A., and Money, J. 1975. Behavior cytogenetics and Turner's syndrome: a new principle in counseling and psychotherapy. *American Journal of Psychotherapy* 29(2):166-178.
6. Money, J., Wiedeking, C., Walker, P., Migeon, C., Meyer W., and Borgaonkar, D. 1975. 47,XYY and 46,XY males with antisocial and/or sex-offending behavior: Antiandrogen therapy plus counseling. *Psychoneuroendocrinology* 1(2):165-176.
7. Money, J., Franzke, A., and Borgaonkar, D.S. 1975. XYY syndrome, stigmatization, social class, and aggression: Study of 15 cases. *Southern Medical Journal* 68(12):1536-1542.
8. Lewis, V.G., and Money, J. 1986. Sexological theory, H-Y antigen, chromosomes, gonads, and cyclicity: Two syndromes compared. *Archives of Sexual Behavior* 15(6):467-474.
9. Kelder, S.H., Perry, C.L., and Klepp, K.I. 1993. Community-wide youth exercise promotion: Long-term outcomes of the Minnesota Heart Health Program and the Class of 1989 Study. *Journal of School Health* 63(5):218-223.
10. Edmundson, E., Parcel, G.S., Feldman, H.A., Elder, J., Perry, C.L., Johnson, C.C., Williston, B.J., Stone, E.J., Yang, M., Lytle, L., and Webber, L. 1996. The effects of the Child and Adolescent Trial for Cardiovascular Health upon psychosocial determinants of diet and physical activity behavior. *Preventive Medicine* 25(4):442-454.

11. Aaron, D.J., and LaPorte, R.E. 1997. Physical activity, adolescence, and health: An epidemiological perspective. *Exercise in Sport Science Review* 25:391-405.

12. Arendt, E., and Dick, R. 1995. Knee injury patterns among men and women in collegiate basketball and soccer: NCAA data and review of literature. *American Journal of Sports Medicine* 23:694-701.

13. Engstrom, B., Forssblad, M., and Tornkvist, H. 1991. Soccer injuries among elite female players. *American Journal of Sports Medicine* 19:372-375.

14. Ireland, M.L., and Wall, C. 1990. Epidemiology and comparison of knee injuries in elite male and female United States basketball athletes. *Medicine and Science in Sports and Exercise* 22:14.

15. Huston, L.J., and Wojtys, E.M. 1996. Neuromuscular performance characteristics in elite female athletes. *American Journal of Sports Medicine* 24:427-436.

16. Varney, H. 1996. *Varney's midwifery*, 3rd ed. New York: Jones & Barlett, p. 796.

17. Rowland, T.H. 1996. *Developmental exercise physiology*. Champaign, IL: Human Kinetics.

18. Haywood, K.M. 1993. *Life span motor development,* 2nd ed. Champaign, IL: Human Kinetics.

19. Malina, R.M. 1978. Growth of muscle tissue and muscle mass. In F. Falkner and J.M. Tanner (eds.), *Human growth, Vol. 2, Postnatal growth.* New York: Plenum Press, pp. 273-294.

20. Green, J.S., Crouse, S.F., and Rohack, J.J. 1998. Peak exercise hemodynamics in exercising postmenopausal women taking versus not taking supplemental estrogen. *Medicine and Science in Sports and Exercise* 30(1):158-164.

21. Krahenbuhl, G.S., Skinner, J.S., and Kohrt, W.M. 1985. Developmental aspects of maximal aerobic power in children. *Exercise and Sport Science Review* 13:503-538.

22. Davies, C.T.M., Barnou, C., and Godfrey, S. 1972. Body composition and maximal exercise performance in children. *Human Biology* 44:195-214.

23. Kempner, H.C.G., Verschuur, R., and deMey, L. 1989. Longitudinal changes of aerobic fitness in youth ages 12 to 23. *Pediatrics and Exercise Science* 1:257-270.

24. Rutenfrans, F., Anderson, K.L., Seliger, V., Klimmer, F., Berndt, I., and Ruppell, M. 1981. Maximum aerobic power and body composition during the pubertal growth period: Similarities and differences between children of two European countries. *European Journal of Pediatrics* 136:123-133.

25. Spiegel, D., Boom, J.R., Kraemer, H.C., and Gottheil, E. 1989. Effect of psychosocial treatment on survival of patients with metastatic breast cancer. *Lancet* ii: 888-891.

26. Shumaker, S.A., and Czajikowski, S.M. (eds.). 1994. *Social support and cardiovascular disease.* NY: Plenum Press.

27. Lever, J. 1976. Sex differences in the games children play. *Social Problems* 23:476-487.

28. Arnold, P.J. 1988. *Education, movement and the curriculum.* NY: Falmer.

29. Lirrg, C. 1992. Girls and women, sport and self-confidence. *Quest* 44:158-178.

30. DeMille, A. 1963. *The book of the dance.* NY: Golden Press, p. 7.

31. Sachs, C. 1937/1963. *World history of the dance.* NY: Norton, p. 3.

32. Hanna, J.L. 1979. *To dance is human: A theory of nonverbal communication.* Austin, TX: University of Texas Press.

33. Ikle, F.C. 1997. Quoted in Rayner, R., Women as warriors, *NY Times Magazine,* June 22, 1997, p. 29

34. Monaghan, E.P., and Glickman, S.E. 1992. Hormones and aggressive behavior. In J.B. Becker, S.M. Breedlove, and D. Crews (eds.), *Behavioral endocrinology.* Cambridge: MIT Press, pp. 261-285.

35. Becker, J.B. 1992. Hormonal influences on extrapyramidal sensorimotor function and hippocampal plasticity. In J.B. Becker, S.M. Breedlove, and D. Crews (eds.), *Behavioral endocrinology.* Cambridge, MA: MIT Press, pp. 325-356.

PART I

ADOLESCENCE

Adolescence is a complicated time for a girl. It is a major life transition for her as a sexual being, a thinking and feeling being, and a social being. The physiological processes involve astonishing physical changes, alterations in mood, increased stress about appearance and acceptance, and the potential for health or disease. Moreover, these processes take place in a complex social setting, where cultural pressures to value interdependency and sensitivity collide with other pressures to develop an aggressive, independent, and emotionally detached identity. Transferring love of parents to oneself and one's peers is another complicated process. A central feature of all these aspects is the self. What adolescent girls do is become women. Why not turn their fitness programs into the study of themselves?

Part I begins with a chapter that discusses the major features of female adolescence as well as physical, mental, and social challenges faced during this period. The next chapter looks at the issues involved in establishing goals and priorities. It recommends short-term, medium-term, and long-term goals of fitness programs for adolescent girls, in addition to priorities. The final chapter in this part of the book describes the types of programs that can be effective in achieving goals and priorities and provides a sample curriculum for such programs.

CHAPTER 2

UNDERSTANDING FEMALE ADOLESCENCE

This chapter focuses on background information about adolescent girls and physical activity. It starts by defining adolescence and several related terms. Then it looks at the physiological processes underlying adolescence in females and some of the major health issues for girls that are associated with these processes. The chapter next examines social issues of adolescence for girls and the importance of physical activity in addressing needs that arise from these issues. A final section of the chapter concerns ways to use this information in creating new models of fitness for adolescent girls.

DEFINING ADOLESCENCE

Adolescence, generally defined as the period of time between childhood and adulthood, includes major physical changes associated with reproductive ability, cognitive leaps, and experimental behaviors that often become lifelong habits. While adolescence is the time when sex differences become visible, often it is the invisible aspects of the process that spell out how a child will emerge from adolescence and whether she will become a healthy, well-adjusted adult.

Puberty is the term usually associated with the change in reproductive status that is part of adolescence. Puberty is generated by genetics, nutrition, and hormones and can also be modified by the psychological state [1]. It is accompanied by an astonishing array of alterations for the female. As indications that women are approaching a fertile reproductive status, changes in the skeleton and genitalia occur, as do internal changes in energy production. The onset of *menarche*—or the start of menstrual cycles—often occurs between the ages of 10 and 12, al-

though it is not uncommon for menstruation to begin as early as 9 and as late as 16. Although a girl may be menstruating, it is *ovulation*—or the release of a mature egg—that marks fertility, and this does not necessarily occur with the first menstrual cycle.

PHYSIOLOGY OF THE ADOLESCENT GIRL

Understanding the physiological functions present in the adolescent female is vital in work with this population. These functions affect cognition, growth, fertility, energy production, and health status. Keep in mind that adolescence is a complex process. Identity is being created on several levels—physical, psychological, and social. Along with these developing functions, each girl responds to the associated changes, and others respond to her as she changes. In the process, a major life transition takes place.

Changes Prior to Puberty

Prior to puberty, events related to sexuality have already occurred. Some of these, such as genetic events and prenatal hormone exposure, we have already covered. But there are other hormonal events that precede the onset of puberty. *Adrenarche*—the turning on of adrenal gland androgen activity beginning at about 6 years of age—may be the first marked step in the process. *Dehydroepiandrosterone* is a weak adrenal androgen that is partially responsible for alterations in behavior, a growth spurt, and changes in complexion that occur at this time. *Androgens*—male steroid hormones such as testosterone and androsterone that control the development and maintenance of traditional male characteristics—are active at neurological sites, including locations in the cerebral cortex and hypothalamus (which participates in regulation of sex hormone activity), implicating these hormones in the development of cognitive skills and emotional and social changes.

The infantile pituitary and ovaries are capable of functioning, but the hypothalamus does not secrete enough *gonadotropin-releasing hormone* (GnRH) for functioning to actually occur. A signal from other brain regions, probably the limbic system, is required to initiate function. The role of brain systems in this part of the process indicates that cognitive changes precede the physical maturation process [2].

Menstrual Cycle

Around the age of 8, the hypothalamus is stimulated to begin releasing much higher levels of GnRH. Eventually, the pituitary releases *follicle stimulating hormone* (FSH), which promotes the maturing of the *follicle,* and *luteinizing hormone* (LH), which promotes ripening of

the ovum. The ovarian hormones, *estrogen* and *progesterone,* are stimulated in response to sufficient levels of FSH and LH.

At the time of *ovulation,* or releasing of the ovum (see figure 2.1) a mature graafian *follicle* ruptures, sending the *ovum* down the *fallopian tube* toward the uterus. The follicle, which produces estrogen and progesterone, is called the *corpus luteum.* This phase of the cycle is the *luteal phase;* a shortening of this phase due to an imbalance between energy intake and output is a dysfunction that can create fertility problems. If the ovum is fertilized (see figure 2.2), the follicle becomes the *corpus luteum of pregnancy* and continues to produce progesterone to help maintain the uterus and prepare it for implantation of the ovum in the *endometrium,* or lining of the uterus. After the fertilized ovum is implanted, placental production of progesterone begins. If the ovum is not fertilized, there is a decline in the corpus luteum, leading ultimately to *menstruation,* or the actual bleeding phase.

Progesterone is one of the *gonadal hormones*—those produced largely by the ovaries, or female gonads (the male gonads are the testes). The influence of progester-

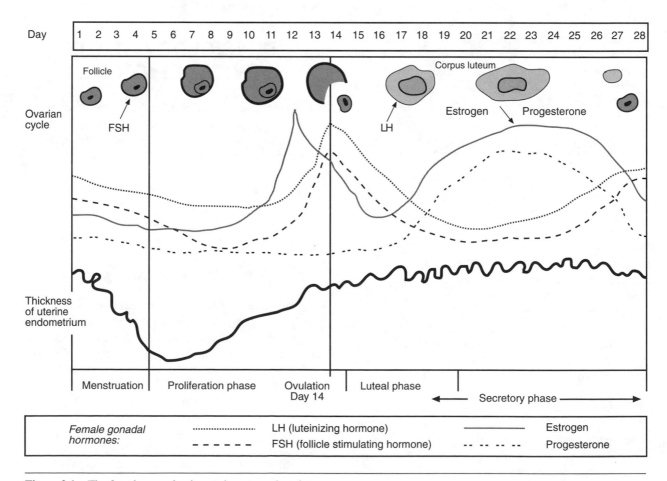

Figure 2.1   The female reproductive cycle or sexual cycle.

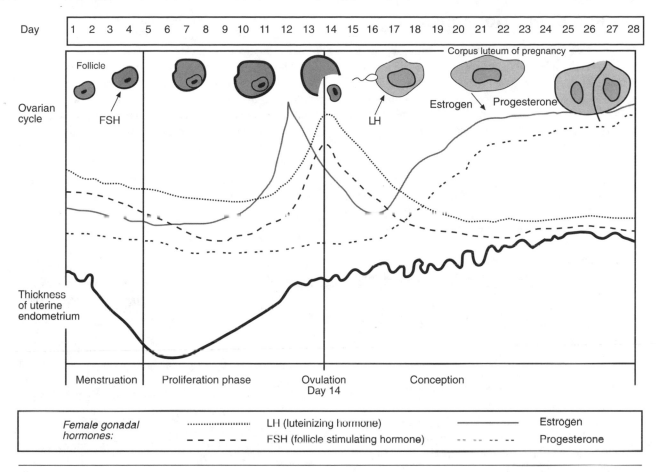

Figure 2.2 Conception.

one is secretory; that is, progesterone stimulates the glands responsible for mucosa and for the nourishment of an embryo. The *secretory phase* is the phase of the cycle in which progesterone is producing this influence. The effect of progesterone on the glands of the breasts is to cause swelling.

Estrogen is a term that applies to a family of hormones—primarily *estradiol, estriol,* and *estrone.* In its various forms estradiol, the most powerful of the three, is also primarily a gonadal hormone and accounts for most of the circulating estrogen during the fertile years. Its function is largely to promote hyperplasia (cell growth and division); it is also produced by the placenta in pregnancy.

Estriol, a weak estrogen, is also secreted by the placenta and/or metabolized from estrone. Estrone is derived mainly from androstenedione (a weak androgen) in fat cells; it accounts for the remaining circulating estrogen and is associated with postmenopausal metabolism, when it is derived with increasing efficiency.

The effect of estrogen on bone is to increase osteoblast activity, which is why puberty produces a growth spurt in girls. The effect of estrogen on the uterus and

sex organs after puberty is about 20 times its prior effect. This leads to an increase in the size of the genitalia, changes the *vaginal epithelium* from a cuboidal to a stratified tissue type (making it more resistant to trauma and infection), and causes an increase in the endometrium. In the breasts, estrogen is responsible for an increase in fat deposits and development of the epithelium and duct system.

Regulation of the reproductive cycle is achieved through several rhythmical mechanisms in the neuroendocrine systems. Neuronal activity in the arcuate nuclei of the mediobasal hypothalamus causes a pulse release of GnRH, which is modified at various limbic brain centers. The *pulsatile secretion* of GnRH occurs for several minutes every 1 to 3 hours. As a consequence LH, and to a certain extent FSH, are released in a pulsatile output as well. *Inhibin,* a hormone produced by the corpus luteum, inhibits FSH and LH. Estrogen and progesterone also inhibit FSH and LH, as does GnRH, though to a lesser extent. A preovulatory surge of LH is required in order for ovulation to occur. The *feedback oscillation process* described here is referred to as the *hypothalamic-pituitary-ovarian* system or the HPO axis.

Sex and Stress Hormones

Gonadal (sex) and adrenal (stress) hormones function throughout the life cycle as regulators of brain development and plasticity. As regulators of gene expression, hormones act on the brain as part of a process that shapes sex and determines the effects of stress. McEwen [3] uses the term *allostasis*—stability through change—to describe the outpouring of hormones and neurotransmitters to help maintain systemic homeostasis. The *allostatic load* is the cost of this adaptation to stress. Extreme and/or continuing stress can result in the inability to shut off this adaptation, which can have adverse effects on metabolism. Many areas of the brain are involved in processing information about potentially stressful life events, and it is the response of the brain through its endocrine and autonomic functions that determines the allostatic load an individual experiences.

During adolescence, sex and stress hormones are affecting both structure and neurochemical function. Gonadal hormones have acted in early development to program groups of neurons to respond in male- or female-typical ways [4] and are now coursing through the blood and setting in motion the cyclical changes of puberty and adolescence. Stress hormones affect cognition, rapidly via catecholamines and more slowly via glucocorticoids [5]. Stress-induced catecholamine responses involve beta-adrenergic receptors and the availability of glucose, and they affect emotionally laden memories most likely through neurohormonal activating regions of the amygdala [5, 6]. Stress-related cognitive impairments of declarative memory (such as loss of memory) derive from glucocorticoid-generated modulations in synaptic plasticity and changes in dendritic structures that may last for weeks, and probably involve changes effected in the hippocampus [5]. Adolescence is a critical period because increases in both sex and stress hormones have an impact on developing cognition and behavior.

An example of how the brain (in this case the adult brain) undergoes changes in structure is seen in the cyclical responses of the CA1 region of the hippocampus of the female rat, where dendrites and accompanying synapses increase during the four- to five-day estrous cycle just prior to ovulation [7]. Their decline occurs rapidly (in 24 hours) and is due to the appearance of progesterone as well as the decline in estrogen. The changes in synaptic density in the hippocampus serve functions related to spatial learning and memory. Similar changes in the hypothalamus are partially responsible for cyclical sexual behaviors. In humans we see similar cyclic fluctuations in performance of various cognitive and motor tasks [7].

For girls, a key mental component of adolescence is the changing identity, brought about by the changes in fertility and the effects of hormonal changes on the physiological response to stress. The life of maturing girls is full of anticipatory angst. When will my period come? Will I be able to maintain my appearance? How will family and friends react? Will I feel okay? Will I be popular, belong to the group? It is important to know how this chronic stress affects girls. Stress has depressive effects on the physiology. One mechanism of chronic stress appears to be an adverse effect on immune function in the spleen [8]. The popular idea that women haven't experienced "real" stress in their lives until they enter the workforce is not viable.

Stress and Exercise

Both vigorous physical activity and stress management exercises can provide outlets for the daily hassles and life stressors that adolescents experience. Stress generates tension in the body, which is alleviated during vigorous activity. And experiences that generate pleasant sensations, positive feelings, and successful outcomes have the potential to alter the body image component of self-image. This brings the role of physical activity into the spotlight, for physical activity can be this kind of experience. It doesn't remove the cause of the stress, but it does help develop coping mechanisms.

Another way in which physical activity may be helpful has to do with self-confidence. We have indications that participating in vigorous aerobic exercise has a positive effect on white girls' self-esteem [9-11]. While the self-esteem issue does not transcend ethnicity, other facets of physical activity—such as skill acquisition and the development of self-efficacy—do [12-14]. Another aspect of physical activity that is helpful is stress management techniques. Relaxation exercises can be tailored to this population. Creative exercises such as theatrical role-playing allow opportunities to discharge difficult feelings. Expressive or fun tasks, as when one contributes one's own arm gestures to a traveling movement, or makes up a funny version of a favorite workout routine, contribute to the release of pent-up tension. Offering simple choices—shall we play basketball or jump rope next?—provides a sense that participants have some control of their lives.

ENERGY BALANCE IN ADOLESCENCE

A key factor in the relationship between exercise and well-being for women is the balance of energy intake (food) and expenditure (physical activity). A body out of balance with energy intake and expenditure—

whether it be too much or too little food or activity—is clearly at risk as early as childhood and certainly by the time of puberty. But, restoring balance is not simple. How do we address food and exercise with adolescent girls? This relationship is complex and includes issues surrounding eating disorders and obesity, many of which emerge in the years around puberty. Adolescents are notorious for the amount of fat they consume. The health and fitness fields may do well to take a fresh look at this. Is it merely the availability of these foods, or could there be another underlying factor? Sex hormones are derived from cholesterol or acetyl coenzyme A. At a time in life that the body is called upon to begin producing sex hormones at increased levels, an innate drive for fat fuels is possible. And simultaneously, attention to appearance and often unattainable body ideals becomes important. This sets the stage for a difficult life transition.

Energy Intake: Eating Disorders and Obesity

The term *eating disorders* includes full-blown pathologies such as *anorexia nervosa, bulimia,* and *binge eating disorder.* There are also subclinical levels of *disordered eating,* a term referring to unhealthy behaviors around food such as chronic dieting and over-eating. Adequate or inadequate nutrition can affect menstruation and fertility.

Prevalence

The scope of the problem of energy expenditure/intake is large. The cultural milieu in which eating disorders and obesity take place has been termed an environment of abundant, "toxic" food combined with ideal, unrealistic body images [15, 16]. While much of the focus for treating eating disorders and obesity has been on the responsibility of the individual to change her behavior through discipline or medical treatment, this approach has been largely ineffective and these problems are increasing. Estimates for the prevalence of eating problems vary. According to one study 2% of the female population are affected by eating disorders, and a third of the female population is obese [17]. Other research implies that virtually all girls are affected to some degree by disordered eating as part of their maturation process [18]. Battle and Brownell suggest a change of emphasis in dealing with these issues from an individual model of treatment to a public health model of prevention; they propose public policy that taxes low-nutrition fast foods much as tobacco is taxed as well as community-wide education promoting healthy behaviors [17].

Why They Start

We also must acknowledge the extent of the stress on girls to achieve an ideal body. In 1984, Rodin, Silberstein, and Striegel-Moore introduced the idea that the cultural attitude toward thinness as beauty prescribes an ideal body weight at odds with the developmental milestones that tend to increase women's body fat (puberty, pregnancy, and menopause) [19]. According to this argument, the focus on appearance that preoccupies women results in large part from social pressure and leads to diminished self-esteem, distorted body image, and frustration, with the inability to attain perfection. A study published in 1997 validates this argument. Comparing chronic dieters, women with medium restraint, and non-dieters, researchers found the chronic dieters had significantly higher scores on body distortion, drive for thinness, body dissatisfaction, feelings of ineffectiveness, depression, and schizophrenia on the Minnesota Multiphasic Personality Inventory-2 [20]. These results also point to the continuity between chronic dieting and the development of eating disorders.

When They Start

When do the roots of these disorders enter the lives of the girls and women who are affected? A 1995 study demonstrated that restrained eating, body dissatisfaction, drive for thinness, self-induced vomiting, laxative use, diet pill use, and alcohol use significantly increased—and physical appearance and self-concept significantly decreased—among adolescent frequent dieters [21]. The authors conclude that dieting may reflect a general pattern of unhealthy behaviors adopted in adolescence. Other researchers place the starting point even earlier, at the child's interaction with important adults as she internalizes working models of body image [22]. Striegel-Moore proposes that female socialization places girls at risk for binge eating, and that understanding the risk requires examining the developmental tasks of female adolescence, including the role of beauty in female identity, the nature of the relational self, and the adjustment to the biological changes of puberty [18]. Eating disorders manifest themselves across the spectrum of races and subcultures. The dominant white models of these problems may limit researchers' understanding of the nature and extent of such problems [23].

Energy Expenditure: Inactivity and Excessive Exercise

Inactivity is associated with cardiovascular and metabolic disorders, including obesity and its sequellae. Physical activity is an accepted component in the prevention and treatment of obesity, and movement therapy can be an

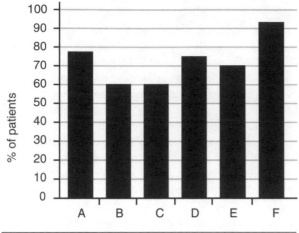

Figure 2.3 Exercise and anorexia nervosa in hospitalized adolescents and adults. A = excessive exercisers, B = competitive athletes prior to illness, C = sport pre-dated dieting, D = claimed physical activity increased when food and weight decreased, E = childhood physical activity levels higher than peers, F = obsessive, ritualized physical activity. From Davis et al. [24].

effective component in the treatment of eating disorders that include mind/body dissociation. There is a relationship between excessive exercise and eating disorders, which can result in menstrual disorders and affect fertility and health. A study by Davis et al. examined the pathogenesis of hospitalized anorexic adolescents and adults. The results suggested that overactivity should not be routinely considered a manifestation of anorexia nervosa as are other behaviors associated with self-starvation, but rather that sport or exercise is often an integral part of the pathogenesis and progression of this disorder (see figure 2.3) [24]. The theoretical basis for Davis et al.'s carefully conducted research rests, in part, on work in animals demonstrating the interrelationship of obsessive activity and restricted eating, and argues for a neuroendocrine connection. Their report contains powerful cautions about pushing structured exercise regimens for younger and younger girls. At particular risk are girls with ritual activity practices (repeating certain actions exactly the same over and over), as well as competitive athletes and dancers, with any degree of disordered eating. Calorie-restriction, interruption of digestive processes through purging, or metabolic sequellae of binge eating/starvation can have grave consequences for health and reproductive function.

Energy Imbalance and Menstruation

Girls who are very active physically and are having regular cycles lasting 25 to 35 days with ovulation and nor-

mal luteal phase are experiencing *eumenorrhea,* or "normal" menstrual cycles. It can be difficult to distinguish between normal cycling and *luteal phase defect,* in which a short luteal phase results in decreased progesterone. Unless there is a significant enough drop in progesterone to cause some midcycle bleeding or if a blood test reveals low levels of progesterone, luteal phase defect may be not be diagnosed. Irregular cycles that occur every 35-90 days are referred to as *oligomenorrhea,* and may be the result of *anovulation* (lack of ovulation), *hypoestrogenism* (low estrogen levels) or other disorders. *Primary amenorrhea* is the delay of menarche until after the age of 16, and *secondary amenorrhea* is cessation of menstruation for at least six months in girls or women who are post-pubertal. All conditions except eumenorrhea are considered menstrual disorders and call into question the balance of energy expenditure and intake, if disease or other medical condition has been ruled out.

Energy Imbalance and Fertility

Warren put forth the idea in 1980 that a chronic condition in which inadequate energy was available played a major part in menstrual disorders of young female athletes and dancers [25]. Since then a number of significant findings have helped bring to light the complex biological issues surrounding energy balance and fertility. The first direct evidence that the availability of metabolic fuels play a part in the control of reproduction came in 1993 when Jenkins et al. reported elevations of cortisol and insulin-like growth factor binding protein 1 (IGFBP-1) as independent predictors of the severity of menstrual disorders in elite athletes [26].

The connection between chronic, high volume exercise in girls and women, unhealthy eating behaviors, and suppression of reproductive functions had been noted for some time [27-36]. These and other findings have led to the identification and description of the syndrome known as the *female athlete triad* [37, 38], characterized by disordered eating, amenorrhea, and *osteoporosis,* or loss of bone mineral density. While secondary amenorrhea probably occurs in only 2-5% of the population [39], athletes and dancers account for a large proportion of those numbers, and there is concern that if no efforts are made to curb unrealistic body images or the propensity of younger and younger girls to begin dieting, this syndrome could become an increasing dilemma.

When energy availability is low, release of GnRH is slowed at the hypothalamus and consequently there is a slowing of the frequency of LH pulsation [40-43]. This indicates that the hypothalamus is a location where reproductive function is altered during low energy availability. Two studies have demonstrated that inadequate energy is the source of the change in reproductive function: a volume of exercise or an increase in training volume was associated with changes in LH pulsatility only when accompanied by insufficient caloric intake [44, 45]. In addition to changes in LH pulsatility, another marker of low energy and reproductive status is the level of the thyroid hormone triiodothyronine, which fluctuates quickly with energy expenditure and intake and reflects the overall energy balance [46].

Activation of the hypothalamic-pituitary-adrenal (HPA) axis can suppress reproductive function through its ability to suppress GnRH secretion. Since physical activity can activate the HPA axis [47], it is possible that HPA involvement is an aspect of the mechanism of exercise-induced menstrual disorders. However, whether it is implicated merely as a signal or as an active mechanism in a stress response has not been evaluated.

Menstrual disorders have an impact on fertility and even though a woman may appear to be cycling normally, subtle changes in the luteal phase can affect ovulation or implantation. In addition, hypogonadotropism (low levels of ovarian estrogen and progesterone) may affect the corpus luteum. Although these difficulties can be reversed, it sometimes requires time to detect and treat them. Young girls who may wish to have families when they are old enough should be encouraged to balance healthy food and physical activity as a preparation for that time.

Dancers and distance runners have long been identified as being at high risk for the female athlete triad. The incidence of anorexia nervosa in dancers is considered to be between 3.5% and 7.6% [48]. Other athletes who may be at risk are swimmers, gymnasts, ice skaters, and cyclists. By and large, those athletes whose sport or art requires a lean aesthetic or high doses of endurance activity are at greater risk than those in other activities. Menstrual dysfunction in competitive swimmers may be a distinct entity. A study by Constantini and Warren indicated that estradiol levels were normal in swimmers with menstrual irregularities following menarche and higher than average in the pre-menarche swimmers [49]. Levels of dehydroepiandrostenedione sulfate and androstenedione (weak androgens or male hormones) were higher than average in all groups of swimmers, leading the researchers to conclude that the delayed puberty and menstrual irregularities in competitive swimmers have a different mechanism, namely mild hyperandrogenism (high levels of male hormones) rather than the hypoestrogenism (low levels of estrogen) associated with other athletes [49].

Female Hormones, Perception, Athletic Performance, and Energy

A complicating issue in the discussion of energy balance in the female is the effect of menstrual cycling on perception, performance, and energy sources. Despite variations noted in early research, the greatest sensitivity to visual, auditory, and olfactory stimuli has been observed at midcycle [50]. Peaks in olfactory sensitivity have been noted in the second half of menses, during midcycle, and midluteally in women both taking and not taking oral contraceptives, leading to the conclusion that mechanisms other than gonadal hormones may be responsible for these changes [50]. Could the midcycle period, when ovulation occurs, represent a period of sensory acuteness and ability to tap energy stores in order to attract the males with the greatest resources? Results of early studies on athletic performance have been difficult to interpret as a consequence of small sample sizes and other confounding variables. However, an investigation by Lebrun et al. does suggest that cyclic increases in endogenous (produced in the body) female hormones may have a slight deleterious effect on aerobic capacity, with substantial variation among subjects [51]. Lebrun's review study indicated that one confounding element may be a perception of performance decrement on the part of individuals [52]. One study has clearly shown that thermoregulation, cardiovascular strain (heart rate), and perceived exertion were adversely affected during the luteal (post ovulation) phase [53].

A related area in which research is scant is the effect of female hormones on substrate (energy source) utilization during exercise. According to one study although there are gender differences in sedentary individuals in substrate utilization during endurance exercise, these differences diminish at the level of highly trained individuals [54]. With what is known about decreases in female hormone production in chronic, excessive exercisers, one is left to speculate about the connection between the diminishing of these substrate differences and diminishing levels of female hormones.

EXERCISE AND DISEASE

Other areas of health are affected by physical activity in adolescence or have an impact on exercise prescription. Bone health, premature puberty, breast cancer, diabetes, and cardiovascular disease are areas in which prior and current research is casting light on the relationship among genetic factors, hormone exposure, lifestyle issues, and health.

Bone Health and Exercise

In the area of bone health, we have a fairly clear understanding of how physical activity in puberty and adolescence, as well as nutrition, relates to bone strength. Peak bone mass [55] along with genetic factors [56] appears to be a major predictor of the rate of postmenopausal bone loss; and peak bone mass probably occurs in the early 20s, with the teen years critical for the attainment of high peak bone mass [57-60]. Athletic amenorrhea can lead to detrimental bone changes [61-63]. Nutritional deficits also adversely affect bone health [28, 64]. It is well accepted that the underlying mechanism in bone loss is hypoestrogenism. While calcium is an important dietary component to good bone health, it appears that weight-bearing exercise and the maintenance of a normal weight in the teen years are the key factors for development of peak bone mass [65].

Bone loss in athletes and dancers may affect the skeleton in unusual ways. For example, in dancers, weight-bearing sites showed higher density than the same areas in anorexic girls matched for age, while at non-weight-bearing sites, deficits were similar [66]. In a comparison of gymnasts and runners, Robinson et al. found that runners had lower lumbar spine bone mineral density than either gymnasts or controls (0.89 ± 0.11, 1.17 ± 0.13, and 1.11 ± 0.11 grams per square centimeter, respectively), as well as lower femoral neck bone mineral density (0.88 ± 0.11, 1.09 ± 0.12, and 0.97 ± 0.10 grams per square centimeter, respectively) [67]. This information supports evidence that bones build at the sites of greatest stress. Bone age is a critical factor in a differential diagnosis of delayed puberty [68].

Premature Puberty, Breast Cancer, and Exercise

Premature puberty is not necessarily just normal puberty occurring early; it may signal reproductive endocrine disturbances over time [69]. An extended duration from puberty to the first pregnancy, as similarly with early menarche, is a risk factor for breast cancer; probable mechanisms involve the more rapid onset of ovulatory cycles in girls menstruating before the age of 12 and thus higher levels of serum estradiol and lower levels of sex hormone-binding globulin even during their 20s. Exposure to increased estrogen production is associated with a high degree of breast epithelial proliferation and possible hyperplasia [70].

Intense physical activity in girls has been associated with a lowered risk of reaching menarche at an early age [71]. We also know that women with an ongoing exercise history may have a lowered risk of breast cancer [72], and that an exercise history often begins in youth. The role of physical activity as a possible primary prevention lies in its ability to reduce the risk of early menarche and reduce exposure to ovarian hormones through reduction of the number of ovulatory cycles [73]. The ability of exercise to reduce the number of breast cancer tumors due to environmental cancer-causing agents has been shown in rats [74]. The authors hypothesize that this effect does not occur due to an effect of exercise on breast tissue, but some other mechanism of exercise [74]. On the other hand, excessive exercise levels may have a negative effect on breast tissue. Exercise-induced menstrual irregularities may be associated with breast cancer when increased levels of free radicals and DNA damage affect breast tissue [75].

Results from large studies that include exercise in adolescence and breast cancer are mixed. Two major studies demonstrate conflicting outcomes. Mittendorf et al. looked at 6888 women with breast cancer between the ages of 17 and 74 and at 9539 controls ages 18 to 74. Women reporting any strenuous physical activity during the ages of 14 to 22 showed a modest reduction in breast cancer, while those who exercised vigorously at least once a day had a 50% reduction in breast cancer [76]. McTiernan et al. examined the relationship between physical activity and risk of breast cancer in middle-aged women and found only a weak correlation, including no association between any duration or intensity of exercise between ages 12 and 21 and the risk of breast cancer [77].

Diabetes, Cardiovascular Disease, and Exercise

Epidemiological evidence strongly supports the theory that sedentary lifestyles are a major factor in the development of non-insulin-dependent diabetes mellitus (NIDDM, type 2 diabetes) [78]. While there are genetic and age factors that influence the development of insulin resistance, hyperinsulinemia, and glucose intolerance, these conditions are also highly susceptible to adult weight gain, particularly in the *android* or *central distribution pattern* (the "apple" shape), in the population aged 20 to 74 [79]. Obesity in girls is linked to overweight in women [80] and is, through this association, suspect as a possible marker for NIDDM in girls whose parents demonstrate this weight gain pattern. While information will be forthcoming on the relationship between physical activity in girls during puberty and NIDDM, Manson has reported that 34- to 59-year-old women who performed vigorous exercise at least once a week had a 16% lower risk of self-reported NIDDM [81].

Adolescent girls with type 1 diabetes represent a special risk, particularly if they show signs of disordered eating. A recent study has indicated that these girls often skip their insulin or underdose themselves [82].

Gutin et al. have found that fasting insulin concentration is associated with cardiovascular reactivity to exercise in young children, supporting the hypothesis that the relationship between hyperinsulinemia and hypertension is mediated by sympathetic nervous tone and that the process begins in childhood [83]. The authors suggest that because body fat is positively associated with both insulin and cardiovascular reactivity to exercise, prevention of childhood obesity may be important as a preventive measure for both NIDDM and cardiovascular disease [83]. Although cardiovascular exercise favorably affects risk factors in adults, there is less evidence that this is true with children and adolescents. Suter et al. has shown no significant relationship between cardiovascular fitness and lipid profiles [84]. Gutin et al. showed that cardiovascular fitness in weight-independent exercise (cycling) did not significantly relate to the level of body fat or major coronary artery disease or NIDDM risk factors, although they did find high levels of body fat related to unfavorable risk factors [85], as have others [86].

On the other hand, Gutin et al. have also shown that the mechanism by which obese children receive cardiovascular benefits through regular physical training over a four-month period may be the favorable reduction in the ratio of sympathetic to parasympathetic activity in cardiac autonomic function [87]. It seems clear that exercise will improve fitness in obese adolescents [88-90] as well as reduce obesity [91, 92], according to studies that include or are limited to girls.

In 1989, Lamon-Fava et al. found that amenorrheic runners had lowered levels of low-density lipoprotein [93]. However, other researchers have found that amenorrheic athletes have elevated low-density lipoprotein levels, although these changes were not statistically significant [92, 94, 95].

SOCIAL ASPECTS OF ADOLESCENT GIRLS AND PHYSICAL ACTIVITY

In addition to the conscious development process that accelerates as a girl's brain undergoes the physiological changes of adolescence, there are social components that affect her psychological state. Two areas in which social issues affect her development can be addressed within physical activity. The first is the social dilemma that surrounds her emerging sense of herself in relation to others. The second is the transference of feelings from parental figures to peers. Both of these areas involve issues of individuation, independence, and identity.

The Social Dilemma of Adolescent Girls

Approaching adolescence, a young girl becomes aware of herself in a social context. What is the social context? The dominant modern worldview is one in which independence and self-assertion have the greatest value [96]. But girls often value the self more in relation to others. As a result, society provides a complex challenge for maturing girls, one that can undermine self-confidence in a number of ways. In Western culture, it appears that white girls' self-esteem plummets drastically after about age 9 [97]. African American girls appear not to be susceptible to this falling self-esteem, but they and girls of many other ethnic backgrounds benefit psychologically from developing self-efficacy [98]. The confidence crisis among girls that accompanies them into adolescence includes vulnerability to a cluster of high-risk behaviors such as smoking, eating disorders, drugs, and unprotected sex [99]. Changing identity also appears to shift the focus of attention from internal concerns to an obsession with appearance [100, 101]. These features point to the delicacy and complexity of the social challenge to girls at this critical point in their development. Just at the time when independence and belief in self are most valued, girls look to others for meaning.

How does this transfer to the playing field? Examining playtime activities of fifth graders in the 1970s, Janet Lever found boys playing outdoors more often than girls, in larger, age-heterogeneous groups highly motivated to play out the game plan [102]. Aggressive legal debates appeared to be enjoyed by the boys as much as the game itself and served as a way to keep the game going. Girls, on the other hand, viewed the rules as open to innovation and saw the game as less significant than keeping harmony among the smaller group.

While much has changed in opportunities for girls since that time, curiously little has changed in girls' social values when it comes to play. Some physically gifted, aggressive girls are now fulfilled through behavior that in the past was acceptable only for boys. Large numbers of girls benefit by learning assertion and developing physical prowess. But for many it is more fulfilling within the context of play to continue to practice social support, stretch the rules to keep the peace, and be rewarded for nurturing behaviors than to dominate others.

Unlike what occurs with their male counterparts, the developmental edge on which girls balance during adolescence takes them in more than one direction at the same time. For young heterosexual men, the drive for adult autonomy, individuation, and conquest so rewarded in Western culture harmonizes with their inner experience. Male puberty signals a time of increasing levels of testosterone, the hormone associated with self-assertion and aggressive behavior, while their brains are developing along a pathway of linear problem-solving so beneficial to the hunter; and the social model encourages them in this path.

But for many young women, such a model can create conflict. If adulthood is defined as aggression, competition, or dominance, what happens to the capacity to care, to see a problem from another's perspective, or to be flexible about the rules of the game so that social fabric stays intact? For girls, whose hormones dictate a cycle of ebb and flow, and whose brains are developing the capacity to work on problems from more than one perspective at the same time, there can be dissonance between inner experience and outer reality. While their world becomes increasingly demanding about the ability to problem-solve with single-minded assertion, their brains are provided with a hemispheric bridge—the *corpus callosum*—larger than the male's [103]. This increases the activity between hemispheres, allowing girls access to more regions of their brains when thinking, and resulting in a multifaceted problem-solving capacity.

The perception of this dissonance for girls is not a new thought. Harvard Professor of Gender Studies Carol Gilligan has discussed this conflict and its impact on women's moral decisions [104]. In psychological research, she found there had long been neglect concerning the importance of intimacy, complex relationships, and caring as lines of development in the adult, and thus that these characteristics appear in the literature not as desirable adult behaviors but as immature stages or as part of that female mystery, *intuition* [104].

Transference of Feelings

The process of transferring attachments in adolescence involves a shifting of object relationships, including moving love and dependency away from parents or authority figures to peers [105]. This situation is one of oscillation, detaching a girl's affection from her parental figures, directing love and attention first to herself and then to peers. But it is not a smooth transition; it involves a lot of testing of feelings and behaviors. It is easy to see why this is a delicate time for the female psyche. Social support is tremendously helpful for reassurance. Feedback from friends and significant adults helps establish behaviors that achieve her needs and desires.

Friends are a key element in transference during this developmental phase. How does this phase play out in the current cultural milieu? A distinct adolescent culture has resulted from modern societal pressures, including compulsory education, child labor laws, and the decreasing presence of working parents [106]. The negative impact of adolescent peer friendships (i.e., experimenting with high-risk behaviors) reaches public attention through the media. A more complete and balanced description of close peer friendships and their import to adolescent development is accessible in academic writing [107-112]. These friendships contribute to cognitive, social, and psychological development and satisfy the desire for intimacy, sensitivity, and understanding, as well as contributing to the development of interpersonal skills; and they do so across racial and socioeconomic groups, although significant differences exist [113-116]. Most striking, for purposes of this text, is the sex difference between European American females and males. Females are more likely to reveal their personal thoughts and feelings to their same-sex friends than are males in this population, who are the one exception to a tendency among adolescent same-sex friends of many races to share confidences [117]. Is this unwillingness to share personal feelings and thoughts related to the need of young white males to develop self-assertion and dominance in order to satisfy the expectations of a male-dominated culture?

In addition to friends, significant nonparent adults play an important role in the transfer process for adolescents, especially for girls [118-123]. One study showed that adults other than parents composed 22.3% of all persons adolescents listed as significant [124], and another showed that nonparent adults composed 27.2% of adolescent girls' social network [125]. These relationships provide emotional support and advice from an adult while allowing a degree of autonomy from parents [120]. Girls more often than boys participate in intergenerational relationships, through which female models other than the mother are available for identification or attachment [126]. Girls of many races and ethnicities exhibit these characteristics [127-131]. It is important to note that such relationships are most effective when they occur naturally, rather than in situations in which an older female may be serving as a volunteer mentor [132]. Teachers and other adults in the adolescent female's environment may be useful in the transference process. Many of us remember that special teacher or coach who inspired us or with whom we formed a bond.

Social Content and Physical Activity

When we move the content focus of physical activities away from the physical education component and onto the cognitive social component, adolescent girls have an opportunity to openly play out experimental social behavior. They can test friendships, try individual actions, and seek advice from teachers or coaches in a safe environment while gaining implicit information about physical fitness. In this model, physical activity provides a practice field, an arena in which to try out schemes for asserting oneself and relating to others. Fitness is the by-product rather than the goal. One can create games that foster avenues of facilitation by identifying where developmental skills might be acquired and finding physical tasks that provide opportunities to work on these behaviors. And the adults who supervise these games have an important responsibility to perceive their own behavior at all times in light of its potential for modeling.

To demonstrate how this information could apply to designing a physical activity session, let's take the example of learning to work one-on-one with various individuals. The commonly used technique of pairing adolescents to do skill drills is an appropriate activity. In applying this method, the instructor would tell the participants what was going on from the start. She would focus on the social processes of pairing and interacting. In order to increase the odds of competency among all members of the group, she would make sure that the physical skills were various—and also make sure that the more vulnerable personalities got extra support if needed. Girls can be paired up for skill drills by a trusted adult in such a way that over the course of the session no preference is shown either for those with close friendships or for those with few friends (e.g., the instructor could call off "1, 2, 1, 2 . . ." and pair the first "1" with the last "2"). Tips for helping each other would be included along with the physical requirements of the drill. The instructor would make sure that each girl congratulated her partner on her execution of the skill. She could then rematch the girls for each of the next several tasks so that there were a number of pairings for each girl.

This method gives each girl an opportunity to interact with different people and to work with people of varying talent and discipline. A girl may also find that someone she wasn't interested in before is more interesting once she has worked with her, or that her usual buddies are fun, but too serious or not serious enough. The instructor would be accessible and helpful, as needed. At the end she would ask the girls what they learned and would be careful not to direct their answers. Probably some girls would talk about the social elements, but others might be struck by mastering new motor skills. They would all get a lot of credit for participating.

INDICATIONS FOR FITNESS PROGRAMS FOR ADOLESCENT GIRLS

How are these practices different from what we are doing now? They involve a shift away from measured performance, winning, or aggression to what might be thought of as more traditional female social characteristics in order to set goals. In assessing the effects of Title IX, we see that they go beyond providing opportunities for girls to play like boys. The major thrust of the entitlement was to make boys' sports accessible to girls on all levels. But as girls have invaded the playing fields, we are feeling an effect on the nature of the arena itself. The competitive male model to which girls now have access turns out to be accessible only to a small group of girls. The rest are somewhat disenfranchised. We need more models.

The legacy of a century in which women have obtained voting rights, and are working to establish control of their bodies and equality in pay for work, is a human arena in which female priorities intrude further and further into the white male concept of the rules of the game. This changing social landscape extends to physical activity, where we see increasing interest in daily activities as a foundation [133]. If we really want to enable adolescent girls to take advantage of fitness programs, these programs have to be connected to the things adolescent girls do. How does our understanding of adolescence in the female affect our ability to provide these girls with beneficial and accessible fitness programs? We are just beginning to put this information together.

Such a curriculum might combine interactive learning sessions around topics of female anatomy and physiology with learning about basic measurement procedures during various physical activities. A brief exercise task successfully completed and including familiarization with peak oxygen uptake and RPE procedures can increase adolescent girls' perceived self-efficacy [134]. We can develop stress management skills by helping girls become aware of their own stressors as well as their preferences for coping, then expanding coping skills to include physical activity, relaxation, and other mind/body techniques. Starting a unit about nutrition by having girls eat various foods, assess individual moods and activity levels, then compare and contrast their findings is another way of bringing together behavior and cognitive learning about oneself. This also provides a way of teaching about individual differences. One girl may feel better if she eats one thing shortly before exercise, while another feels better eating different types of food a couple hours before she exercises.

The step of awareness that precedes any behavior change in adults is active in adolescence really for the first time. Let us open up the adolescent process in the female to herself, allowing her to gain whatever self-awareness she needs. In this chapter, we have reviewed information about female adolescence in an academic fashion. To make it accessible to adolescent girls through physical activity, we need to take other steps. What do we want to achieve? What is the best setting? How do we design effective programs? In the next chapter—to further this process—we delineate outcome goals and establish priorities for the implementation of beneficial fitness programs for adolescent girls.

REFERENCES

1. Rogol, A.D. 1996. Delayed puberty in girls and primary and secondary amenorrhoea. In O. Bar-Or (ed.), *The child and adolescent athlete,* Vol. VI, *The encyclopaedia of sports medicine.* London: Blackwell Scientific, pp. 304-317.

2. Guyton, A.C., and Hall, J.E. 1997. *Human physiology and mechanisms of disease,* 6th ed. Philadelphia: Saunders.

3. McEwen, B.S. 1997. Hormones as regulators of brain development: Life-long effects related to health and disease. *Acta Paediatrica Supplement* 422:41-44.

4. McEwen, B.S. 1994. How do sex and stress hormones affect nerve cells? (Review). *Annals of the New York Academy of Sciences* 734:1-16; discussion 17-18.

5. McEwen, B.S., and Sapolsky, R.M. 1995. Stress and cognitive function (Review). *Current Opinion in Neurobiology* 5(2):205-216.

6. Schulkin, J., McEwen, B.S., and Gold, P.W. 1994. Allostasis, amygdala, and anticipatory angst. *Neuroscience and Biobehavioral Reviews* 18(3):385-396.

7. McEwen, B.S., and Woolley, C.S. 1994. Estradiol and progesterone regulate neuronal structure and synaptic connectivity in adult as well as developing brain. *Experimental Gerontology* 29(3-4):431-436.

8. Spencer, R.L., Miller, A.N., Moday, H., McEwen, B.S., Blanchard, R.J., Blanchard, D.C., and Sakai, R.R. 1996. Chronic social stress produces reductions in available splenic type II corticosteroid receptor binding and plasma corticosteroid binding globulin levels. *Psychoneuroendocrinology* 21(1):95-109.

9. Jaffee, L., and Wu, P. 1996. After-school activities and self-esteem in adolescent girls. *Melpomene Journal* 15(2):18-24.

10. Jaffee, L., and Ricker, S. 1993. Physical activity and self-esteem in girls: The teen years. *Melpomene Journal* 12(3):19-26.

11. Edwards, P., and Capella, A. 1992. *Self-esteem and adolescent women.* Ottawa, ON: Canadian Teachers Federation and Canadian Association for the Advancement of Women and Sport and Physical Activity.

12. Dzewaltowski, D.A. 1994. Physical activity determinants: A social cognitive approach. *Medicine and Science in Sports and Exercise* 26:1395-1399.

13. Gottlieb, N.H., and Chen, M. 1985. Sociocultural correlates of childhood sporting activities: Their implications for heart health. *Social Science and Medicine* 21:533-539.

14. Sallis, J.F., Hovell, M.F., Hofstetter, C.R., Faucher, P., et al. 1989. A multivariate study of determinants of vigorous exercise in a community sample. *Preventive Medicine* 18:20-34.

15. Brownell, K.D. 1991. Dieting and the search for the perfect body: Where physiology and culture collide. *Behavior Therapy* 22:1-12.

16. Brownell, K.D. 1994. Get slim with higher taxes (Editorial). *New York Times,* December 15, p. A29.

17. Battle, E.K., and Brownell, K.D. 1996. Confronting a rising tide of eating disorders and obesity: Treatment vs. prevention and policy. *Addictive Behaviors* 21(6):7

18. Striegel-Moore, R. 1995. Psychological factors in the etiology of binge eating. *Addictive Behaviors* 20(6):713-723.

19. Rodin, J., Silberstein, L., and Striegel-Moore, R. 1984. Women and weight: A normative discontent. *Nebraska Symposium Motivation* 32: 267-307.

20. Cachelin, F.M., Striegel-Moore, R., and Paget, W.B. 1997. Comparison of women with various levels of dietary restraint on body image, personality and family environment. *Eating Disorders: Journal of Treatment and Prevention* 5(3):205-215.

21. French, S.A., Perry, C.L., Leon, G.R., and Fulkerson, J.A. 1995. Changes in psychological variables and health behaviors by dieting status over a three-year period in a cohort of adolescent females. *Journal of Adolescent Health* 16(6):438-447.

22. Kearney-Cooke, A., and Striegel-Moore, R. 1997. The etiology and treatment of body image disturbance. In D.M. Garner and P.E. Garfinkel (eds.), *Handbook of treatment for eating disorders,* 2nd ed., New York: The Guilford Press, pp. 295-306.

23. Striegel-Moore, R., and Smolak, L. 1996. The role of race in the development of eating disorders. In L. Smolak, M.P. Levine, and R. Striegel-Moore (eds.), *The developmental psychopathology of eating disorders: Implications for research, prevention, and treatment.* Mahwah, NJ: Lawrence Erlbaum, pp. 259-284.

24. Davis, C., Kennedy, S.H., Ravelski, E., and Dionne, M. 1994. The role of physical activity in the development and maintenance of eating disorders. *Psychological Medicine* 24(4):957-967.

25. Warren, M.P. 1980. The effects of exercise on pubertal progression and reproductive function in girls. *Journal of Clinical Endocrinology and Metabolism* 51:1150-1157.

26. Jenkins, P.F., Obanez-Santos, X., Holly, J., Cotterill, A., Perry, L., Wolman, R., Harries, M., Grossman, A. 1993. IGFBP-1: A metabolic signal associated with exercise-induced amenorrhea. *Neuroendocrinology* 57(4):600-604.

27. Brooks-Gunn, J., Warren, M.P., and Hamilton, L.H. 1987. The relation of eating problems and amenorrhea in ballet dancers. *Medicine and Science in Sports and Exercise* 19(1):41-44.

28. Calabrese, L.H., and Kirkendall, D.T. 1983. Nutritional and medical considerations in dancers. *Clinical Sports Medicine* 2(3):539-547.

29. Calabrese, L.H., Kirkendall, D.T., Floyd, M., et al. 1983. Menstrual abnormalities, nutritional patterns and body composition in female classical ballet dancers. *Physician and Sports Medicine* 11:86-98.

30. Dale, E., Gerlack, D.H., and Wilhite, A.L. 1979. Menstrual dysfunction in distance runners. *Obstetrics and Gynecology* 54:47-53.

31. Erdelyi, G.J. 1962. Gynecological survey of female athletes. *Journal of Sports Medicine and Physical Fitness* 2:174-197.

32. Feicht, C.B., Johnson, T.S., Martin, B.J., Sparkes, K.E., Wagner, Jr., W.W. 1978. Secondary amenorrhea in athletes. *Lancet* 2:1145-1146.

33. Frisch, R.E., Gotz-Welbergen, A.V., McArthur, J.W., Witschi, J., Bullen, B.A., Birnholz, J., Reed, R.B., and Herman, H. 1980. Delayed menarche and amenorrhea of college athletes in relation to age of onset of training. *Journal of the American Medical Association* 246:1559-1563.

34. Frisch, R.E., Wyshak, G., and Vincent, L. 1980. Delayed menarche and amenorrhea in ballet dancers. *New England Journal of Medicine* 303:17-18.

35. Loucks, A.B., and Horvath, S.M. 1985. Athletic amenorrhea: A review. *Medicine and Science in Sports and Exercise* 17(1):56-72.

36. Stager, J.M., Robertshaw, D., and Miescher, E. 1984. Delayed menarche in swimmers in relation to age at onset of training and athletic performance. *Medicine and Science in Sports and Exercise* 16:550-555.

37. Otis, C.L., Drinkwater, B.L., Johnson, M., Loucks, A.B., and Wilmore, J.H. 1997. American College of Sports Medicine stand: The female athlete triad. *Medicine and Science in Sports and Exercise* 29(5):i-ix.

38. Yeager, K.K., Agostini, R., Natiiv, A., and Drinkwater, B. 1993. The female athlete triad. *Medicine and Science in Sports and Exercise* 25:775-777.

39. Drew, F.L. 1961. The epidemiology of secondary amenorrhea. *Journal of Chronic Disorders* 14:396-401.

40. Loucks, A.B. 1989. Alterations in the hypothalamic-pituitary-ovarian and hypothalamic-pituitary-adrenal axes in athletic women. *Journal of Clinical Endocrinology and Metabolism* 68:402-411.

41. Velduis, J.D., Evan, W.S., Demer, L.S., Thorner, M.O., Wakat, D., and Rogol, A.D. 1985. Altered neuroendocrine regulation of gonadotropin secretion in women distance runners. *Journal of Clinical Endocrinology and Metabolism* 61:557-563.

42. Cumming, D.C., Vickovic, M.M., Wall, S.R., and Fluker, M.R. 1985. Defects in pulsatile LH release in normally menstruating runners. *Journal of Clinical Endocrinology and Metabolism* 60:810-812.

43. Laughlin, G.A., and Yen, S.S.C. 1996. Nutritional and endocrine-metabolic aberrations in amenorrheic athletes. *Journal of Clinical Endocrinology and Metabolism* 81:4301-4309.

44. Loucks, A.B., Brown, R., King, K., Thruman, J.R., and Verdun, M. 1995. A combined regimen of moderate dietary restriction and exercise training alters luteinizing hormone pulsatility in regularly menstruating young women. *Endocrine Society Abstracts* #P3-360:558.

45. William, N.I., Young, J.C., McArthur, J.W., Bullen, B.A., Skrinar, G.S., and Turnbull, B.A. 1995. Strenuous exercise with caloric restriction: Effect on luteinizing hormone secretion. *Medicine and Science in Sports and Exercise* 27(10):1390-1398.

46. Danforth, E. 1989. The impact of nutrition on thyroid hormone physiology and action. *Annual Review of Nutrition* 9:201-207.

47. Farrell, P.A., Garthwaite, T.L., and Gustafson, A.B. 1983. Plasma adrenocorticotropin and cortisol responses to submaximal and exhaustive exercise. *Journal of Applied Physiology* 55:1441-1444.

48. Nelson, D.P., and Chatfield, S.J. 1998. What do we know from the literature about the prevalence of anorexia nervosa in female ballet dancers? *Journal of Dance Medicine & Science* 2(1):6-13.

49. Constantini, N.W., and Warren, M.P. 1995. Menstrual dysfunction in swimmers: A distinct entity. *Journal of Clinical Endocrinology and Metabolism* 80(9):2740-2744.

50. Doty, R.L., Snyder, P.J., Huggins, G.R., and Lowry, L.D. 1981. Endocrine, cardiovascular and psychological correlates of olfactory sensitivity changes during the human menstrual cycle. *Journal of Comparative and Physiological Psychology* 95(1):4-60.

51. Lebrun, C.M., McKenzie, D.C., Prior, J.C., and Taunton, J.E. 1995. Effects of menstrual cycle phase on athletic performance. *Medicine and Science in Sports and Exercise* 27(3):437-444.

52. Lebrun, C.M. 1993. Effect of the different phases of the menstrual cycle and oral contraceptives on athletic performance. *Sports Medicine* 16(6):400-430.

53. Pivarnik, J.M., Marichal, C.J., Spillman, T., and Morrow, J.R. 1992. Menstrual cycle phase affects temperature regulation during endurance exercise. *Journal of Applied Physiology* 72(2):543-548.

54. Ruby, B.C., and Roberts, R.A. 1994. Gender differences in substrate utilization during exercise. *Sports Medicine* 17(6):393-410.

55. Ott, S.M. 1990. Attainment of peak bone mass. *Journal of Clinical Endocrinology and Metabolism* 71:1028A-C.

56. Decqueker, J., Nijs, J., Verstraeten, A., Guesens, P., and Gevers, G. 1987. Genetic determination of bone mineral content at the spine and radius: A twin study. *Bone* 8:207-209.

57. Takahashi, Y., Minamitani, K., Kobayashi, Y., Minagawa, M., Yasuda, T., and Niimi, H. 1996. Spinal and femoral bone mass accumulation during normal adolescence: Comparison with female patients with sexual precocity and with hypogonadism. *Journal of Clinical Endocrinology and Metabolism* 81:1248-1253.

58. Kroger, H., Kotaniemi, A., Kroger, L., and Alhava, E. 1993. Development of bone mass and bone density of the spine and femoral neck—A prospective study of 65 children and adolescents. *Bone and Mineral* 23:171-182.

59. Theintz, G., Buchs, B., Rizzoli, R., Slosman, D., Clavien, H., Sizonenko, P.C., and Bonjour, J.-P.H. 1992. Longitudinal monitoring of bone mass accumulation in healthy adolescents: Evidence for a marked reduction after 16 years of age at the levels of lumbar spine and femoral neck in female subjects. *Journal of Clinical Endocrinology and Metabolism* 75:1060-1065.

60. Bonjour, J.-P.H., Theintz, G., Buchs, B., Slosman, D., and Rizzoli, R. 1991. Critical years and stages of puberty for spinal and femoral bone mass accumulation during adolescence. *Journal of Clinical Endocrinology and Metabolism* 73:555-563.

61. Drinkwater, B.L., Bruemner, B., and Chestnut, C.H. 1990. Menstrual history as a determinant of current bone density in young athletes. *Journal of the American Medical Association* 263:545-558.

62. Lloyd, T., Myers, C., Buchanan, J.R., and Demers, L.M. 1988. Collegiate women athletes with irregular menses during adolescence have decreased bone density. *Obstetrics and Gynecology* 72:639-642.

63. Warren, M.P., Brooks-Gunn, J., Hamilton, L.H., Warren, L.F., and Hamilton, W.G. 1986. Scoliosis and fractures in young ballet dancers. *New England Journal of Medicine* 314:1348-1353.

64. Nelson, M.E., Fisher, E.C., Catos, P.H., Meredith, C.N., Turksoy, R.N., and Evans, W.J. 1986. Diet and bone status in amenorrheic runners. *American Journal of Clinical Nutrition* 43:910-916.

65. Welten, D.C., Kemper, H.C.G., Post, G.B., Van Mechelen, W., Twisk, J., Lips, P., and Teule, G.J. 1994. Weight-bearing activity during youth is a more important factor for peak bone mass than calcium intake. *Journal of Bone and Mineral Research* 9(7):1089-1096.

66. Young, N., Formica, C., Szmukler, G., and Seeman, E. 1994. Bone density at weight-bearing and non weight-bearing sites in ballet dancers: the effects of exercise, hypogonadism and body weight. *Journal of Clinical Endocrinology and Metabolism* 78:449-454.

67. Robinson, T.L., Snow-Harter, C., Taaffe, D.R., Gillis, D., Shaw, J., and Marcus, R. 1995. Gymnasts exhibit higher bone mass than runners despite similar prevalence of amenorrhea and oligomenorrhea. *Journal of Bone and Mineral Research* 10(1):26-35.

68. Rosenfield, R.L., and Barnes, R.B. 1993. Menstrual disorders in adolescence. *Endocrinology and Metabolism Clinics of North America* 2(3):491-505.

69. Rosenfield, R.L. 1994. Normal and almost normal precocious variations in pubertal development, premature pubarche and premature thelarche revisited. *Hormone Research* 41 (Suppl 2):7-13.

70. Apter, D. 1996. Hormonal events during female puberty in relation to breast cancer risk. *European Journal of Cancer Prevention* 5(6):476-482.

71. Moisan J., Meyer, F., and Gingras, S. 1991. Leisure physical activity and age at menarche. *Medicine and Science in Sports and Exercise* 23(10):1170-1175.

72. Kramer, M., and Wells, C. 1996. Does physical activity reduce the risk of estrogen-dependent cancer in women? *Medicine and Science in Sports and Exercise* 28:322-334.

73. Friedenreich, C.M., and Rohan, T.E. 1995. A review of physical activity and breast cancer. *Epidemiology* 6(3):311-317.

74. Whittal, K.S., and Parkhouse, W.S. 1996. Exercise during adolescence and its effects on mammary gland development, proliferation, and nitrosomethylurea (NMU) induced tumorigenesis in rats. *Breast Cancer Research and Treatment* 37(1):21-27.

75. DeCree, C., Van Kranenburg, G., Geurten, P., Fujimori, Y., and Keizer, H.A. 1997. 4-hydroxycatecholestrogen metabolism responses to exercise and training: Possible implications for menstrual cycle irregularities and breast cancer. *Fertility and Sterility* 67(3):505-516.

76. Mittendorf, R., Longnecker, M.P., Newcomb, P.A., Dietz, A.T., Greenberg, E.R., Bogdan, G.F., Clapp, R.W., and Willett, W.C. 1995. Strenuous physical activity in young adulthood and risk of breast cancer. *Cancer Causes & Control* 6(4):347-353.

77. McTiernan, A., Stanford, J.L., Weiss, N.S., Daling, J.R., and Voigt, L.F. 1996. Occurrence of breast cancer in relation to recreational exercise in women age 50-64 years. *Epidemiology* 7(6):598-604.

78. Kriska, A.M., Blair, S.N., and Pereira, M.A. 1994. The potential role of physical activity in the prevention of non insulin-dependent diabetes mellitus: The epidemiological evidence. *Exercise and Sports Review* 22:121-143.

79. Harris, M.I., Hadden, W.C., Knowler, W.C., and Bennett, P.H. 1987. Prevalence of diabetes and impaired glucose tolerance and plasma glucose levels in US population aged 20-74 yr. *Diabetes* 36:523-534.

80. Wing, R.R. 1993. Obesity and related eating and exercise behaviors in women. *Annals of Behavioral Medicine* 15: 124-134.

81. Manson, J.E., Rimm, E.B., Stampfer, M.J., Colditz, G.A., Willett, W.C., Krolewski, A.S. et al. 1991. Physical activity and incidence of non-insulin-dependent diabetes mellitus in women. *Lancet* 338:774-778.

82. Rydall, A.C., Rodin, G.M., Olmsted, M.P., Devenyi, R.G., and Daneman, D. 1997. Disordered eating behavior and microvascular complications in young women with insulin-dependent diabetes mellitus. *New England Journal of Medicine* 336(26):1849-1854.

83. Gutin, B., Islam, S., Treiber, F., Smith, C., and Manos, T. 1995. Fasting insulin concentration is related to cardiovascular reactivity to exercise in children. *Pediatrics* 96(6):1123-1125.

84. Suter, E., and Hawes, M.R. 1993. Relationship of physical activity, body fat, diet, and blood lipid profile in youths 10-15 yr. *Medicine and Science in Sports and Exercise* 25(6):748-754.

85. Gutin, B., Owens, S., Treiber, F., Islam, S., Karp, W., and Slavens, G. 1997. Weight-independent cardiovascular fitness and coronary risk factors. *Archives of Pediatrics and Adolescent Medicine* 151(5):462-465.

86. Zonderland, M.L., Erich, W.B., Erkelens, D.W., Kortlandt, W., Wit, J.M., Huisveld, I.A., and DeRidder, C.M. 1990. Plasma lipids and apoproteins, body fat distribution and body fatness in early pubertal children. *International Journal of Obesity* 12(12):1039-1046.

87. Gutin, B., Owen, S., Slavens, G., Riggs, S., and Treiber, F. 1997. Effects of physical training on heart-period variability in obese children. *Journal of Pediatrics* 130(6):938-943.

88. Epstein, L.H., Coleman, K.J., and Myers, M.D. 1996. Exercise in treating obesity in children and adolescents. *Medicine and Science in Sports and Exercise* 28(4):428-435.

89. Ignico, A.A., and Mahon, A.D. 1995. The effects of a physical fitness program on low-fit children. *Research Quarterly of Exercise and Sport* 66(1):85-90.

90. Gutin, B., Cucuzzo, N., Islam, S., Smith, C., Moffatt, R., and Pargman, D. 1995. Physical training improves body composition of black obese 7-to-11-year old girls. *Obesity Research* 3(4):305-312.

91. Epstein, L.H., Valoski, A.M., Vara, L.S., McCurley, J, Wisniewski, L., Kalarchian, M.A., Klein, K.R., and Shrager, L.R. 1995. Effects of decreasing sedentary behavior and increasing activity on weight change in obese children. *Health Psychology* 14(2):109-115.

92. Gutin, B., Cucuzzo, N., Islam, S., Smith, C., and Stachura, M.E. 1996. Physical training, lifestyle education and coronary risk factors in obese girls. *Medicine and Science in Sports and Exercise* 28(1):19-23.

93. Lamon-Fava, S., Fisher, E.C., Nelson, M.E., Evans, W.J., Millar, J.S., Ordavas, J.M., and Schafer, E.J. 1989. Effects of exercise and menstrual cycle status on plasma lipids, low density lipoprotein protein size and apolipoproteins. *Journal of Clinical Endocrinology and Metabolism* 68:17-21.

94. Friday, K.E., Drinkwater, B.L., Bruemmer, B., Chestnut, C, and Chait, A. 1993. Elevated plasma low-density lipoprotein cholestrol levels in amenorrheic athletes: Effects of endogenous hormone status and nutrient intake. *Journal of Clinical Endocrinology and Metabolism* 77:1605-1609.

95. Kaiserauer, S., Snyder, A.C., Sleeper, M., and Sierath, J. 1989. Nutritional, physiological and menstrual status of distance runners. *Medicine and Science in Sports and Exercise* 21 (2):120-125.

96. Taylor, J.M. 1995. *Philosophical arguments.* Cambridge, MA: Harvard University Press.

97. Hancock, E. 1990. *The girl within.* NY: Ballantine.

98. Brown, K.M., McMahon, R.P., Biro, F.M., Crawford, P., Schreiber, G.B., Similo, S.L., Waclawiw, M., and Striegel-Moore, R. 1998. Changes in self-esteem in black and white girls between the ages of 9 and 14 year. *Journal of Adolescent Health* 23:7-19.

99. Ozer, E.M., Brindis, C.D., Millstein, S.G., Knopf, D.K., and Irwin, C.E. 1998. *America's adolescents: Are they healthy?* San Francisco, CA: UCSF. National Adolescent Health Information Center.

100. Brumberg, J.J. 1997. *The body project.* NY: Random House.

101. Hesse-Biber, S. 1996. *Am I thin enough yet?* NY: Oxford University Press.

102. Lever, J. 1976. Sex differences in the games children play. *Social Problems* 23:476-487.

103. De Lacoste-Utamsing, C., and Holloway, R.L. 1982. Sexual dimorphism in the human corpus calliosum. *Science* 216:1431-1432.

104. Gilligan, C. 1982/1993. *In a different voice.* Cambridge, MA: Harvard University Press.

105. Blos, P. 1967. The second individuation. *Psychoanalytic Study of the Child* 22:162-182.

106. Fasick, F.A. 1994. On the "invention" of adolescence. *Journal of Early Adolescence* 14:6-23.

107. Laursen, B, (ed.). 1993. *Close friendships in adolescence.* San Francisco: Jossey Bass.

108. Jessor, R. 1993. Successful adolescent development among youth in high-risk settings. *American Psychologist* 48(2):117-126.

109. Savin-Williams, R.C., and Berndt, T.J. 1990. Friendship and peer relations. In S.S. Feldman and G.R. Elliott (eds.), *At the threshold: The developing adolescent.* Cambridge, MA: Harvard University Press.

110. Youniss, J., and Smollar, J. 1985. *Adolescent relations with mothers, fathers, and friends.* Chicago: University of Chicago Press.

111. Selman, R. 1980. *The growth of interpersonal understanding: Developmental and clinical analyses.* NY: Academic Press.

112. Youniss, J. 1980. *Parents and peers in social development: A Sullivan-Piaget perspective.* Chicago: University of Chicago Press.

113. Hamm, J.V. 1994. Similarity in the face of diversity? African-American, Asian-American, European-American, and Hispanic-American Adolescents' best friendships in ethnically diverse high schools. Paper presented at the biennial meetings of the Society for Research on Adolescence, February, San Diego.

114. Gallagher, C., and Busch-Rossnagel, N.A. 1991. Self-disclosure and social support in the relationships of black and white female adolescents. Paper presented at Society for Research on Child Development, March, Seattle.

115. Dubois, D.L., and Hirsch, B.J. 1990. School and neighborhood friendship patterns of Blacks and Whites in early adolescence. *Child Development* 61: 524-536.

116. Clark, M.L. 1989. Friendships and peer relations in black adolescents. In R. Jones (ed.), *Black adolescents.* Berkeley, CA: Cobb and Henry.

117. Jones, D.C., Costin, S.E., and Ricard, R.J. 1994. Ethnic and sex differences in best friendship characteristics among African-American, Mexican-American, and European-American adolescents. Poster presented at the Society for Research on Adolescents, February, San Diego.

118. Gotlieb, B.H., and Sylvestre, J.C. 1994. Social support in the relationships between older adolescents and adults. In F. Nestmann and K. Hurrelman (eds.), *Social networks and social support in childhood and adolescence.* Berlin: de Gruyter.

119. Hirsch, B.J., Boerger, R., Levy, A.E., and Mickus, M. 1994. The social networks of adolescents and their mothers: Influences on

Blacks and Whites in single- and two-parent families. In F. Nestmann and K. Hurrelman (eds.), *Social networks and social support in childhood and adolescence.* Berlin: de Gruyter.

120. Allen, J.P., Aber, J.L., and Leadbeater, B.J. 1990. Adolescent problem behaviors: The influence of attachment and autonomy. *Psychiatric Clinics of North America* 13:455-467.

121. Coates, D.L. 1987. Gender differences in the structure and support characteristics of black adolescents' networks. *Sex Roles* 17:667-686.

122. Konopka, G. 1986. *Young girls: A portrait of adolescence.* Englewood Cliffs, NJ: Prentice-Hall.

123. Strommen, E.A. 1977. Friendship. In E. Donelson and J. Gullahorn (eds.), *Women: A psychological perspective.* NY: Wiley, pp. 154-167.

124. Garbarino, J., Burston, N., Raber, S., Russell, R., and Crouter, A. 1978. The social map of children approaching adolescence. *Journal of Youth and Adolescence* 7:417-428.

125. Blyth, D.A., Hill, J.P., and Thiel, K.S. 1982. Early adolescents' significant others: Grade and gender differences in perceived relationships with familial and nonfamilial adults and young people. *Journal of Youth and Adolescence* 11:425-450.

126. Chodorow, N. 1992. *Feminism and psychoanalysis.* San Francisco: Jossey-Bass.

127. Collins, P.H. 1987. The meaning of motherhood in black culture and black mother/daughter relationships. *Sage* 4:3-10.

128. Wilson, M.N. 1986. The black extended family: An analytical consideration. *Developmental Psychology* 22:246-258.

129. Dore, M.M., and Dumois, A.O. 1990. Cultural differences in the meaning of adolescent pregnancy. *Journal of Contemporary Human Services* 2:93-105.

130. Ramirez, O. 1989. Mexican American children and adolescents. In Gibbs and Huang (eds.), *Children of color: Psychological interventions with minority youth.* San Francisco: Jossey-Bass.

131. Escobar, J.I., and Randolph, E.T. 1982. The Hispanic and social networks. In Becerra et al. (eds.), *Mental health and Hispanic Americans, clinical perspectives.* NY: Grune and Stratton.

132. Rhodes, J.E., and Davis, A.B. 1996. Supportive ties between nonparent adults and urban adolescent girls. In B.J.R. Leadbeater and N. Way (eds.), *Urban girls.* NY: NYU Press, pp. 213-225.

133. Corbin, C.B., and Pangrazi, R.P. 1998. Physical activity pyramid rebuffs peak experience. *ACSM's Health and Fitness Journal* 2(1):12-17.

134. Pender, N.J., Bar-Or, O., Wilk, B., and Mitchell, S. 2002. Self-efficacy and perceived exertion of girls during exercise. *Nursing Research* 51(2):86-91.

CHAPTER 3

GOALS AND PRIORITIES OF FITNESS PROGRAMS FOR ADOLESCENT GIRLS

This chapter deals with setting goals and priorities of fitness programs for adolescent girls. It starts by recapping information about adolescent girls that was presented in previous chapters, which bears on this process. The chapter then focuses on the associations among physical activity, adolescent girls' health, and long-term health in order to suggest how emphasis on the public health sector—as opposed to the competitive or performance measurement sector—affects the setting of goals. Subsequent sections address what is meant by goals and priorities and identify and elaborate on each of the major goals (increasing participation in girl-centered programs, helping girls develop active lifestyles, and promoting long-term health) and priorities (safety, self-efficacy, and community). The final section of the chapter introduces ideas about how establishing these goals and priorities affects program design, the subject of the next chapter.

DESCRIBING ADOLESCENT GIRLS

In the previous chapters we discovered that adolescent girls often value the social network above the hierarchical objectives of games; that they are in a critical period of identity building made complex by a combination of physiological and societal forces; and that they may be sabotaged physically and emotionally by the settings in which they encounter activities, by what they are taught about their bodies, and by the methods used to measure their performance. The male military models that prevail in the fitness field rely on a male concept of the body, as well as aggressive, single-minded, rules-dominated measurement of performance—all of which run counter to physical and cultural characteristics of the archetypical female life cycle. During adolescence, the number of females participating in physical activities drops off, never to recover. As we see in figure 3.1, prepubescent girls are capable of very vigorous play—complex spontaneous expression within a festive social setting. As girls grow into adolescence, we are not harnessing this innate joy, the emotionally transcendent behavior, that emerges from girls when they are allowed to generate their own forms of activity.

We have also seen that by altering the actual physical movements girls and women are asked to make in supervised activities (e.g., through adjusting stance and posture, utilizing their lower center of gravity, and developing strong three-dimensional movement in the hip joint) and also by being sensitive to hormone cycles, we may be able to reduce injury and provide a satisfying female movement vocabulary. Changes in the psychosocial design of programs (e.g., through altering our concept of fitness to one that is less linear and more circular, altering our methods of evaluation to include more female-friendly components like verbal feedback, using more

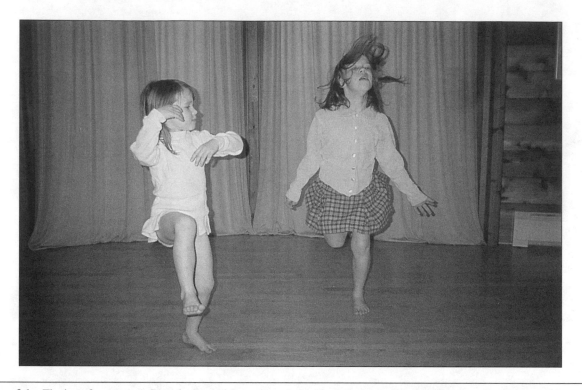

Figure 3.1   The joy of movement. Prepubescent girls at play at a family gathering—why does this joy of movement disappear in adolescence?

activities of daily living, and being creative about adolescent developmental issues) may help us attract and retain more adolescent girls in health-promoting physical activities.

PHYSICAL ACTIVITY AND ADOLESCENT GIRLS' HEALTH

We are setting our goals and priorities in relation to current public health issues such as obesity, eating disorders, increasing rates of adult-onset diabetes, and other disorders preventable through a healthy lifestyle, as well as psychosocial issues around educating women as one avenue to increased national health. In choosing goals and priorities, we are assuming that there is a public value to be gained if we reach our goals. What might that value be? Physical activity is a component of healthy behavior, and healthy behavior reduces lifetime health care costs. Investing in fitness for adolescent girls as a way to improve health and reduce costs can potentially give us value in return. Is there a relationship between physical activity and adolescent girls' health that warrants this investment?

A positive association between physical activity and health for adults is well established [1]. But for adoles-

cent girls, there is less to go on. It seems that obesity, NIDDM, and other adverse consequences of a sedentary lifestyle are on the rise in children and adolescents as well as adults. One avenue to reverse this "trend" would be the application of high volumes of vigorous exercise, which research has shown to have a positive effect for children and adolescents with genetic predispositions and other high risk markers for cardiovascular diseases [2-10]. How practical is this? In the case of girls, puberty signals the start of a decline in willing participation in physical activity [11]. For a portion of this population, high levels of ritualized, vigorous physical activity carries the risk of eating disorders, as noted previously. Primary preventions and treatments for eating disorders and obesity (a number of which include physical activity) have been woefully disappointing [12]. And, Aaron and LaPorte have pointed out that the data does not support the notion that adolescents who are physically active are in better health than those who are inactive [13].

As a result, from the public health perspective, we must ask questions about our intentions. Are we primarily focused on promoting high levels of physical activity in the component of this population at high risk of obesity or diseases that are considered preventable in adults? What if we focused primarily on achieving a healthy quality and level of physical activity within this overall population as a by-product of doing activities that enhance their development? Looking at other public health concerns for adolescents may better enable us to answer these questions.

The National Adolescent Health Information Center has delineated six major public policy goals for adolescent health. Included are improving access to health care for adolescents; improving adolescent environments; increasing the role of schools in improving adolescent health; promoting positive adolescent health; improving the adolescent transition to adulthood; and improving collaborative relations among government, public, private, community-based, and professional groups and individuals working in this area [14]. A companion report reviewing statistical information tells us that this group has the least access to health care; is increasingly living in poverty; dies most frequently from accidents, homicide, and suicide; and increasingly initiates risky behavior at younger ages [15].

Does physical activity help with any of these issues? Altering the sociopolitical climate to improve living conditions and access to health care for adolescents is a complicated task, but—assuming that girl-centered fitness programs include cognitive components—there is a place for these programs within this large, complex policy shift. Yale economics professor T. Paul Schultz has noted that when developing nations spend more money educating girls than educating boys, the rate of return is higher in a number of ways: birthrates drop; infant and maternal mortalities drop; overall health increases; the incidence of AIDS (acquired immunodeficiency syndrome) drops; more women enter the workforce; wages increase 10% to 20% for each additional year of school; educated mothers are more likely to have educated children; and all of these factors contribute to a stronger economy [16]. When women learn how to generate health, they pass this information on to their families and communities. In the United States, it is clear that commercial forces are aware of this phenomenon, because they point health-related advertising toward women. Reframing girls' and women's fitness programs to take advantage of their contribution to the improvement of national health is possible and desirable.

Promoting positive adolescent health and improving the transition to adulthood are areas in which new gender-based models of physical activity might also be helpful. Teaching girls how physical activities promote health and using activity to facilitate developmental processes are girl-centered methods we have already identified. What about behavior issues among adolescents? Aaron and LaPorte note that physically active adolescents are not less likely than others to engage in risky behaviors [13]. On the other hand, Pate et al. have reported that sport participation is prevalent among U.S. high school students and is associated with numerous positive health behaviors and few negative health behaviors [17]. Could

it be that existing health promotion and physical education rely on taking something away—such as smoking or alcohol or sex—and on requiring specific, uniform levels and amounts of exercise, and that this strategy is less effective than sport? Instead, sport can provide an activity-based social setting capable of generating survival strategies. Maybe it is the lens through which we view the issue of physical activity and adolescent health that needs a change. Rather than asking what we can do to make young people behave in a certain way, we might ask: How do we give them survival skills?

Another public health concern for adolescent girls is the controversial idea that girls, especially African American girls, may be entering puberty at an earlier age than their mothers [18, 19]. A complex of influences has been implicated—including body fat associated with dietary intake [20], leptin [21] and estrogen simulators in the environment (chemicals and plastics) also associated with breast cancer [22], the possibility that the absence of a biological father in the household affects biological cues in female puberty [23, 24], and the visual cues to girls via sexualization of children in the media [25]. Although there is disagreement about whether early puberty is an actual trend, this research does give us insight into possible causes for early puberty. And dealing with the sequellae of this phenomenon within the physical activity setting certainly seems reasonable. A situation in which girls can finish their developmental tasks of childhood through play, while addressing the developmental challenges of maturation through teamwork, is achievable.

Obesity, risky behaviors, environmental influences, and socioeconomic factors are the major health issues for adolescents. Activity models that rely on quantity have some effect, but are not practicable. Data from two large studies [26, 27] and the Surgeon General's report [11] do not support the idea that American teenagers are a particularly inactive portion of the population or are becoming a more inactive portion of the population. However, as with other populations, the need for increased physical activity is clear. We know that over time, regular physical activity is part of a healthy lifestyle that promotes health and prevents some disorders—a valuable goal for the long term. But, in the short and the medium term with this population, we clearly need a new tack. From a public health perspective, the greatest appeal of physical activity may be that it has the immediate (albeit momentary) benefit of preventing unhealthy behaviors. While they are in a socially oriented activity session, adolescent girls are not engaged in unhealthy behaviors. Moreover, the setting can be one in which trusted adults have an opportunity to steer those at risk away from unhealthy behaviors or adverse environmental influences toward resources that provide support for such problems as eating disorders, smoking, drug abuse, pregnancy, poverty, or sexual abuse. In a safe, efficacious, community-building program, girls have opportunities to learn about themselves, become involved in a supportive network, develop coping skills, and participate in physical activities in tune with their needs. By defining appropriate goals and priorities we develop guidelines for translating these findings into practical programs.

DEFINING GOALS AND PRIORITIES

Goals are the end to which an effort is aimed. If we make gender-based alterations in our models of fitness for adolescent girls, outcomes may also change. If we have assessed the available evidence correctly, these outcomes will match our goals. In a community program or school exercise class, one might identify a specific program goal, such as "each student will make at least one more free throw than she thinks she can." But in this text, we are identifying broad goals that all fitness programs for girls could ultimately and cumulatively be working toward. Our major goals include the short-term goal of increasing participation in girl-centered fitness programs, the medium-term goal of helping adolescent girls develop active lifestyles, and the long-term goal of promoting health and preventing some disorders.

There are also immediate concerns that program designers and leaders need to keep in mind to help them achieve goals. These are the *priorities* of fitness programs for adolescent girls. For instance, safety has long been considered a priority of fitness programs. If we do not provide a safe program (a priority), we cannot expect the program to develop the habits that promote health and prevent disorders (a long-term goal). We want to reach our long-term goal, but we must maintain our priorities in the everyday running of our programs. Our priorities are safety, self-efficacy, and community.

SHORT-TERM GOAL: INCREASE PARTICIPATION IN GIRL-CENTERED FITNESS PROGRAMS

In the short term, there are three gender-based strategies in programming that can potentially help increase participation in girl-centered physical activity. The first is to focus more on the whole girl than on measured physical performance elements. The second is to properly prepare instructors—make sure they understand female bio-

mechanics and are creative in making movement appropriate for girls. The third strategy is to develop lesson plans based on things girls value.

Focus on the Whole Girl

The health of the whole girl—physical, mental, emotional, and social—is the immediate outcome concern of each activity session. It is ideal when girls come out of an activity session feeling positive, physically capable, and cognizant of what they have gained, as well as of its application to real life. Programs that achieve positive physical, emotional, and cognitive results have the best chance to develop a charismatic reputation in the local girl culture. If we are to draw more and more girls into participation in physical activities, positive information must turn up in their informal communication network.

To stay focused on girls' overall health rather than on whether they perform at a prescribed level, we need, first, to use physical activity as the tool rather than the end; second, to consider what we measure and how we measure; and third, to promote the development of physical activity as a life skill.

Physical Activity as a Tool

Because movement can carry content on several levels at once ("The wind is moving past my face . . . pushing on the ground helps me run faster . . . I like playing with these people . . ."), it can be used to teach many things. A quiet session following a specific activity or workout can be used to relate a physical activity to some other practical aspect of participants' lives. For example, after a session on how to carry weighted objects in a biomechanically correct manner, the instructor could ask junior high or high school girls what they discovered while doing the exercise. She could then inquire what pieces of furniture they have in their room and how they would carry each one if they were rearranging their room. Why would they rearrange their room? As they grow up, they may want to change their room as a way of restating their identity. Rearranging the furniture is vigorous physical activity that allows a girl to control her immediate environment and express herself. Or, following a step aerobics session with pregnant adolescents, the instructor could ask them how this activity compares and contrasts with being a cheerleader, playing on a soccer team, or cleaning their rooms at home—what's the same and what's different? She could then ask the girls what they do to help themselves get through difficult movements, plays, or decisions and how they might use those strategies getting through labor. One girl might say it helps her to stay focused and not fuss about things, whereas another says she's a team player so she relies on her teammates. Each now has a strategy she can use in real life, and this strategy connects her mind to her body.

What and How Do We Measure?

If we are not going to quantify performance, how are we going to decide what is working? It's not that measurement is banished, but rather that how it is accomplished, what we evaluate, and why we evaluate are different. Girls should do any measuring themselves, because that gives them knowledge and control. Everything must be explained to them so that there is no hidden agenda. If a grant or the continuation of a program is at stake, we should tell them. To say, "We are doing this because the state will give us money to do more classes if they have the numbers to show you are healthy" provides a perfectly acceptable motivation for learning to measure how many curl-ups members of the class can do. This message is reality based, and has no more effect on outcome than not telling the class the reason or purpose for evaluation, which sometimes leads to fear or anger and affects outcome.

But, even more importantly, subjective methods of evaluation—especially letting girls talk about their response to an activity or experience—must be used and must be given primary importance. Not only does this give the girls a chance to talk; it also provides the leader with information about how well a project is working and how it might be improved. Talking about what they like best allows the participants to verbalize or identify something they have experienced that elicited positive feelings. Unlike achievement goals based on performance measures, the use of experiences or activities that can be subjectively evaluated by the girls themselves allows the instructor or facilitator an opportunity to listen to what each girl values. Girls who are achievement or performance oriented can express their satisfaction with a performance result, but without the added negative connotations that accrue to those whose performance is less effective in situations where performance *is* the goal. If a paper trail is needed, discussion can always be followed up with Likert-type scales assessing how much a girl agrees or disagrees with statements about the experience, or some assessment of what she learned, or both.

Take the case of learning to do free throws in basketball. In the measurement-oriented male model, we have as our specific objective that each student will make 3 out of 10 free throws. In the female model we have as our objective that each student will make one more free throw than she thinks she can. In the male model, we start out by structuring the population (get in lines, take turns, etc.) and teach them skills for improving their free throws. Then we test them. In the female model, we start out by asking each girl whether she has ever played bas-

ketball, how important she thinks basketball is in the real world (however she defines this), and what she perceives is the most important action to accomplish in the game. Next, if she is not curious yet about whether she can get the ball in the hoop, we ask her if she can think of how shooting a basketball will improve her posture (or make her appear taller, or give her upper arms a good shape). And, of course, we explain the answers to her. Even girls who are initially negative can be drawn into participation when they see that opinions are important and they are not threatened by demands. Then, we put the girls into small groups and let them try free throws. We adjust the distance, if necessary, and continue making minor adjustments until they start teaching each other how to get the ball into the hoop. We continue this process until there is some interest in moving on. Then we ask how many free throws each girl thinks she can make in about a minute. Next we let her do free throws until she makes one more than she thinks she can. Girls with talent and interest will make themselves known, and they can move into more structured or competitive programs. Others will have the experience of succeeding at a physical skill, and this may lead them to work on this skill because they can do it, or it is fun, or it can be done in a group, or they can teach it to someone else, or because it just feels good to move around. This process could constitute a single session, or it could cover several weeks of activity. It also ends up including a lot of low- and moderate-intensity aerobic activity and some skill building—walking and running after balls, shooting, and dribbling. It includes a lot of discussion about what the girls like. This kind of instruction can always be followed up by a brief written quiz or a Jeopardy-type game to reinforce what was learned.

The instructor, meanwhile, is busy keeping the social flow going like a well-run party. She is thinking on her feet about how to develop some of the girls' answers into relevant applications, making sure in subtle ways that all the girls are physically active, observing who the effective peer leaders are and pairing them up with those who may benefit from the association, carefully adding information that may help the girls make progress, noting things that girls might want to share in a debriefing session, encouraging as much interaction as possible, and listening to what produces positive feelings.

Developing Life Skills

Listening to what makes girls feel positive avoids a dilemma concerning differences in female and male perceptions of success and the potential for danger inherent within competitive success. This is how Carol Gilligan has articulated the problem that particularly afflicts white American women:

. . . the findings of the images of violence study suggest that men and women may perceive danger in different social situations and construe danger in different ways—men seeing danger more often in close personal affiliation than in achievement and construing danger to arise from intimacy, women perceiving danger in impersonal achievement situations and construing danger to result from competitive success. [28, p. 42]

When we provide a strategy that takes into account the complex influences at work on adolescent girls' health, we can better control such problems as fearing achievement for its ability to mark and thus separate a girl from her social setting. If girls can comfortably express what is satisfying for them—no matter their racial or cultural background—they can confirm their personal identities without removing themselves from the social fabric that often gives meaning to their lives. Additionally, we must connect activities with their real-life applications through cognitive components. We might even consider putting physical activity into the setting of a life skills class, where a combination of learning about female anatomy and physiology along with manipulation of space, time, and energy provides an opportunity to develop a living relationship with the laws of physics, math, geometry, and biology. Working on social and physical skills together can lead to creative problem-solving.

Properly Prepared Instructors

With what we know about female anatomy, an instructor skilled in female biomechanics is a critical variable. Those leading activity programs have a responsibility to promote healthy female biomechanics to avoid injury, attrition, and other adverse outcomes. Adequate training in female anatomy and physiology are clearly needed. Skeletal and muscular differences between females and males, the physiology of the female reproductive cycle, and a method (such as effort/shape analysis) for differentiating movement preferences among individuals are topics that need to be added to the educational curriculum for those who work with girls and women. It may also be helpful to screen instructors for their natural abilities to turn the laws of physics into healthy biomechanics [29].

Instructors also need to be skilled in the area of creativity with movement and in the ability to adapt motion to appropriate size, shape, speed, flow, and effort for individual participants' capabilities. The capacity to adapt daily movements to fitness purposes is another area in which creativity is needed. Assessing how well instructors can do these skills [30] may be an avenue for under-

standing why some programs and interventions are more successful with girls than others.

The developmental issues for adolescent girls concerning identity, interdependency, and individuation constitute another critical area with which instructors and facilitators need to be familiar. While greater depth is required for those designing programs, a basic understanding of the dichotomy faced by girls as they become women is important for the people who lead programs. The oscillation between single-minded assertion of self versus the value of self in relation to others creates conflicts that an instructor will see acted out regularly. Of course, it is important for instructors to know such things as how to compute body mass index (BMI) and why it is a significant indicator of health status; but it is equally important to know if, when, and how to introduce this concept to a group of adolescent girls. Sensitivity to the characteristics of this population tells us that you don't introduce the topic until they are already interested in knowing the information for their own enlightenment and well-being. Also, it is important to acknowledge that— no matter how careful one might be with the information—the girls must be ready to deal with the reality that others will gain information about their bodies.

Develop Lesson Plans Based on Things Girls Value

We have already seen evidence of what girls value: social process, opportunities to experiment with identity (or self-schema), feelings, and appearance. We also know that they vary in the extent to which they are interested in competition. In addition, we have some evidence that girls in a wide range of ages like physical activity [31] and that adolescent girls understand the health value of exercise [32]. As part of a Girl Scouts of the USA study entitled *Strength in Diversity* [31], findings were taken from data on 362 girls, ranging in age from 6 to 18, with a mean age of 12.4 (standard deviation = 2.6), concerning what made them feel good. The cohort included 77 Native American, 94 African American, 41 Anglo-European, 76 Asian Pacific, and 74 Latina girls. When asked what made them feel good, 46% of all girls named physical activities; 19% mentioned activities involving arts and crafts; 14% indicated activities involving service to others; and 13% mentioned playing. Asked what aspect of the activity made them feel good about themselves, 28% indicated mastery or competence; 25% said they enjoyed the activity; 14% said it helped people; 10% said it was an opportunity to be with friends; and 6% indicated that it was a means of self-expression. Although this is a small cohort, a large percentage of the girls named physical activity as something that made them feel good, lending support to the idea that it is not being active that sabotages girls' participation, but rather what they are asked to participate in. We also see that mastering skills, having fun and feeling good, helping others, and expressing themselves are values that girls hold in relation to activities in general.

In this study, preference patterns relating to ethnicity, socioeconomic status (SES), and urbanization of residence, as well as interactions among these variables, led the researchers to conclude that cultural context and opportunity played significant roles in determining what activities made girls feel good about themselves and why. Clearly, the cultural milieu will extend its influence onto an individual girl. Findings on gender inequities between boys and girls regarding self-esteem [33-35], as well as findings that appear to establish loss of a positive sense of self for girls during puberty and adolescence [36, 37], actually reflect the situation of white high- and middle-SES girls who predominate in early studies. Looking at longitudinal data on black and white girls aged 9 to 14, Brown et al. found clear evidence that self-esteem does not follow the same declining pattern in black girls as in whites [38]. Subculture expectations and ideals regarding black women's appearance may suggest broader support for black girls' physiques [39, 40]. For girls of color such factors as gender, BMI, and puberty issues may be only part of their struggle for survival.

So, how do these findings help us determine what to include in a lesson plan that has a likelihood of attracting girls? Two things pop out: first, we want to offer activities structured around process-oriented projects that provide a high level of social interaction; and second, we want to permit choice so that there is more than one avenue through which a girl may participate. To build lessons that allow these things to happen, one good strategy is to divide the class or meeting session into more than one focus period. The first part of class might include doing something vigorous together, or a choice of activities (jumping rope or aerobic kick-boxing); the second part could include working on activity projects. The various activity projects can involve conducting experiments (e.g., learning to take a pulse, assess perceived exertion, and relate the two during a variety of activities) or expression (e.g., choreographing aerobic steps to a favorite song). Several projects can be started at the beginning of a course, and over time participants are allowed to complete the projects in the sequence they wish, in small groups or on their own. This requires some flexibility, as well as the availability of additional projects that the more advanced students can do for extra credit.

Presenting more than one activity for the whole group can resolve several difficulties. Choices allow for options of high or low intensity, competition or cooperation, teamwork or individuality, sheer athleticism or aesthetic considerations, and so on. In a setting where boys and girls are in the same class, the choice could be between a typically male activity and a typically female one. Pate and his colleagues have found, in high school settings where the choices might be football and aerobic dancing, that most of the boys choose football and most of the girls choose aerobic dance but that some of each will cross over and for a variety of reasons [41]. If the population is racially mixed, it is essential to offer choices and activities that reflect sensitivity to the specific situation. If instructors need ideas for projects, the PE Central Web site [42] offers a large and ever evolving variety.

MEDIUM-TERM GOAL: HELP GIRLS DEVELOP ACTIVE LIFESTYLES

What turns an experience into a memory or a habit? Think about occasions in your life, major family events, movies you have seen, books you have read, games you have played, events that constitute critical memories, learning experiences that define your life, times that stay vital in your mind, or skills you can do with your eyes closed. Consider also your state of being and the setting surrounding the event or the impact of the images that were created as part of your response. Great joy—your first kiss. Great sadness—the death of a parent, sibling, child, or friend. Great panic—a fire. Great satisfaction—first prize. Great, seemingly endless, repetition and boredom, but also great motivation—swimming 10 miles a week for eight years. Great learning—that amazing teacher you had in third grade. Great sense of identity building—the first time you saw professional women's basketball or *Swan Lake* live. These experiences are neurologically assimilated into your hard-wiring through the combination of intense energy and resulting neurochemical responses that occur during these events. This is the biological basis of learning. Whether we call these things memories or habits depends on whether they are going on only in the brain or whether physical behavior is also present.

The underlying mechanism in turning experiences into memories and habits are the plastic changes at synapses that cause a predictable chain of neurons to fire [43]. In 1949, Hebb hypothesized that cell assemblies—pairs or groups of neurons that become associated because they are repeatedly active at the same time—are physical pathways that constitute learning and memory at the cell level [44]. Since Hebb first proposed that neuron A can develop this type of functional relationship with neuron B, research has not only demonstrated the validity of the concept but also uncovered the conditions at pre- and postsynaptic sites that are necessary for assembly to occur. To fully explain all the details of this situation is outside the scope of this text, but a few fundamental features are helpful. The state of arousal of the organism is critical. A system that is highly energized has a positive effect on the bonding process. A high level of excitability at both the pre- and postsynaptic sites is required, and the presence of naturally occurring opiates is associated with this process. A body in motion, interacting with others, is full of energy, creating exactly the kind of biological setting that makes neurological learning and memory possible. Remarkable events occurring during this high-energy state are embedded at the cell level as neural assemblies. From a biological perspective, when we refer to lifestyle habits we are really referring to a complex neuromuscular buildup of these types of neural assemblies that turns them into reflex movements and rhythmic patterns initiated by associated stimuli.

Habituation, as delineated by neurobiology, involves a decrease in the behavioral reflex that occurs with repeated presentations of a stimulus. This phenomenon helps explain the nature of addiction, in which increasing levels of stimulus are required to achieve a given response. It also helps explain why making gains in fitness measures requires greater and greater stress on the adaptive systems involved. And it explains why changing habits as an adult is a difficult procedure. Over time, behaviors become more spinal and less cerebral. Instituting effective change requires bringing the behavior cycle into the conscious realm—to work on such issues as intrinsic or extrinsic motivation, perceived benefits and barriers, and self-efficacy—before neural networks can be altered and eventually sunk back to an unconscious level.

With adolescents, who are involved in experimental actions that may become habits, we are more concerned with providing the environmental conditions that promote biological learning for the first time. To construct an environment in which healthy habits are created, it is essential to understand this relationship among learning, memory, and habituation at the cell level. Ultimately, it is habituation on the cell level that drives the healthy behavior. Once we have a good sense of how people learn on this biological level, we have the keys to what turns an experience into a memory or a habit. We want to create activities that get girls' attention in the sense of producing these neurological assemblages. If our goal in the medium range is to help girls develop an active lifestyle because they are aware that they feel enhanced (i.e., attractive, well, and embedded in a meaningful social network), this is a modest and obtainable aim. Over time, they move from physical activity as a pleasure-inducing experimental behavior to physical activity as a lifestyle habit, and eventually to physical activity as a pathway to disease prevention.

LONG-TERM GOAL: PROMOTE HEALTH AND PREVENT DISEASE

The long-term practice of healthy habits, including regular physical activity, provides a female with her best possibility of outsmarting opportunistic illnesses and disorders. Genetics can predispose individuals to disorders, but behaviors, as well as environmental factors, can determine whether genetic potentials will be realized. By reducing allostatic load—the metabolic consequences of stress—on the immune system, a woman who habitually engages in healthy behavior positively affects the health potential of her life over time. By strengthening her body, she accretes resources and defenses such as a strong heart, lungs, blood, bones, nutrient stores, and so on.

There is still much to be learned about how developing health and fitness behaviors centered on the natural self-interest of adolescence can lead to the health and fitness habits of adulthood. For now, at least time will have been spent creating cell assemblages predisposed to health-inducing behaviors. A woman may need to reinvent motivations to remain active as her life progresses and takes on different meanings; but then, pregnancy and menopause, as well as other events, will provide her with new central issues around which to do so.

FIRST PRIORITY: SAFETY

Always, in any movement program of any type, the first priority is safety. Such factors as maintaining equipment, using liability releases, and employing trained personnel are implicit in operating a safe fitness program. The American College of Sports Medicine has published standards and guidelines for health/fitness facilities [45] that are useful for understanding in detail what constitutes a safe place for exercise. Budgets, especially for school systems and community centers, may not allow for state-of-the-art facilities. However, it is important to know what is recommended so that priorities can be established for selecting or equipping a space.

There are also a few safety issues that pertain specifically to adolescent girls. Some of these come under the heading of physical safety, whereas others constitute psychological safety; both types of issues are discussed in the remainder of this section.

Physical Safety

Injuries are a common measure of the safety of a sport or physical activity. Studies of high school athletics indicate that major injuries and upper-body injuries are most likely in football and baseball, sports girls rarely play, with the greatest number of injuries occurring in football [46, 47]. Although absolute numbers of sport-related injuries among high school students are greater in males, research suggests that basketball and soccer may have the greatest injury rates for adolescent girls, and higher rates for girls than for boys [46-49]. Knee injuries and anterior cruciate ligament surgeries appear to be higher for girls in these sports than for boys in these sports, or for girls in other sports [46, 50]. Other lower limb injuries and spinal injuries are distributed among both boys' and girls' sports at much lower rates.

In the first chapter of this text, we noted the high levels of anterior cruciate ligament injuries for female college and professional athletes in soccer and basketball, as well as the possibility that hormonal changes around the time of ovulation, which soften connective tissue, contribute to injury rates. In contrast, researchers looking at lower-body pain in pregnant and postpartum women—where effects of hormones might be expected to most greatly affect joint laxity and therefore vulnerability—concluded that biomechanics, not hormonal changes, contributed most greatly to lower leg pain and injury [51]. It may be true that the rate of female knee injuries in activities that place the knee in jeopardy—such as basketball, soccer, slide or step aerobics—can be partially attributed to vulnerability due to hormones. However, the likelihood that male-based biomechanics imposed on female anatomy contributes to damage is just as great and is more within our control. In fact, this is a huge, uncharted area in need of research.

During adolescence, when female anatomy is emerging, changing physiology and movement mechanics deserve a great deal of attention. The center of gravity and lever lengths within a growing body are shifting and may require muscle strength that is not yet present for adequate movement control [48, 52]. To ensure safe movement in adolescent girls, we must give them accurate information about their bodies and allow them to develop their own biomechanical movement preferences. Preventing injuries through traditional training methods can be augmented by somatic training techniques, that is, by directing attention toward sensory education, anatomical knowledge, release of tension, and biomechanical balance during movement. This method, employing associative mental focus, not only produces beneficial (and measurable) postural changes over time, but also develops kinesthesia and sensory awareness of detrimental body tensions [53]. One method of somatic training, known as centering, is described in the next chapter. It is critical that those facilitating movement technique be able to accurately observe what is happening at the bone level within each individual. To ensure that muscles are not pulling on bone that is out of alignment with gravity, and to help girls adjust their alignment accordingly, instructors must have the capacity to visualize action within the joints while watching the body from the outside.

Another area that needs attention is modification of space and equipment for biomechanical appropriateness, as well as greater opportunity for experimentation. For adolescent girls, especially during puberty, this is an age of transition, with the body changing in shape as well as size. Leverage and balance are affected. Giving girls opportunities to choose equipment, try out varying sizes, change their minds, and do other appropriate experimentation with equipment acknowledges this transition phase and helps them learn to be empirical. Chase et al. looked at the effects of modifying the basketball size and basket height on shooting performance and self efficacy of girls and boys 9 to 12 years old. The youngsters made more baskets at the 8-foot level than at the 10-foot level, and this was especially true for girls and for 9- and 10-year-olds [54]. The children's self-efficacy was higher prior to shooting than after, with boys having higher self-efficacy than girls; and self-efficacy was higher when the participants shot at the 8-foot basket than at the higher basket [54]. These findings point to the possibility that our attention to equipment may affect not only girls' performance, but also their beliefs.

Aaron and LaPorte have pointed out that improvements in screening, training, and equipment have yet to be shown to reduce the risk of accidental injury in the course of sport or exercise for this population [13]. These are areas in which we may need to refocus. When we screen, train, and alter equipment, we are trying to change the gate through which injury enters the picture and at the same time continue the game. Trying out various pieces and sizes of equipment is a way for young people to become familiar with the mechanisms of sport and other physical activities. But we often consider this familiarization process as a way into the activity. Instead, we might consider familiarization with an activity in itself an activity that may need frequent repetition as a girl grows. Providing new points of screening and training, as well as opportunities for girls older than 10 or 12 to merely experiment with equipment, could extend both physical and psychological safety.

Psychological Safety

The exercise environment as a place that should be psychologically safe is a relatively new topic of discussion. Most often, the discussion of psychological factors regarding exercise concerns antecedents, motivation, perceived benefits and barriers, and other issues that arise from the application of the transtheoretical model of intentional behavioral change to lifestyle behaviors, including exercise. The first step in this process was Prochaska and DiClemente's extension of the model to smoking cessation [55, 56]: when the negative, or con, factors of smoking become sufficiently unappealing, contemplation of change moves to action. Marcus found that this version of the model translated to exercise adoption by demonstrating that when pro (rather than con) factors became sufficiently significant, the action of behavior change took place [57]. In this model, the perceived benefits-barrier differential that results from contemplating the pros and cons of a behavior will influence outcome. The psychological stages of exercise adoption in the model—precontemplation, contemplation, preparation, action, and maintenance—correspond to concepts we discussed previously regarding habituation and change, namely, that to alter neurologically patterned behaviors, one must first bring them into the conscious realm in order to affect the neural assemblages.

With adolescents, however, we are working at a different point in the process (i.e., initial experimental behavior that may become habit). We want to know what influences adolescents to participate in exercise and make it part of their self-schema. Garcia et al. have looked at the potentiality for exercise participation in preadolescents and adolescents and have mapped findings on exercise antecedents that may help predict participation [58]. Such factors as school grade, perceived health, self-efficacy, social support, and exercise norms affect the benefits-barriers differential just described, which has a direct influence on exercise participation. But two other antecedents also have a direct effect on adolescent participation in exercise. They are race, which affects access to exercise, and gender [58]. Here we have uncovered a new vein of questioning: What is it about racial and sexual identity that so affects adolescent exercise participation? Could it be that the psychological safety zone for exercise is aimed at the white male? How do we change the safety zone for girls?

So a new topic enters our discussion of the psychological landscape surrounding physical activity for adolescent girls: Is this setting psychologically safe? How do we know? The most practical way to determine whether or not a program permits participants to feel psychologically safe may be to look at attendance, participation, and attrition. Whatever models one may use regarding beliefs, motivations, or barriers to exercise, ultimately either girls participate or they don't. Their level of comfort is clearly reflected in whether or not it is valuable for them to attend and participate on a regular basis. Because we know that adolescence is a time when girls' participation drops off, we have to ask ourselves what makes girls uncomfortable in the exercise settings we offer. Part of the answer lies in the discussion of fitness models described in chapter 1. Just at the time girls are turning into women, we ask them to act the most like men—and not just regular men, but hypermasculine men. Although this works for some girls, for many it does not.

We also need to look at settings in which participation and retention levels are high, and ask gender-based questions about the psychological environment and why these programs are successful. Is everyone acquainted? Are new girls introduced and allowed to tell and learn personal histories? Does everyone have a buddy, big sister, or some option for developing helpful relationships? Does everyone know how to play the game at hand? Are the peer leaders positive, setting a tone that is encouraging? Do the girls have self-calming abilities to deal with the emotional upheavals that beset adolescent girls, or do they need to learn such techniques? Some children did not have the opportunity or inclination to develop this ability (self-calming) as an infant; and adolescence can provide a second chance through the learning of centering, relaxation, and imagery exercises. Are there options about clothing, so that girls who prefer not to wear revealing costumes aren't afraid? And another component might seem obvious, but needs emphasis: Are there bathrooms nearby? Are sanitary supplies available, as well as extra clothing?

Because our criterion for success in programming for adolescent girls is not victory over others, but enhancement of this phase of the female life cycle, psychological safety is a critical issue. If girls are not comfortable in the environment in which we are asking them to develop an active lifestyle, can they possibly develop such a habit? It's a shame to lose those girls who are at risk of becoming sedentary because they do not know for sure there are sanitary napkins within a few steps or that it's okay not to wear a uniform—but it happens all the time.

SECOND PRIORITY: SELF-EFFICACY

Increasingly, perceived self-efficacy is seen as a highly reliable predictor of exercise behavior in many populations [59-62], including adolescents [63, 64] and women [65]. The concept of self-efficacy emerges from Bandura's social cognitive theory of behavior regulation [66-68] and involves more than knowledge and skills, including the perception that one is capable of effectively executing the intended act [62]. In this sense, self-efficacy is belief in one's ability to perform behaviors that produce certain outcomes, and it is derived to the largest extent from active mastery [69]. Structuring activities so that girls accomplish acts promoting their perception of self-efficacy is the second priority of individual sessions. In every class, there can be something for each girl that contributes to this result. Sometimes it may be repeating a skill that she knows well; at other times, it may be reflecting on something she did for the first time. These individual personal acts of completion can be very small tasks, but the continued practice of accomplishing and acknowledging them increases the perception of self-efficacy. Finding out what activities a girl does, has abilities in, or has done in the past is critical. Talent and know-how help to tap her existing beliefs about what she can do [70, 71].

To put self-efficacy into perspective, it is useful to look at Pender's revised Health Promotion Model [72]. This model, shown in figure 3.2, seeks to place all of the many

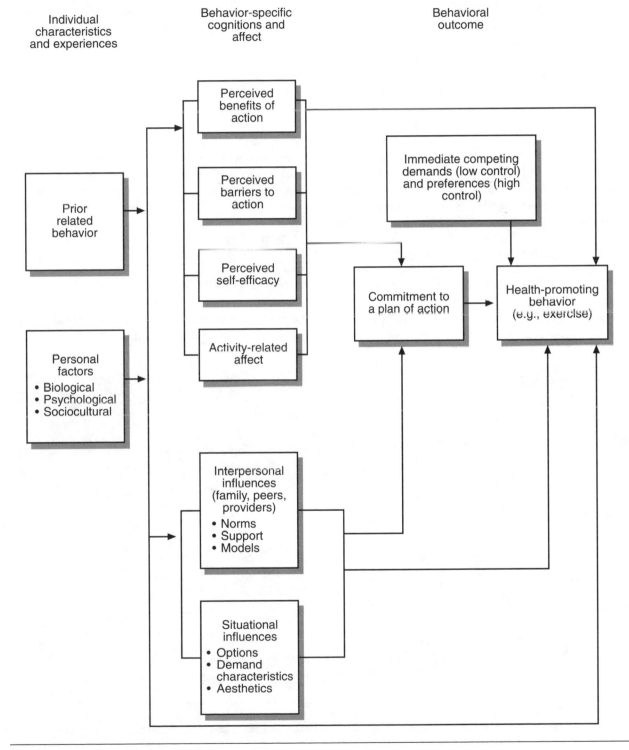

Figure 3.2 Pender's revised Health Promotion Model.

findings on factors affecting health behaviors into a pattern of influence. Individual characteristics and experiences, on the left, are preexisting components that contribute to action, including prior related experiences, which are among the best predictors of the same or similar behaviors. Other characteristics in this column are personal factors including biological, psychological, and sociocultural variables. Biological variables include age, gender, BMI, maturation status, $\dot{V}O_2$ maximum, strength, balance, and so on. Psychological factors include such variables as self-esteem, self-motivation, personal competence, perceived health status, and definition of health. Sociocultural factors include variables such as race, ethnicity, acculturation, education, and SES.

The category of behavior-specific cognitions and affect, in the middle, is the critical area in which interventions are most effective. Included are perceived benefits of and perceived barriers to actions, perceived self-efficacy, and activity-related affect (subjective feeling states that occur prior to, during, and following behaviors and that relate to the activity, oneself, and the environment). The fact that perceived self-efficacy is emerging as a major factor in physical activity behavior in all populations and that it is amenable to manipulation through intervention [73, 74] makes it an important element in program design. Also included are interpersonal variables (including norms, social support, and peer models,) and situational variables or factors that make an activity more or less appealing (such as updated equipment, a clean space).

The third set of characteristics that affect health-promoting behaviors is behavioral outcomes, on the right. The commitment to a plan of action begins a behavioral event. Commitment is what drives an individual through completion unless competing demands (e.g., family, school, work), over which an individual has little control, become overbearing or unless preferences (e.g., talking on the phone, shopping), over which one has a high degree of control, intrude into one's thoughts and derail intentions.

Pender's Health Promotion Model can be used to design activities that center on promoting the growth of perceived self-efficacy. Creative projects that combine expressive with physical activities can bring together many aspects of this model. One such project is the "Who Am I?" project, in which participants make an artful sociogram of their roles in life—such as student, daughter, friend, cousin, cook, athlete (see figure 3.3)—and then perform a simple self-directed strength test that involves activities at various sites in the room or building (see figure 3.4).

The "Who Am I?/Strength Test" project was developed by the author, working with adolescent mothers to help them see that they do have complex lives, but also their own coping styles. The initial artwork component

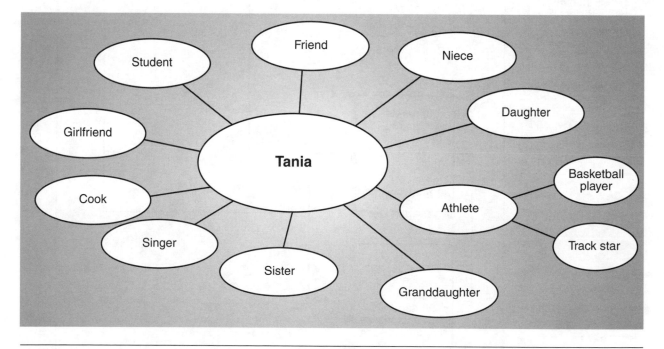

Figure 3.3 Sociogram for the "Who Am I" project. Each girl makes a list of her life roles and turns it into a sociogram, such as the one shown here. She then selects colors, shapes (abstract or realistic), and other design factors to create an expressive version. Examples of finished projects are shown in figure 11.15.

Sign by stairs
(typical 13-step
flight of stairs)

Strength training
Heart
(stair climb)

Sign by
chairs

Strength training
Legs
(stand up and sit down)

Sign on
wall

Strength training
Arms
(wall push-ups)

Sign by
abdominal
roller

Strength training
Abdomen
(curl-ups)

Strength Training Worksheet

ID# (or Name):_____ Date:_____

I can climb _____ times up *and* down the stairs.

I can do _____ wall push-ups.

I can do _____ stand-ups and sit downs.

I can do _____ curl-ups.

Figure 3.4   Strength test supplies for strength training of the heart, arms, legs, and abdomen accompanied by a worksheet.

turns out to be mildly active, as the girls move about choosing materials, working on their drawings, and helping each other accomplish their desired results. It serves as a warm-up. The strength test employs utilitarian objects—walls, chairs, stairs, and the floor—and is very simple. By associating these two tasks, the girls learn that within their self-schema are self-directed capacities—they know who they are and can execute acts of strength. This is an example of a creative solution to a situation in which there are few resources; it has been so successful that we have extended it to other populations.

Any physical education project can be opened up and an avenue found to incorporate this type of self-creating knowledge. For example, we often teach squats or other resistance movements to adolescents by showing them what to do, explaining carefully, and trying to perfect their technique. However, when they see the action of iliofemoral, knee, and ankle flexion on a skeleton first, they can use the visual image-homunculus connection to internalize the action before they even watch a model do it. If they see the action on the skeleton, then close their eyes and "watch" their own bones moving, their own minds become powerful teaching tools before they even try the action.

Running is full of learning opportunities: how fall and rebound becomes forward motion, how to go faster by increasing stride versus increasing turnover (and who prefers which system), how to keep your feet on the ground as long as possible to make your stride lengthen out, plus any discoveries the girls themselves make. A half-hour of trying various experiments with running gives the girls many things to think about the next time they are running. Learning to think in concepts derived from experience and knowledge is one of the tasks of adolescence. Connecting the two phenomena—running and thinking—helps them become mindful movers and develops belief and awareness that they can do things.

THIRD PRIORITY: COMMUNITY

The third priority in a movement program is building community. What does this mean? The author first became attuned to the communal or tribal nature of women's exercise groups when she began working with pregnant and postpartum women. Not being prepared for this side effect provided a perfect opportunity to observe it. It was clear that as much health was being derived from women's social support as from the exercise itself and that the support system was self-organizing.

The instructor's job was simply to create an atmosphere that did not stifle the tribe.

Early program evaluations held the key to why this community building was happening. Typical comments were "I'm so far away from my parents at this important time of life"; "Nobody at work wants to hear about my pregnancy, but at least I have friends in the class who understand what I'm going through"; and "It's so reassuring to talk with other women who have been through this before." In a mobile society, in which we no longer experience important life transitions within the safety of extended family, these classes were actually taking the place of an important cultural institution for women.

We have already seen that girls share this tribal trait. Whether it is inborn or learned seems of little consequence. It is valuable and worth nurturing. How might we do this? It is important to recognize that this is a largely self-organizing phenomenon. The instructor or facilitator can provide an environment in which community building will develop on its own. The preconditions are those we have already outlined: we want the projects to be about skill mastery and self-discovery rather than performance; we want to use social networking techniques such as peer leaders, activity choices, and small groups; and we want to focus on cognitive development and learning about health and fitness as well as spending time on physical skills.

An example with a slightly younger population will help illustrate the use of physical activity to do community building. The 1997-1998 Peer Health Education Kids Club for 9- to 10-year-olds—an activity-based club made up of a lower-middle-class mixed-race population, predominantly girls, at the Clinton Avenue Elementary School in New Haven, Connecticut—was facilitated by Karen Klein, PNP, MSN. The group participated in after-school activities that ranged from playing games such as praise and phrase tag (the same as freeze tag except that you get unfrozen if you say something nice about the person), meditation, singing, storytelling, reading aloud, taking one's own pulse, measuring each other's heights, plotting one's own growth charts, African dancing and drumming, and studies on gangs and abuse of power. By the end of the school year, Klein reports that the children had learned to associate feelings with behavior. When they read stories out loud they had begun to talk about what motivated characters' actions and what characters must be thinking and feeling to act as they did. Attendance was good, with no attrition. As an end-of-the-year project, the club created a video, *Take Care of Yourself, Take Care of Each Other* [75]. In this way, they not only built a meaningful community for themselves, but are contributing in an ongoing way to the health of the larger community they live in.

DEVELOPING CURRICULUMS BASED ON GIRL-CENTERED GOALS

By shifting our focus from developmental tasks primarily associated with male models of physical activity to developmental tasks of adolescent females, we are able to delineate goals and objectives that are more in keeping with the concerns of this population. Rather than emphasizing performance of aggressive acts that establish a physical hierarchy, a girl-centered model emphasizes expression, functional acts, biomechanics based on balance rather than immobility, and the recognition that our national health is, in part, in the hands of our women. We must do our best to educate young women about the health problems that result from inactivity, poor nutrition, and lack of self-care—such issues as obesity, heart disease, diabetes, and smoking.

Our programs—both school and community based—need to focus on the health of the whole girl, properly preparing our instructors and developing lesson plans based on things girls value. The goals for these programs include the short-term goal of bringing more adolescents into girl-centered programs, the medium-term goal of helping girls develop active lifestyles, and the long-term goal of health promotion and disease prevention. Our first priority, as always, is safety—both physical and psychological safety. Our second priority is helping girls develop perceived self-efficacy, and our third priority is community building. In the next chapter, we look at the nature of programs that can enable us to reach these goals and priorities, as well as a sample curriculum based on achieving these ends.

REFERENCES

1. Blair, S.N., Kohl, H.W., 3rd, Paffenbarger, R.S., Clark, D.G., Cooper, K.H., and Gibbons, L.W. 1989. Physical fitness and all-cause mortality: A prospective study of healthy men and women. *Journal of the American Medical Association* 262:2395-2401.

2. Armstrong, N., and Simons-Morton, B. 1994. Physical activity and blood lipids in adolescents. *Pediatric Exercise Science* 6:381-405.

3. Alpert, B.S., and Wilmore, J.H. 1994. Physical activity and blood pressure in adolescents. *Pediatric Exercise Science* 6:361-380.

4. Bryant, J.G., Garrett, H.L., and Dean, M.S. 1984. The effects of an exercise programme on selected risk factors to coronary heart disease in children. *Social Science and Medicine* 19:765-766.

5. Nizankowska-Blaz, R., and Abramowicz, T. 1983. Effects of intensive physical training on serum lipids and lipoprotein. *Acta Paediatrica Scandinavica* 72:357-359.

6. Hagberg, J.M., Goldring, D., Ehsani, A.A., Heath, G.W., Hernandez, A., Schechtman, K., and Holloszy, J.D. 1983. Effect of exercise training on the blood pressure and hemodynamic features of hypertensive adolescents. *American Journal of Cardiology* 52:763-768.

7. Brownell, K.D., and Kaye, F.S. 1982. A school-based behavior modification, nutrition education and physical activity program for obese children. *American Journal of Clinical Nutrition* 35:277-283.

8. Sasaki, J., Shindo, M., Tanaka, H., Ando, M., and Arakawa, K. 1987. A long-term aerobic exercise program decreases the obesity index and increases the high density lipoprotein cholesterol concentration in obese children. *International Journal of Obesity* 11:339-345.

9. Aaron, D.J., Dearwater, S.R., Anderson, R., Olsen, T., Kriska, A.M., and LaPorte, R.E. 1995. Physical activity and the initiation of high-risk behaviors in adolescents. *Medicine and Science in Sports and Exercise* 27:1639-1645.

10. Wing, R.R. 1993. Obesity and related eating and exercise behaviors in women. *Annals of Behavioral Medicine* 15:124-134.

11. U.S. Dept. of Health and Human Services. 1996. *Physical activity and health: A report of the Surgeon General.* Atlanta: USDHHS, CDC, NCCDPHP.

12. Battle, E.K., and Brownell, K.D. 1996. Confronting the rising tide of eating disorders and obesity: Treatment vs. prevention and policy. *Addictive Behaviors* 21(6):755-865.

13. Aaron, D.J., and LaPorte, R.E. 1997. Physical activity, adolescence, and health: An epidemiological perspective. In J.O. Holloszy (ed.), *Exercise and Sport Sciences Reviews,* vol. 25. Baltimore: Williams & Wilkins, pp. 391-405.

14. Brindis, C.D., Irwin, C.E., Ozer, E.M., Handley, M., Knopf, D.K., and Millstein, S.G. 1997. *Improving adolescent health: An analysis and synthesis of health policy recommendations.* San Francisco, CA: UCSF. National Adolescent Health Information Center.

15. Ozer, E.M., Brindis, C.D., Millstein, S.G., Knopf, D.K., and Irwin, C.E. 1998. *America's adolescents: Are they healthy?* San Francisco, CA: UCSF. National Adolescent Health Information Center.

16. Schultz, T.P. 1989. Investments in women, economic development, and improvements in health in low-income countries. *Annals of New York Academy of Sciences* 569:288-310.

17. Pate, R.R., Trost, S.G., Levin, S., and Dowda, M. 2000. Sports participation and health-related behaviors among U.S. youth. *Archives of Pediatrics and Adolescent Medicine* 154(9):904-911.

18. Herman-Giddens, M.E., Slora, E.J., Wasserman, R.C., Bourdony, C.J., Bhapkar, M.V., Koch, G.G., and Hasemeier, C.M. 1997. Secondary characteristics and menses in young girls seen in office practice: A study from the Pediatric Research in Office Settings network. *Pediatrics* 99(4):505-512.

19. Kaplowitz, P.B., and Oberfield, S.E. 1999. Reexamination of the age limit for defining when puberty is precocious in girls in the United States: Implications for evaluation and treatment. *Pediatrics* 104(4):936-941.

20. Berkey, C.S., Gardner, J.D., Frazier, A.L., and Colditz, G.A. 2000. Relation of childhood diet and body size to menarche and adolescent growth in girls. *American Journal of Epidemiology* 152(5):446-452.

21. Ahmed, M.L., Ong, K.K., Morrell, D.J., Cox, L., Drayer, N., Perry, L., Preece, M.A., and Dunger, D.B. 1999. Longitudinal study of leptin concentrations during puberty: Sex differences and relationship to changes in body composition. *Journal of Clinical Endocrinology and Metabolism* 84(3):899-905.

22. Davis, D.L., Bradlow, H.L., Wolff, M., Woodruff, T., Hoel, D.G., and Anton-Culver, H. 1993. Medical hypothesis: Xenoestrogens as preventable causes of breast cancer. *Environmental Health Perspectives* 101(5):372-377.

23. Ellis, B.J., McFadyen-Ketchum, S., Dodge, K.A., Pettit, G.S., and Bates, J.E. 1999. Quality of early family relationships and individual differences in the timing of pubertal maturation in girls: A longitudinal test of an evolutionary model. *Journal of Personality and Social Psychology* 77(2):387-401.

24. Moffit, T.E., Caspi, A., Belsky, J., and Silva, P.A. 1992. Childhood experience and the onset of menarche: A test of a sociobiological model. *Child Development* 63(1):47-58.

25. Belkin, L. 2000. The making of an 8-year-old woman. *NY Times Magazine* (December 24):43.

26. Aaron, D.J., Kriska, K.A., Dearwater, S.R., Anderson, R.L., Olsen, T.L., Cauley, J.A., and Laporte, R.E. 1993. The epidemiology of leisure physical activity in an adolescent population. *Medicine and Science in Sports and Exercise* 25:847-853.

27. Ross, J.G., Dotson, C.O, Gilbert, G.G. et al. 1984. After physical education: Physical activity outside of school physical education programs. *Journal of Physical Education, Recreation and Dance* 56:77-81.

28. Gilligan, C. 1982/1993. *In a different voice.* Cambridge, MA: Harvard University Press.

29. Baehr, M.E. 1959. *Intuitive mechanics (weights and pulleys): Interpretations and research manual.* Park Ridge, IL: London House.

30. Torrance, E.P. 1981. *Thinking Creatively in Action and Movement (TCAM).* Bensenville, IL: Scholastic Testing Service.

31. Erkut, S., Fields, J.P., Almeida, D., DeLeon, B., and Sing, R. 1994. *Strength in diversity.* NY: Girl Scouts of the USA.

32. Cowlin, A.F. 2000. Unpublished data concerning attitudes of pregnant adolescents toward exercise.

33. Minnesota Women's Fund. 1990. *Reflections of risk: Growing up female in Minnesota: A report on the health and well-being of adolescent girls in Minnesota.* Minneapolis, MN: Women's Fund.

34. Phillips, D.A., and Zimmerman, M. 1990. The developmental course of perceived competence and incompetence among competent children. In R. J. Sternberg and J. Kolligan, Jr. (eds.), *Competence considered.* New Haven, CT: Yale U. Press.

35. Gans, J., and Blyth, D. 1990. *America's adolescents: How healthy are they?* Chicago: American Medical Association.

36. Brown, L.M., and Gilligan, C. 1992. *Meeting at the crossroads: Women's psychology and girls' development.* NY: Random House.

37. American Association of University Women. 1991. *Shortchanging girls, shortchanging America.* Washington, DC: AAUW, Analysis Group, Greenberg-Lake.

38. Brown, K.M., McMahon, R.P., Biro, F.M., Crawford, P., Schreiber, G.B., Similo, S.L., Waclawiw, M., and Striegel-Moore, R. 1998. Changes in self-esteem in black and white girls between the ages of 9 and 14 years. *Journal of Adolescent Health* 23:7-19.

39. Melnyk, M.G., and Weinstein, E. 1994. Preventing obesity in black women by targeting adolescents: A literature review. *Journal of American Dietetic Association* 94:536-540.

40. Kumanyika, S., Wilson, J., Guilford-Davenport, M. 1993. Weight-related attitudes and behaviors of black women. *Journal of American Dietetic Association* 53:416-422.

41. Pate, R.R. 2000. *Lessons from LEAP: Promotion of physical activity in high school girls.* Presented at the 3rd Yale Conference on Women's Health and Fitness, October 27.

42. **http://pe.central.vt.edu**.

43. Shepherd, G.M. 1988. *Neurobiology,* 2nd ed., ch. 29. NY: Oxford University Press.

44. Hebb, D.O. 1949. The *organization of behavior.* NY: John Wiley.

45. Tharrett, S.J., and Peterson, J.A. (eds.). 1997. *ACSM's health/fitness facility standards and guidelines,* 2nd ed. Champaign, IL: Human Kinetics.

46. Powell, J.W., and Barber-Foss, K.D. 2000. Sex-related injury patterns among selected high school sports. *American Journal of Sports Medicine* 28(3):385-391.

47. Axem N.H., Newcomb, W.A., and Warner, D. 1991. Sports injuries and adolescent athletes. *Delaware Medical Journal* 63(6):359-363.

48. Backous, D.D., Friedl, K.E., Smith, N.J., Parr, T.J., and Carpine, Jr., W.D. 1988. Soccer injuries and their relation to physical maturity. *American Journal of Diseases in Children* 142(8):839-842.

49. McLain, L.G., and Reynolds, S. 1989. Sports injuries in a high school. *Pediatrics* 84(3):446-450.

50. Baker, M.M. 1998. Anterior cruciate ligament injuries in the female athlete. *Journal of Women's Health* 7(3):343-349.

51. Vullo, U.J., Richardson, J.K., and Hurvitz. E.A. 1996. Hip, knee and foot pain during pregnancy and the postpartum period. *Journal of Family Practice* 43(1):63-68.

52. Timmerman, M.G. 1996. Medical problems of adolescent female athletes. *Wisconsin Medical Journal* 95(6):351-354.

53. Gamboian, N., Chatfield, S.J., and Woollacott, M.H. 2000. Further effects of somatic training on pelvic tilt and lumbar lordosis alignment during quiet stance and dynamic dance movement. *Journal of Dance Medicine & Science* 4(3):90-98.

54. Chase, M.A., Esing, M.E., Lirgg, C.D., and George, T.R. 1994. The effects of equipment modification on children's self-efficacy and basketball shooting performance. *Research Quarterly of Exercise in Sport* 65(2):159-168.

55. Prochaska, J.O., and DiClemente, C.C. 1982. Transtheoretical therapy: Toward a more integrative model of change. *Psychotherapy: Theory and Research Practice* 20:161-173.

56. Prochaska, J.O., and DiClemente, C.C. 1983. Stages and processes of self change in smoking: Toward an integrative model. *Journal of Consulting and Clinical Psychology* 51:390-395.

57. Marcus, B.H., Rakowski, W.B., and Rossi, J.S. 1992. Assessing motivational readiness and decision making for exercise. *Health Psychology* 11(4):257-261.

58. Garcia, A.W., Broda, M.A.N., Frenn, M., Coviak, C., Pender, N.J., and Ronis, D.L. 1995. Gender and developmental differences in exercise beliefs among youth and prediction of their exercise behavior. *Journal of School Health* 65(6):213-219.

59. King, T.K., Marcus, B.H., Pinto, B.M., Emmons, K.M., and Abrams, D.B. 1996. Cognitive-behavioral mediators of changing multiple behaviors: Smoking and a sedentary lifestyle. *Preventive Medicine* 25(6):684-691.

60. Dzewaltowski, D.A. 1994. Physical activity determinants: A social cognitive approach. *Medicine and Science in Sports and Exercise* 26(11):1395-1399.

61. Marcus, B.H., Selby, V.C., Niaura, R.S., and Rossi, J.S. 1992. Self-efficacy and the stages of exercise behavior change. *Research Quarterly of Exercise in Sport* 63(1):60-66.

62. Willis, J.D., and Campbell, L.F. 1992. *Sports psychology,* ch. 5. Champaign, IL: Human Kinetics.

63. Allison, K.R., Dwyer, J.J., and Makin, S. 1999. Self-efficacy and participation in vigorous physical activity by high school students. *Health Education and Behavior* 26(1):12-24.

64. Reynolds, K.D., Killen, J.D., Bryson, S.W., Maron, D.J., et al. 1990. Psychosocial predictors of physical activity in adolescents. *Preventive Medicine* 19(5):541-551.

65. Sternfeld, B., Ainsworth, B.E., and Quesenberry, C.P. 1999. Physical activity patterns in a diverse population of women. *Preventive Medicine* 28(3):313-323.

66. Bandura, A. 1986. *Social foundations of thought and action: A social cognitive theory.* Englewood Cliffs, NJ: Prentice-Hall.

67. Bandura, A. 1982. Self-efficacy mechanism in human agency. *American Psychologist* 37(2):122-147.

68. Bandura, A. 1977. Self-efficacy: Toward a unifying theory of behavioral change. *Psychological Review* 84(2):191-215.

69. Lirgg, C.D. 1993. Effects of same-sex versus coeducational physical education on the self-perceptions of middle and high school students. *Research Quarterly of Exercise in Sport* 64(3):324-334.

70. Gottlieb, N.H., and Chen, M. 1985. Sociocultural correlates of childhood sporting activities: Their implications for heart health. *Social Science and Medicine* 21:533-539.

71. Sallis, J.F., Hovell, M.F., Hofstetter, C.R., Faucher, P., Elder, J.P., Blanchard, J., Caspersen, C.J., Powell, K.E., and Christenson, G.M. 1989. A multivariate study of determinants of vigorous exercise in a community sample. *Preventive Medicine* 18:20-34.

72. Pender, N.J., Murdaugh, C.L., and Parsons, M.A. 2002. *Health promotion in nursing practice,* 4th ed. Upper Saddle River, NJ: Prentice Hall.

73. Bandura, A., Barbaranelli, C., Caprara, G.V., and Pastorelli, C. 1996. Multifaceted impact of self-efficacy beliefs on academic functioning. *Child Development* 67(3):1206-1222.

74. Caruso, C.M., and Gill, D.L. 1992. Strengthening physical self-perceptions through exercise. *Journal of Sports Medicine and Physical Fitness* 32(4):416-427.

75. Peer Health Education Kids Club. 1998. *Take care of yourself, take care of each other* (video). New Haven, CT: Fair Haven Health Clinic.

CHAPTER 4

PROGRAM DESIGN FOR ADOLESCENT GIRLS

This chapter focuses on the design of programs that meet the goals and priorities outlined in the previous chapter. To begin, it is helpful to know where things currently stand. So, this chapter starts with a brief look at research findings of physical activity interventions that have included adolescent girls, as well as recommendations from the Centers for Disease Control and Prevention (CDC), aimed at increasing physical activity in young people. The next section of the chapter delineates core characteristics — that is, program structure, content, and ambience— that can be effective in achieving the designated goals and priorities on the basis of the information gathered so far. Subsequent sections describe intake procedures and program evaluations that help in meeting participant needs and assessing program outcomes, and lastly present a sample physical activity program for adolescent girls.

PHYSICAL ACTIVITY INTERVENTIONS

Results of intervention studies of school-based programs including girls in or near adolescence are mixed. Early studies focused largely on knowledge-based classroom lessons. Two of these studies, Know Your Body and the Stanford Heart Health Program, demonstrated gains in knowledge and attitude changes; but the Know Your Body intervention did not stop the decrease in levels of physical activity [1], and long-term outcomes were not examined in the Stanford study [2].

Increasing the Amount of Physical Activity in Schools and in the Community

The Sports, Play and Active Recreation for Kids study in San Diego combined a health-related physical education curriculum with in-service programs on quality and quantity of physical education classes. The study demonstrated that improving curriculum through training of physical education specialists and classroom teachers can substantially increase the amount of physical activity students receive in the course of their school day [3].

The Class of 1989 study, part of the Minnesota Heart Health Program, showed that multiple intervention components, such as in-school behavioral education and complementary community-wide strategies, can produce lasting improvement in adolescent physical activity, especially in female students [4]. Other findings were that over time (the study began with sixth graders and ran seven years), the value placed on physical appearance increased in both the intervention and reference communities, that girls in the intervention community tended to value the kinds of food they ate to a greater degree than the reference community did, and that a positive value regarding physical education was maintained by the intervention group but decreased in the reference group [5]. A positive attitude toward physical education is correlated with adolescent participation in physical activity [6, 7].

Effects on Self-Perception and Heart Health Predictors

In a related study, a cross-sectional analysis to assess the relationship of self-esteem and body mass index (BMI) in middle-class white seventh to ninth graders at baseline, French et al. found an inverse association between physical appearance self-esteem and BMI in both females and males [8]. In females, BMI was inversely associated with global self-esteem, close friendship, and behavioral conduct self-esteem [8]. The authors conclude that there is a modest association in this age group between self-esteem concerning physical appearance and BMI, but that low self-esteem did not necessarily predict obesity over time [8]. However, prospectively, females' physical appearance and social acceptance self-esteem at baseline were inversely related to BMI three years later [8]. Previously we noted that this relationship does not hold for African American girls.

The Child and Adolescent Trial for Cardiovascular Health (CATCH) was a three-year multisite study of a school-based intervention to reduce or prevent the development of risk factors for cardiovascular disease. As part of the study, an innovative health-related physical education program was started in the third grade. In the lunches in the intervention school, the percentage of energy intake from fat fell significantly more than in the control schools, and the intensity and duration of physical education classes significantly increased in the intervention schools compared with control schools. Although blood pressure, body size, and cholesterol measures did not differ significantly between the two types of schools [9], the study did demonstrate effectiveness in changing the psychosocial variables likely to influence a reduction in unhealthy behavior for cardiovascular disease [10]. In assessing the CATCH results, Stone et al. conclude that the study provided more scientific evidence of the importance of schools in the population approach to health promotion [11]. They also suggest that the strategies may be useful in other similar settings for research purposes.

The Cluster Nature of Health Behaviors

Through the work of Jessor and others, we have also learned that health behaviors in adolescents tend to occur in clusters [12, 13]. That is, several behaviors that have an impact on health and fitness often occur at the same time, such as school truancy, inactivity, smoking, alcohol intake, and poor nutrition, all of which place the student's health at risk. The National Heart, Lung, and Blood Institute is presently supporting research on the effectiveness of interventions aimed at increasing levels of physical activity while decreasing health-risk behaviors in adolescent girls.

Coed Versus Same-Sex Programs

Lirgg has examined the effects of coed versus same-sex physical education on several self-perception variables in learning basketball in middle school and high school students. Variables examined on both the individual and group levels included perceived self-confidence about learning basketball, perceived usefulness of basketball, and perceived gender appropriateness of basketball. Variability in groups for self-confidence could be explained by grade, class type, and the interaction between gender and class type [14]. At the individual level, males in same-sex classes were significantly less confident in their ability to learn basketball than were males in coed classes [14]. In general, however, middle school students preferred same-sex classes [14].

These findings raise questions: Are adolescent females viewed as less competent as a group? Do males feel more confident in a coed setting because they can compare themselves to less aggressive players, whereas in a same-sex setting there is a greater sense of competition? This bears on issues raised previously about the changing nature of the playing field deriving merely from the presence of women. The research also raises questions about the perception of women's skills, expectations for their performance, and the measure of outcome. And for adolescent girls, this research also clarifies the point that many girls prefer same-sex settings at this transitional time in their lives.

Centers for Disease Control Guidelines

The CDC's "Guidelines for School and Community Programs to Promote Lifelong Physical Activity Among Young People," issued in 1997, makes recommendations for physical activity programs. These recommendations focus on the importance of both school- and community-based programs and on providing a safe and supportive setting, working on knowledge and skills, improving self-confidence, setting programs within the greater context of health education, involving parents and training staff, extending the scope and quantity of health-related counseling and services, and doing regular evaluation (of outcomes, instruction, and facilities) [15].

The CDC's recommendations acknowledge the central role of physical activity in healthy behavior. It is clear that health issues are complex for young people. Healthy behavior is actually a cluster of various behaviors, including appropriate physical activity; good nutrition; and avoidance of drugs, alcohol, tobacco, and unprotected sex. Risky behavior not only is unhealthy, but also threatens the academic potential of youngsters engaged in such behavior. Reviewing the literature concerning this relationship, Symons et al. have drawn the link between student health-risk behavior and education outcomes, behavior, and attitudes, and conclude that healthy children learn better [16].

CORE CHARACTERISTICS OF PROGRAMS DESIGNED SPECIFICALLY FOR ADOLESCENT GIRLS

Clearly, improving the health and fitness of adolescent girls is a worthy area for investment of resources—both research and energy for program development. Although models are still few and the evolution of interventions for this population is in its infancy, there are indications of how to proceed with implementing school and community programs to achieve this end. The existing research tells us that girls do respond to the attention provided in special programs that include more physical activity within the physical education curriculum, the regular classroom, and the community.

Effective program design starts with current research and experience, translating this knowledge into concrete activity. Programs aimed at increasing adolescent participation in girl-centered programs and helping adolescent girls develop active lifestyles, as well as the long-term goal of health promotion and disease prevention, will share common features—the core characteristics of these programs. Based on the information we have gathered, these core characteristics fall into three categories in which we should see major differences from male models in design and implementation: structure, content, and ambience.

Structure

Physical activity is embedded within school-based and community-based programs. Community centers, churches, health clinics, and other venues that already have access to this population all contribute. The quality of social interaction is the organizing factor, as opposed to learning behaviors that lead to others' losses. New enterprises may emerge. Much as the burgeoning industry of pregnancy and mother-baby programs has developed over the past 20 or 30 years, programs that create new community associations promoting health and fit-

ness education for adolescent girls should develop in the next decades. Ongoing short-duration programs (6 to 10 weeks), with participants grouped by interest rather than by age, might be the norm. Repeating sessions could include brief review, then greater detail—so girls can perpetually join in, and peer models/teachers can emerge. Same-sex format, and/or activity choices that include female-based preferences, would be used.

Content

Components of physical fitness (i.e., cardiovascular endurance, strength, flexibility, balance, and coordination) are both topic and method. Through a combination of exercise, sports, dance, enhancement of daily activities, and interactive learning, the interdependence of physical activity, basic nutrition, personal hygiene, stress management, female physiology, safe sex and abstinence, and avoidance of drugs and alcohol is reinforced as a valuable part of self-interest. Creative and expressive approaches to motor skills are used, and cognitive connections are made to real-life applications; physical activity is used as a means to accomplish various tasks, from moving furniture to looking good. And, perhaps most importantly, programs designed for adolescent girls use female anatomy, biomechanics, imagery, and models.

Ambience

Nurturing, flexibility, and consensus are valued; socializing is built in; and working in small groups is facilitated. The facilities and environment are comfortable and correctly sized for girls. Circles are used more often than rows with a military-style leader. And, instructors hear girls out rather than enforce specific behaviors.

INTAKE PROCEDURES

Intake procedures and program evaluation are necessary to determine the extent to which a program meets a girl's needs or impacts outcomes. For school or community programs, complex instruments or data collection may not be appropriate. Even so, tracking illness, injury, exercise history, nutrition, preferences, and so on will help instructors develop effective strategies for working with adolescent girls. The information-gathering procedures used when girls come into a program and at the end should be designed to ensure safety and determine outcomes. During the intake process, interviewing or screening participants for prior injuries or adverse health histories, as well as needs and interests, is important for safety and for comparison in the evaluation of results.

Successful research efforts rely on asking the right questions. In girl-centered programs we are asking how physical activity, and especially increased confidence in the female body, affect or enhance adolescent development in girls. As a result, psychosocial instruments need to be wedded to those that measure the quantity of activity, strength, endurance, and so on, and many need to be adapted for use with programs based on girl-centered values. Readers interested in developing research questions may also wish to examine existing research tools, including those that cover demographic questions in relation to adolescent health factors [17-21]; assessments of awareness, knowledge, motivation, and behavior in relation to adolescent health and physical activity [22-29]; assessments of support, stress and life events, coping abilities, and gender identity in young people [30-40]; and assessment of issues surrounding female maturation [41-50]. In addition, it is helpful to be familiar with tools that currently guide fitness testing [51-54] and those that are used for injury screening and inventory [54-57], as well as physical activity questionnaires that quantify amounts of activity [58-66] and assess perceptual and motor skills [67-71].

Health Screening: Illness, Injury, and Exercise History

It is essential to discover whether there is an underlying illness or injury that would prohibit participation in the planned activity. It is also advisable to keep a log of any injuries. Should there be a pattern of injury in the group or to an individual, it is vital to determine the cause. The form, "Health Screening" given on page 57, is an example of a health screening form that includes illness, injury, and exercise history.

Nutrition Diary

As we have seen, eating behavior is critically important for this population, but getting accurate information entails challenges. Obtaining a food recall requires great patience, and many girls do not know how to break down the food they eat into components. One alternative is to find a listing of food items that gives protein, carbohydrate, fat, calories, and micronutrients for each item. Another method is to break down foods into their individual components with the students as part of a class activity. The form titled "Food Log" on page 58 facilitates this process. Software programs that analyze diet are also available from a number of sources.

In situations where funding is limited and we wish to log food intake, the author and her colleagues use the form "Weekly Young Adult Food Diary" on pages 59-60. Within a listing based on the food pyramid, students only have to place a check on each serving line. This can also be worked on in the classroom setting. Conveniently, serving information is provided on the back of the food diary. Although this system is not as detailed or precise as some, its simplicity is an advantage, as is the fact that it is a good tool for teaching about food servings and sizes.

Age at Menarche

For purposes of program design, age at menarche is the most convenient marker of biological development. Whether obtaining this information retrospectively or prospectively, one prefers to obtain both the accurate birth date of the girl and the date of the onset of the first menstruation. At the start of a program, a girl will be considered pre- or postmenarche. Technically, a prepubertal girl is one who is at Tanner stage 1 for pubic hair, genitalia, and breast development; has not entered a growth spurt; and has low levels of estrogen and no menses. But, for the sake of simplicity, an initial designation as pre- or postmenarche is sufficient for many settings.

This information may be considered delicate or private, and at least one research group reports that they were unable to do the biological assessment component of their project because parents objected to the collection of data on pubertal status [72]. However, it is desirable to have some accurate information about girls' biological status when designing programs. Although we frequently use chronological age to delineate a group, not all 11-year-olds are at the same stage of physical or mental development. Observing girls at various stages—and changing stages—of adolescence will explain a great deal about the shifting dynamics and motivations of an individual or a group. As is obvious by now, girls' cognitive, emotional, and physical development are intertwined. The right mix of activities familiar and new will vary from girl to girl, group to group, and time to time. For example, in a group where 3 or 4 girls out of 15 11-year-olds are menstruating, an instructor might need an extra activity for these girls—such as being the assistant coaches—on days they might not feel like vigorous participation. Later in the year, the instructor may need additional activities of these types as more girls begin to menstruate.

Despite the cultural taboos surrounding menarche, we have found that most girls are willing to talk with someone they trust and they feel respects them; we have also found that careful listening is fruitful. It is important not to equate menstruation with illness, so that girls learn to differentiate between the sensations of menses and being sick. Talking about these matters is not given much play in Western society, and consequently learning to be

Health Screening Form—Illness, Injury, Exercise History

ID# (or Name): _____ Age: _____ years _____ months

Ethnic background: ☐ White ☐ Hispanic ☐ Native American ☐ African American
☐ Hispanic/African American ☐ Asian ☐ Other

Height: _____ Weight: _____ [BMI_____]*

Today's date: _____ Your birth date: _____ Grade: _____ (in school)

A. Do you have any of these diseases that require constant medical attention?

Heart disease	☐ Yes	☐ No
Asthma	☐ Yes	☐ No
Diabetes	☐ Yes	☐ No
Severe anemia	☐ Yes	☐ No
Thyroid disease	☐ Yes	☐ No
Other	☐ Yes	☐ No If yes, name: _____

B. Do you have any injuries or broken bones? ☐ Yes ☐ No

Did you have any in the past? ☐ Yes ☐ No   If yes, check those that apply.

☐ Spine	☐ Thigh	When?_____
☐ Neck	☐ Knee	
☐ Shoulder	☐ Lower leg	Describe injury: _____
☐ Upper arm	☐ Ankle	_____
☐ Lower arm/elbow	☐ Foot	_____
☐ Pelvis/hip/buttocks	☐ Head	_____

C. Which of these activities did you do at least once a week (in the months you did them) in the last year?

☐ Aerobics or aerobic dancing	☐ Soccer
☐ Running (cross country/track)	☐ Ballet, creative dance, African dance, etc.
☐ Walking	☐ Weightlifting
☐ Basketball	☐ Cheerleading
☐ Softball	☐ Drill team
☐ Volleyball	☐ Jump rope
☐ Bicycling	☐ Other: _____
☐ Swimming	

D. How many days per week do you participate in sports, dance, cheerleading, gym class, exercise, or other physical activity? ☐ 0 ☐ 1 ☐ 2 ☐ 3 ☐ More than 3

E. How many days per week do you exercise, breathe hard, and raise your pulse for at least 20 minutes? _____

---

*BMI = weight in kg/height in meters squared. (1 lb. = 0.454 kg   1 ft. = 0.304 m   1 in. = 0.025 m)

© 1996 Ann Cowlin. Used by permission.

A.F. Cowlin, 2002, *Women's fitness program development* (Champaign, IL: Human Kinetics).

Food Log

ID # (or Name: _____ Date: _____

Day (circle): Monday Tuesday Wednesday Thursday Friday Saturday Sunday

Food	Amount	Calories (gms)	Protein	Carbohydrates	Fat
Examples					
Bagel	1	180	4	35	2
Orange juice	1 cup	110	2	25	0

A.F. Cowlin, 2002, *Women's fitness program development* (Champaign, IL: Human Kinetics).

"If it's messy, eat it over the sink."

—Tom Robbins
Even Cowgirls Get the Blues

ID# (or Name): _____

Food by servings (check off each day)

Monday Date: _____

Fats, oils, sweets (1) ☐

Milk, cheese, yogurt (2-3) ☐ ☐ ☐

Meat, poultry, fish, beans, eggs, nuts (2-3) ☐ ☐ ☐

Fruits and vegetables (3-5) ☐ ☐ ☐ ☐ ☐

Grains: Cereal, pasta, bread, rice (6-11) ☐ ☐ ☐ ☐ ☐ ☐ ☐ ☐ ☐ ☐ ☐

Tuesday Date: _____

Fats, oils, sweets (1) ☐

Milk, cheese, yogurt (2-3) ☐ ☐ ☐

Meat, poultry, fish, beans, eggs, nuts (2-3) ☐ ☐ ☐

Fruits and vegetables (3-5) ☐ ☐ ☐ ☐ ☐

Grains: Cereal, pasta, bread, rice (6-11) ☐ ☐ ☐ ☐ ☐ ☐ ☐ ☐ ☐ ☐ ☐

Wednesday Date: _____

Fats, oils, sweets (1) ☐

Milk, cheese, yogurt (2-3) ☐ ☐ ☐

Meat, poultry, fish, beans, eggs, nuts (2-3) ☐ ☐ ☐

Fruits and vegetables (3-5) ☐ ☐ ☐ ☐

Grains: Cereal, pasta, bread, rice (6-11) ☐ ☐ ☐ ☐ ☐ ☐ ☐ ☐ ☐ ☐ ☐

Thursday Date: _____

Fats, oils, sweets (1) ☐

Milk, cheese, yogurt (2-3) ☐ ☐ ☐

Meat, poultry, fish, beans, eggs, nuts (2-3) ☐ ☐ ☐

Fruits and vegetables (3-5) ☐ ☐ ☐ ☐ ☐

Grains: Cereal, pasta, bread, rice (6-11) ☐ ☐ ☐ ☐ ☐ ☐ ☐ ☐ ☐ ☐ ☐

Friday Date: _____

Fats, oils, sweets (1) ☐

Milk, cheese, yogurt (2-3) ☐ ☐ ☐

Meat, poultry, fish, beans, eggs, nuts (2-3) ☐ ☐ ☐

Fruits and vegetables (3-5) ☐ ☐ ☐ ☐ ☐

Grains: Cereal, pasta, bread, rice (6-11) ☐ ☐ ☐ ☐ ☐ ☐ ☐ ☐ ☐ ☐ ☐

Weekly Young Adult Food Diary *(continued)*

(continued)

Saturday Date: _____

  Fats, oils, sweets (1) ☐

  Milk, cheese, yogurt (2-3) ☐ ☐ ☐

  Meat, poultry, fish, beans, eggs, nuts (2-3) ☐ ☐ ☐

  Fruits and vegetables (3-5) ☐ ☐ ☐ ☐ ☐

  Grains: Cereal, pasta, bread, rice (6-11) ☐ ☐ ☐ ☐ ☐ ☐ ☐ ☐ ☐ ☐ ☐

Sunday Date: _____

  Fats, oils, sweets (1) ☐

  Milk, cheese, yogurt (2-3) ☐ ☐ ☐

  Meat, poultry, fish, beans, eggs, nuts (2-3) ☐ ☐ ☐

  Fruits and vegetables (3-5) ☐ ☐ ☐ ☐ ☐

  Grains: Cereal, pasta, bread, rice (6-11) ☐ ☐ ☐ ☐ ☐ ☐ ☐ ☐ ☐ ☐ ☐

Serving Sizes

Fats, oils, sweets

This category includes foods high in fat and/or sugar, items such as ice cream, sour cream, salad dressing, butter or margarine, mayonnaise, French fries, chips, sausage, hot dogs, cake, cookies, pastries, pies, corn syrup, and sugar. One item per day: 1 cup ice cream; 2 or 3 cookies; a dozen French fries; a small bag of chips; 1 hot dog; 2 slices of regular cheese; 2 tablespoons butter, margarine, mayonnaise, or salad dressing; 1 candy bar.

Milk, cheese, yogurt

  1 cup low-fat, nonfat, or soy milk

  1 cup low-fat yogurt or pudding

  1 1/2-2 oz. low-fat hard cheese

  1 1/2 cups cottage cheese

Meat, poultry, fish, beans, eggs, nuts

  2 oz. beef, veal, lamb, chicken, turkey, pork, fish, shellfish

  1 c. tofu or dry beans (kidney, lima, soy, lentil, navy, mung, black, peas)

  1/4 c. peanut butter

  1/2 c. nuts or seeds

  2 med. eggs

Fruit

  1 orange, tangerine, mango, pear, papaya, apple, banana, peach

  2 apricots, nectarines, plums

  1 c. grapes

  2/3 c. raisins

  1/2 c. strawberries, cantaloupe, grapefruit, pineapple, cherries

Vegetables

1 c. raw or 2/3 c. cooked celery, tomato, cauliflower, corn, lettuce, carrots, broccoli, peas, zucchini, squash, potato, cabbage, spinach, yams, greens

Grains: Cereal, pasta, bread, rice

  1 slice whole grain bread

  1 med. muffin, biscuit, tortilla

  1/2 bagel, hamburger bun, English muffin

  1/2 c. pasta, rice, cooked cereal

  3-4 crackers

  3/4 c. dry cereal

comfortable discussing these issues may take a while. One should ascertain the policy on such matters at the local level and perhaps be prepared to meet with parents and/or administrators, well ahead of the start of a program, to discuss how data collection will be handled.

Screening as Part of the Curriculum

The simple screening procedures we have reviewed can be handled as group projects and can form part of the health education curriculum. Taking a straightforward but gentle approach to information about women's bodies allows girls to see that they can be comfortable with their growing sexual identity. Maintaining privacy lets girls know that the instructor or leader respects the girls and supports them in their effort to become more self-aware.

Other information that might be gathered, such as resting pulse, BMI, and so on, depends on the purpose of the activity program. As much as possible, taking the time to allow each girl to learn how to do a procedure shows her that she is respected and viewed as an individual capable of performing measurement tasks. A willingness to listen to her talk about these experiences encourages her to perceive her own feelings about events and skills.

SAMPLE PHYSICAL ACTIVITY PROGRAM FOR ADOLESCENT GIRLS, GRADES 7 TO 10

All the issues discussed so far help one imagine a successful environment in which health and fitness programs may flourish for girls in puberty. The transformation of data into practical, effective settings in the real world is the province of those who design and implement programs. This is a particular art form, as it involves not only organizational skills, knowledge of the subject, and the capacity to adjust, but also vision. The process entails grasping the import of available research, adapting models and theories to a new population, and deriving a curriculum that is effective. This takes time. To ensure that a given program is effective and can grow and change as its designers and instructors gain information, it is necessary to standardize intake and evaluation procedures.

Intake

Screening may take place prior to the start of the program or at the first meeting. The form "Health Screening," already described, covers health and exercise history. A second form, "Menses Information," covers details regarding the woman's or girl's menses. It is important to have all of this information for a number of reasons. The first is self-awareness on the part of the girls. If they are to develop self-images as healthy human beings, they need to see, hear, and work with words that enable them to understand the nature of health. A second reason relates to protection for the instructors and program administrators. Having knowledge helps prevent putting a girl into inappropriate activities. And third, this information is for evaluation purposes. Whatever curriculum is being used can be modified when items are found that do or don't work satisfactorily with a specific group or individual.

Assessment of needs and interests is also part of the intake procedure. Including questions regarding demographics, such as ethnic background, aids in determining broad concerns. An instructor may be less concerned about self-esteem issues with African American adolescent girls than with whites or Latinas, although one is concerned about self-efficacy issues with all of these

Menses Information

ID # (or Name): _____

Birth date: _____

Date of first period: _____

Today's date: _____

How many days between periods? _____

Do you know how old your mother was when she started? ☐ Yes ☐ No

If yes, how old was she? _____

Sisters? ☐ Yes ☐ No   If yes, how old was she?   1. _____   2. _____   3. _____

A.F. Cowlin, 2002, *Women's fitness program development* (Champaign, IL: Human Kinetics).

groups. Asking about motivations—finding out whether a given girl is interested in skill acquisition, helping others, aesthetic or expressive concerns—permits the instructor to tailor instructions or descriptions so they make sense to various girls who may be interested in doing the same activity, but for different reasons.

In some instances, demographics and motivations can intersect. For example, values that girls learn in Hawaiian culture include many subtle types of helping and community building, which are important motivations for this population. There are a number of words that delineate these subtleties, including *kokna* (help), *laulima* (many hands, cooperation), *malama* (care for), *malama'ola* (care of life), *aloha* (love), *lokahi* (unity), and *ohana* (family) [73]. The concept of family does not necessarily mean only blood relatives, but may include those who contribute to the unity or caring of a group. Working with girls in this population effectively means respecting these subtleties and learning to design projects that fulfill specific aspects of helping others.

Curriculum

The following curriculum, entitled the Creative Physical Activity curriculum, can be used as a 10-week or 12-week program. It is presented here in its 10-week format. For a 12-week format, the first week is separated into two weeks: week 1—screening, the juggling game, and pretesting; week 2—repetition of the juggling games and presentation of the remainder of the material. In the 12-week format, the last week is separated into review and relaxation (week 11) and posttest and closure (week 12).

Ideally, the program takes place two or three times a week for 40 to 50 minutes per session. The content for the week can be repeated each day of the week the program meets, or part can be done the first day and the rest added on the second or third day of the week. The program is designed to be additive, so that once learned, skills are repeated regularly. For example, once the activity log has been introduced, it can be done each week.

The focus of this curriculum is on the quality of physical activity experiences rather than only measured activities. No attempt is made in the classroom to separate cognitive content and behavior. Rather, these are incorporated together as activities. This plan capitalizes on the fact that physical activity carries content on several levels at the same time. The curriculum is outlined in the form "10-Week Creative Physical Activity Curriculum for Girls in Puberty." Worksheets that form part of the curriculum are presented separately as the given segment of the plan is described in the text.

Week 1

The first sessions—*Hello*—can be done in one week or in two. *Say your name and make a movement* is a simple way to greet each girl, allow her to express herself, give the other girls a chance to observe her (so they can learn names by association), and put everyone on equal footing. Starting in a circle, the leader(s) demonstrate by saying her (their) name(s) and making a simple movement. They can give examples ahead of time to ease any possible apprehension for those unused to inventing movement. Simple arm or leg gestures, turns, jumps, and so on can be shown to allow girls to choose something for when their turn comes. Leaders make it clear that girls can choose a movement or invent something, whatever suits them. After each person says her name and does her movement, the whole circle says the name and does the movement. Once everyone in the circle has had a chance, a general celebration is in order.

The *juggling game* starts as the leader says one girl's name and then throws her a ball (beach balls work well); that girl then says another girl's name and throws her the ball. If group members are not familiar with each other, some prompting and gentle coaching will be necessary. The leader encourages creative helping and associations. There will be a quickening of the rhythm of the game when a critical point is reached and everyone knows everyone's name. At that point, another element is added such as a book, toy, or article of clothing, which is passed around the circle clockwise at the same time that the naming and ball throwing continue. Again, a critical point is reached when the group accommodates to the demands of the game, at which point another item is added, traveling counterclockwise. Items are added until the point at which there are enough items that occasionally someone could be overwhelmed with items, but the climate is kept humorous. Others can help the individual. When the "joke" has gotten old, the game can be stopped and it can be pointed out to the girls how differently each person handles having several tasks to do at once. Some people pass everything off quickly, whereas others wait for things to collect and then deal with them. The leader encourages observations and lets the girls point out features they found interesting or fun.

Once the group is acquainted in this way, the leader can administer a *pretest for fitness* and a *pretest for knowledge* (see forms "Pretest/Posttest—Fitness" on page 65 and "Pretest/Posttest—Knowledge", page 66). Allowing the group to do some bonding before the pretest undoubtedly affects the outcome to a small extent; however, this is also the situation with the posttest in any case, and it is the aim of this intervention for the procedures to be girl centered. An interesting study in its own right would be to look at pretest results among girls who are acquainted and those who are strangers.

Activity component	Behavior/purpose	Cognitive content	Description
Screening*			
Week 1: Hello			
Say your name and make a movement	Introductions Start in a circle	Self	Say your name and make a movement
Juggling game	Learn names Do complex task	Others Life's complex	Say another's name and throw ball; add objects
Pretest*			
Centering and abdominals	Well-being Torso strength Posture	Kinesthesia Anatomy	Seated ab exercises Look at a pelvis
Relaxation	Well-being	Calm	Seated, breathing
Week 2: Heart			
Review	Reinforcement	Recall	Repeat favorite things
Heart rate (HR)	Self-care	How heart works	Take own pulse
Intensity	RPE and HR	Why HR changes	Take pulse at various intensities*; note RPE
Arms and legs	Connect body parts	Kinesthesia	Creative strength
Activity Log	Data collection	Keeping track	Fill in activity log*
Relaxation	Well-being	Calm	Seated, breathing
Week 3: Flexibility			
Review	Reinforcement	Preferences	Repetition
Aerobic work	Sweat and continuity	Stay focused	Creative aerobics
Stretching	Proprioception	Discomfort of 3 on 1-10 scale	Whole body and parts stretches; flexibility test
Relaxation	Well-being	Calm	Supine or lateral
Week 4: Fit Food			
Warm-ups	Warm-up	Fun ways to warm up	Add-a-pearl games
Act like food	New view of food	Imagination	Act like foods (e.g., bacon frying, raisins)
Running aerobics	Aerobic	New view—running	Creative running
Intro to food 101	New view of food	Nutrients	Food types* Play with NDC cards
Relaxation	Well-being	Calm	Seated, breathing
Week 5: Food Diaries			
Review	Reinforcement	Recall	Decided in process
Food recall	Learn to use forms	Think about food	Fill in Food Diary*
Aerobic choice	Students decide	Have choices	Creative, run, games
Relaxation	Well-being	Calm	Seated or supine

(continued)

Activity component	Behavior/purpose	Cognitive content	Description
Week 6: Girl Stuff			
Workout	Make a package	What is aerobic, strength, flexibility, etc.	Do examples
Cooperation game	Help each other	Support system good	Group task (e.g., build a bridge)
Menstruation	Be okay with it	Self-esteem	Explain charts* (figures 2.1 and 2.2)
Self-care	Provide a guide*	Learn elements	Discuss healthy mind/body behavior
Relaxation	Well-being	Calm	Seated
Week 7: Exercise Aesthetics: Space, Time, and Energy			
Workout	Make a package	Self-efficacy	Do it
Labanotation	New view	Beauty in movement	Very basic Laban
Relaxation	Well-being	Calm	Seated or supine
Week 8: Who Am I?			
Workout	Make a package	Self-schema	Do it
Who am I art project	Self-esteem	Self-esteem	Draw self-gram*
I can do this strength test	Independence	Self-efficacy	Stair, chair, wall, floor strength test*
Relaxation	Well-being	Calm	Seated or supine
Week 9: Review/Complete			
Review and complete	Complete projects	How to finish	Finish, ask questions
Workout	Each girl has own	Everything	Controlled chaos
Cheer for us	Feel good	Reward	Make a cheer
Relaxation	Well-being	Calm	Seated
*Week 10: Review/Posttest**			
Review	Reinforcement	Recall	What needs attention
Posttest*			
Relaxation	Well-being	Calm	Seated or supine
Closure			

*Worksheets are included.

A.F. Cowlin, 2002, *Women's fitness program development* (Champaign, IL: Human Kinetics).

Pretest/Postest—Fitness

ID # (or Name): _____   Date: _____

1. 1-mile run/jog/walk time: _____ min. _____ sec.

   pulse at finish line: _____/10 sec.   5 minutes later: _____/10 sec.

   bpm: _____   bpm: _____

2. Number of push-ups: _____

3. Number of sit-ups: _____

4. Flexibility: seated reach to   ☐ knees

   [ankle flexed]   ☐ mid calf

                                   ☐ ankle (lateral malleolus)

                                   ☐ 2 inches past ankle

                                   ☐ 6 inches past ankle

A. F. Cowlin, 2002, *Women's fitness program development* (Champaign, IL: Human Kinetics).

Centering is the next activity. With this population, we have found that sitting on chairs in a circle is the most acceptable method for making them comfortable to learn centering. Another option is for participants to sit on exercise balls. Once they have kinesthetically located their *ischial tuberosities,* or *sitsbones,* at the base of the pelvis, girls are asked to sit directly on these bones, not on their tailbone. In this position, the pelvis is neutral. Next, they learn to balance their heads at the top of their spines rather than hold their head up with tension in the neck or shoulders. The image of balancing a spinning basketball on the finger or a spinning plate on top of a stick is useful and prompts participants to achieve a vertical torso. Then, girls learn to inhale and exhale while relaxing and contracting the transverse abdominal muscle, respectively. Through repetition, they acquire the basic skills for centering—or balancing and relaxing their bodies in a neutral position. Keeping the directions simple and being sure to repeat exactly the same steps each time are key to allowing girls over time to develop their own system for achieving the calm but alert sense that accompanies centering. Centering is described in greater detail in chapter 8.

Seated on their sitsbones, with the torso vertical and the head balanced on top, and breathing from the abdomen, girls can kinesthetically sense their transverse muscle, learning to "pull in" with this deep muscle, saving the surface muscles (rectus abdominis and obliques) for movement of the torso. We find that hissing or blowing through the mouth (pretend you are blowing through a straw) aids in innervating the deep muscle action. From here, *abdominal exercises* for the surface muscles can be added, including curl-ups and spiral actions. Returning to chairs, the girls can resume a centered posture and listen to some peaceful music and directions for progressive *relaxation.*

Week 2

Activity components in the second week—*Heart*—are mostly self-explanatory, except for the creative strength activity. Asking the girls what they enjoyed most from the previous week is the entree into getting them to *review* and, when possible, demonstrate items from the previous sessions. They may wish to repeat activities, which we generally take as a good sign. When starting the new material, be sure that in the process of taking an initial *heart rate* and rates at various activity levels, the issue of why the heart beats faster when one is working harder is clear to the girls. The form "Cardiovascular Fitness Worksheet" on page 67 is a worksheet on heart rate and intensity. Another form, "Activity Log," page 68, is for tracking the activity level of participants. This activity log is a modification of the Godin-Shephard Physical Activity Survey [74], which we have altered to be appropriate for girls in puberty.

For the *creative strength* activity, everyday objects familiar to girls and having a variety of weights can be lifted, carried, handed off, put down, picked up, dragged, pushed with the feet, and so on. Such objects as books, purses, potted plants, paperweights or tape holders, gallon jugs of liquid, sport equipment, and bags of groceries can be weighed ahead of time and used in place of free weights. Over time, girls can progress from lifting

ID # (or Name: _____ Date: _____

A. What are the three (3) major elements of physical fitness? (Circle three.)

Strength	Weight	Speed
Size	Endurance	Flexibility

B. Circle five (5) aerobic endurance activities from the list below.

Basketball	Bicycling	Drawing
Hip hop dancing	Running	Stretching
Swimming	Weightlifting	Yoga

C. What is the target heart rate (pulse) for aerobic exercise for teens? (Circle one.)

90-125	100-250	120-180 beats per minute (bpm)

D. Food match-ups: Carbohydrate   Fat   Protein   (types of food)

   1. Match the type of food to its function. (Put each on the correct line.)

   Growth and repair: _____

   Energy for activity: _____

   Stored energy: _____

   2. Match the type of food to these examples. (Put each on the correct line.)

   Spaghetti, muffin, banana, orange juice, salad: _____

   Steak, peanut butter, fish, rice & beans, skim milk: _____

   Potato chips, mayonnaise, butter, chocolate candy: _____

E. Creative movement: Space   Time   Energy (elements of movement)

   Which elements of movement above belong to which descriptions below? (Put the element on the correct line.)

   _____   _____   _____

Speed	Size	Dynamics
Rhythm	Shape	Intensity
Flow	Direction	Attack
	Level	

A.F. Cowlin, 2002, *Women's fitness program development* (Champaign, IL: Human Kinetics).

Cardiovascular Fitness Worksheet

How Hard Does My Heart Work?

ID # (or Name): _____ Date: _____

1. Sit quietly for 2 to 3 minutes.

    My sitting pulse: ___ (for 10 sec.) × 6 (60 sec. = 1 min.) = ___ beats per minute (bpm)

    How hard am I working? (Circle one.)

    Very light   Light   Fairly light   Somewhat hard   Hard   Very hard   Very, very hard

2. Play some music, stretch, do a dozen squats (no weights) with legs turned out, do the Texas two-step in a circle—for 3 minutes.

    My warming-up pulse: ___ × 6 = ___ beats per minute (bpm)

    How hard am I working? (Circle one.)

    Very light   Light   Fairly light   Somewhat hard   Hard   Very hard   Very, very hard

3. Climb stairs (13-stair flight, up and down, repeating) or jog for 3 minutes.

    My aerobic pulse: ___ × 6 = ___ bpm

    How hard am I working? (Circle one.)

    Very light   Light   Fairly light   Somewhat hard   Hard   Very hard   Very, very hard

Aerobic activity provides cardiovascular fitness = heart health.

For teens, the "aerobic zone" is 120 to 180 bpm.

For preteens, the "aerobic zone" is 120 to 200 bpm.

A. F. Cowlin, 2002, *Women's fitness program development* (Champaign, IL: Human Kinetics).

or carrying at an initial appropriate weight for longer periods to lifting or carrying heavier objects. Care must be taken to ensure safety, healthy biomechanics, and appropriate weights. At some point, free weights can be introduced, depending on the girls' interest. Initially, however, the focus is on how working against resistance affects kinesthetic awareness of the *arms and legs* in relationship to the center of the body. *Relaxation,* as always, closes the session.

Week 3

The third group of activities—*Flexibility*—again starts with the "What did you like?" *review.* Building on the prior week's work, sustained cardiovascular or *aerobic work* is introduced. Having the girls design or choreograph the sequence of activities for this section (15 minutes) is helpful in getting them used to the idea that they can take responsibility by using their imagination. Anything reasonable is good as long as they work hard. They can walk the stairs for 3 minutes followed by dancing to

a favorite song, followed by jogging, then more stair walking, double Dutch jump rope, and so on. The leader can have them make a list of what activities to do and how long to do each.

Stretching follows a cool-down period. These are simple stretches, with the caution that 3 on a scale of 1 to 10 is the most discomfort the girls should feel. All the principles of careful stretching apply: alignment, slow movement, holding the stretch, deep breathing. This is an opportunity to discover who is very flexible and who is not. If the girls are comfortable, they can do the *relaxation* lying down, either in the constructive rest position (lying supine, with knees bent and feet on floor) or the lateral recumbent position (lying on the side, in a loose fetal position).

Week 4

The fourth group of activities centers on *Fit Food. Warm-ups* are given form. Add-a-pearl is an old dance trick in which each person adds a movement, making a choreo-

Activity Log

ID # (or Name): _____ Date: _____

1. How many times in the last week did you do mild activity for at least 15 minutes? _____

   (Examples: painting or drawing, singing, playing a musical instrument, vacuuming, laundry, cooking, walking at the mall.)

2. How many times in the last week did you do moderate activity that made you feel warm for at least 15 minutes? _____

   (Examples: walking fast, washing windows, dancing, softball, volleyball, cheerleading.)

3. How many times in the last week did you do strenuous activity that made you sweat and breathe hard for at least 15 minutes? _____

   (Examples: running, riding a bike, jumping rope, basketball, swimming, track, soccer.)

Level	METs	× # of times/week	= Amount
1	3	× _____	= _____
2	5	× _____	= _____
3	9	× _____	= _____
		Total	= _____

A.F. Cowlin, 2002, *Women's fitness program development* (Champaign, IL: Human Kinetics).

graphed sequence. Girls may use their original movement or make a new movement. The first person shows her movement, followed by the second person; then the two movements are done in sequence. The third person shows her movement and it is added onto the sequence, and so on. An observant teacher can coach by saying such things as, "Do something for the left leg; no one did anything for the left leg!" and thus make sure that all the body parts are used. Movements may be taken from life (e.g., brushing your teeth), sports (e.g., shooting a basket), or the imagination (e.g., jumping with fancy feet).

Act like food—another old dance trick—removes food from its ordinary frame of reference. The leader provides examples such as bacon frying or raisins or peanut butter and sees what develops. An easy transition into the *running aerobics* section is to ask the girls to be the food running ("Be raisins or peanut butter running down the street . . ."). Following a cool-down period, food types and their jobs in the body can be discussed. Figure 4.1 shows three signs with very simple explanations of protein, carbohydrate, and fat. These can be used to stimulate discussion through questions such as "Can you name some foods with protein and fat in them?" The National Dairy Council offers Food Model Comparison Cards *(NDC cards)* [75] and a leader guide that can be used in conjunction with the signs for a variety of activities, in-

cluding creating a balanced meal. As always, *relaxation* closes the sessions.

Week 5

In the fifth series of activities—*Food Diaries*—students learn to use the *food log* and the *food diary*. The form "Food Log" may be used as part of the pretest/posttest materials or may be introduced at this time. The food diary system, which may be easier for this population, is shown in the form "Weekly Young Adult Food Diary." By this time, the girls have developed a repertoire of aerobic activities, and having them plan their own sessions reinforces what they know. *Aerobic choice* can involve all the ideas of the group. The girls may also enjoy having choices about how to do their *relaxation.*

Week 6

The sixth series is *Girl Stuff,* a package of activities aimed at both community and identity. Having girls design an entire *workout,* followed by a *cooperative game* in which they must create something tangible (it needs to be something they can do in a relatively brief time, and the necessary supplies must be on hand), gives them a lot of practice working together. Learning about *menstruation* (see figure 2.1 as a teaching aid) and *self-care* (see the

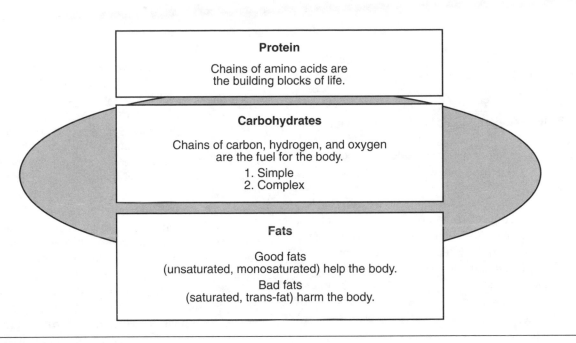

Protein

Chains of amino acids are
the building blocks of life.

Carbohydrates

Chains of carbon, hydrogen, and oxygen
are the fuel for the body.
1. Simple
2. Complex

Fats

Good fats
(unsaturated, monosaturated) help the body.
Bad fats
(saturated, trans-fat) harm the body.

Figure 4.1

Self-Care Guidelines

1. Care for my body.

   • Eat protein to grow, carbohydrates for energy, and a little fat so things work right.

   • Get plenty of exercise or creative activity.

   • Get enough rest and relaxation.

   • Stay away from unhealthy things.

   • Practice good hygiene.

2. Care for my mind.

   • Take time to read, think, and have feelings about life.

   • Treat myself with respect.

   • Treat others with respect.

A.F. Cowlin, 2002, *Women's fitness program development* (Champaign, IL: Human Kinetics).

form "Self-Care Guidelines") makes this a fairly serious and work-intensive week, and the *relaxation* component may require especially careful guidance.

Week 7

The seventh group of activities—*Exercise Aesthetics: Space, Time, and Energy*—builds on the *workout* designed by the girls in the preceding week. Using the movements that occur in this activity, sessions introduce spatial elements of direction, level, size, and shape; the time ele- ments of speed and flow (sustained or legato and quick or staccato) and rhythm; and the energy elements of dy- namics, intensity, and attack. These are the fundamen- tals of *Labanotation*. If time permits, the eight basic ef- fort/shapes from Laban's work may also be introduced. For an instructor not already skilled in the use of Laban's movement notation and analysis, more information is available in Hutchinson's text [76], from Laban's work itself [77, 78], at the Web site **www.dancenotation.org,** and in chapter 8 of this book. *Relaxation* closes each ses- sion.

Week 8

The eighth set of activities is called *Who Am I?* The *workout* section now includes individualizing activities and sequences. The *"Who Am I"* project described in chapter 3, figure 3.3, is an example of a project we have seen in the past. Each girl makes a list of potential roles she plays in her life, such as daughter, student, friend, sister, cousin, church member, athlete, dancer, singer. Placing her name at the center of her sociogram and her roles around the center, she may express her life. Paper, markers, crayons, paste-ons, glue, scissors, and the like are needed to complete this project (see figure 11.16). Once each girl has finished her project, she is given the *I can do this strength test* (figure 3.4). Girls may work in pairs or groups to get the test done. Each item is repeated until the girl decides to quit, so the instructor needs to keep an eye open to prevent the overachievers from injuring themselves. As always, *relaxation* closes the sessions.

Week 9

The sessions in week 9 comprise *Review/Complete* activities. There are inevitably projects that don't get finished or girls who miss a class and have something to catch up on. This series provides an opportunity to finish things. It is also a chance to let the girls direct their own programming. The author finds it very helpful to make a list of items that are supposed to be done by the end of the marking period or program and to give the girls rein to work on their own. They are expected to do a *workout* in the process as well, since this represents real life. Toward the end of the week, creating the *Cheer for us* is a fun way to celebrate. Of course, *relaxation* closes each meeting.

Week 10

The final sessions may take one or two weeks. *Review/Posttest* can be split into two sets of activities for weeks 11 and 12 if that format is desired and the first week has been split into weeks 1 and 2. Girls may wish to take turns leading portions of the workout. Talking about their favorite parts of the program and what they learned is a good way to review the information. The *posttest* should be given at the last meeting, but it is important to leave adequate time for *closure* and reassurance of girls who may need a proper detachment from the group.

Evaluation

Reviewing by participatory means and taking a written posttest help the instructor and each girl assess the extent of her change in skills and development. Likert-type scales can be used to find out which activities were most successful or appreciated by the group and individuals. In a school-based program where grading may be part of the evaluation process, many factors will help determine the grade outcome. Individual projects, participation, and improvements in physical, cognitive, and interpersonal skills all provide evidence of effort.

Instructors will be aided in the process of improving their program by making notes of their own observations on a regular basis. Comments from participants during informal verbal evaluations in the course of the program also provide powerful feedback. Making accurate notes following these sessions is important if one wants to collect evidence of what is effective from the girls' perspectives. For some girls, an opportunity to write down comments in answer to open-ended questions is also an important and meaningful part of the process. On more than one occasion, the author has found that a girl—unable to say something in front of others, but wanting to communicate about her experience in written form—has made major conceptual breakthroughs in the course of such a program.

Other Topics

There is no boundary to how much one can cover in the manner described in this program curriculum plan. In setting an overall structure for the program outlined here, the objective was simply to cover a basic movement repertoire that illustrates many of the principles we have been discussing. At its most simple, a once-a-week program can cover one or two movement skills and self-care topics. At the other end of the spectrum, as part of a school's daily-life skills course, several instructors with different qualifications could team teach. One instructor might cover topics such as health education—nutrition, tobacco, alcohol, drugs, pregnancy, and sexually transmitted diseases—whereas another covered anatomy and physiology of the female body, and still another taught movement or sport skills adapted to the female body. But, as we have noted many times, it is key to draw all of these components together so that the girls see them as intertwined, meaningful, and consonant with their own self-interest—and also so that the girls feel they are receiving special attention.

Physical fitness components, games, sports, health education topics, creative movement, dance styles, and social skills are all topics that can be adapted to this curriculum format. To work in greater depth on individual activities, the format can be stretched in one area and reduced in others. If girls wanted to work on volleyball or modern dance, elements of either of these activities could become target skills or topics of study for as many weeks as needed to satisfy the girls' interests. The format can be reproduced from one marking period to another (or one community course to another) over the course of a year through a change of topics or an increase in depth and detail. As girls approach their later teens, game strategies or expressing feelings while dancing might replace learning how to execute basic skills.

LOOKING AHEAD

The challenge of bringing more adolescent girls into the realm of the physically active is very interesting and complex. In the United States, despite laws and policies providing girls greater access to competitive sports, only a fraction of them have benefited. Evidence suggests that what may be needed is a new approach to increasing physical activity for girls by creating new forms of instruction, based on the circular thinking, social identity, and multitask abilities of females. Classes in which sex education, physics, chemistry, nutrition, and deep breathing techniques are combined might seem an unusual arrangement for increasing a girl's level of physical activity. But because all these topics are critical to her daily survival, she can experience how these elements work together to improve her strength, endurance, range of motion, and other physical characteristics that enhance her physical existence. By examining the adolescent female, the importance of physical activity to her short- and long-term well-being, and ideas for how new programs might increase exercise participation by adolescent girls, this part of the text has made a step in highlighting this challenge. The next part deals with the phenomenon of pregnancy, along with its special relationship to physical activity and the ways in which this relationship affects what may be a woman's most profound experience, giving birth.

REFERENCES

1. Bush, P.J., Zuckerman, A.E., Taggart, V.S., Theiss, P.K., Peleg, E.O., and Smith, S.A. 1989. Cardiovascular risk factor prevention in black schoolchildren: The Know Your Body evaluation project. *Health Education Quarterly* 16:215-227.
2. Killen, J.D., Telch, M.J., Robinson, T.N., Maccoby, N., Taylor, C.B., and Farquhar, J.W. 1988. Cardiovascular disease risk reduction for tenth graders: A multiple-factor school-based approach. *Journal of the American Medical Association* 260:1728-1733.
3. McKenzie, T.L., Sallis, J.F., Faucette, N., Roby, J.J., and Kolody, B. 1993. Effects of a curriculum and inservice program on the quantity and quality of elementary physical education classes. *Research Quarterly for Exercise and Sport* 64:178-187.
4. Kelder, S.H., Perry, C.L., and Klepp, K.I. 1993. Community-wide youth exercise promotion: Long-term outcomes of the Minnesota Heart Health Program and the Class of 1989 Study. *Journal of School Health* 63(5):218-223.
5. Prokhorov, A.V., Perry, C.L., Kelder, S.H., and Klepp, K.I. 1993. Lifestyle values of adolescents: Results from Minnesota Heart Health Youth Program. *Adolescence* 28(111):637-647.
6. Zakarian, J.M., Hovell, M.F., Hofstetter, C.R., Sallis, J.F., and Keating, K.J. 1994. Correlates of vigorous exercise in a predominantly low SES and minority high school population. *Preventive Medicine* 23:314-321.
7. Ferguson, K.J., Yesalis, C.E., Pomrehn, P.R., and Kirkpatrick, M.B. 1989. Attitudes, knowledge, and beliefs as predictors of exercise intent and behavior in schoolchildren. *Journal of School Health* 59(3):112-115.
8. French, S.A., Perry, C.L., Leon, G.R., and Fulkerson, J.A. 1996. Self-esteem and change in body mass index over three years in a cohort of adolescents. *Obesity Research* 4(1):27-33.
9. Luepker, R.V., Perry, C.L., McKinlay, S.M., Nader, P.R., Parcel, G.S., Stone, E.J., Webber, L.S., Elder, J.P., Feldman, H.A., and Johnson, C.C. 1996. Outcomes of a field trial to improve children's dietary patterns and physical activity. The Child and Adolescent Trial for Cardiovascular Health. *Journal of the American Medical Association* 275(10):768-776.
10. Edmundson, E., Parcel, G.S., Feldman, H.A., Elder, J., Perry, C.L., Johnson, C.C., Williston, B.J., Stone, E.J., Yang, M., Lytle, L., and Webber, L. 1996. The effects of the Child and Adolescent Trial for Cardiovascular Health upon psychosocial determinants of diet and physical activity behavior. *Preventive Medicine* 25(4):442-454.
11. Stone, E.J., Osganian, S.K., McKinlay, S.M., Wu, M.C., Webber, L.S., Luepker, R.V., Perry, C.L., Parcel, G.S., and Elder, J.P. 1996. Operational design and quality control in the CATCH Multicenter Trial. *Preventive Medicine* 25(4):389-399.
12. Jessor, R. 1991. Risk behavior in adolescence: A psychosocial framework for understanding and action. *Journal of Adolescent Health* 12:597-605.
13. Donovan, J.E., Jessor, R., and Costa, F.M. 1993. Structure of health-enhancing behavior in adolescence: A latent-variable approach. *Journal of Health & Social Behavior* 34(4):346-362.
14. Lirgg, C.D. 1993. Effects of same-sex versus coeducational physical education on the self-perceptions of middle and high school students. *Research Quarterly for Exercise and Sport* 64(3):324-334.
15. Centers for Disease Control and Prevention. 1997. Guidelines for School and Community Programs to Promote Lifelong Physical Activity Among Young People. *Journal of School Health* 67(6):202-219.
16. Symons, C.W., Cinelli, B., James, T.C., and Groff, P. 1997. Bridging student health risks and academic achievement through comprehensive school health programs. *Journal of School Health* 67(6):220-227.
17. Ford-Gilboe, M. 1997. Family strengths, motivation, and resources as predictors of health promotion behavior in single-parent and two-parent families. *Research in Nursing & Health* 20:205-217.
18. Barr, S.I. 1994. Associations of social and demographic variables with calcium intakes of high school students. *The Journal of the American Dental Association* 94:260-266, 269.
19. Lettieri, D.J., Nelson, J.E., and Sayers, M.A. (eds.). 1985. *NIAA treatment handbook series 2: Alcoholism treatment assessment research instruments.* Rockville, MD: National Institute on Alcohol Abuse and Alcoholism.
20. Jackson, C., Bee-Gates, D.J., and Henriksen, L. 1994. Authoritative parenting, child competencies, and initiation of cigarette smoking. *Health Education Quarterly* 21:103-116.
21. Poivka, B.J. 1996. Rural sex education: Assessment of programs and interagency collaboration. *Public Health Nursing* 13:425-433.
22. Krowchuk, D.P., Kreiter, S.R., Wods, C.R., Sinal, S.H., and DuRant, R.H. 1998. Problem dieting behaviors among young adolescents. *Archives of Pediatrics and Adolescent Medicine* 152:884-888.
23. Mosback, P.A.A., and Leventhal, H. 1988. Peer group identification and smoking: Implications for intervention. *Journal of Abnormal Psychology* 97:238-245.

24. Rahdert, E.R. (ed.). 1991. *The Adolescent Assessment/Referral System*. Rockville, MD: National Institutes of Health, National Institute on Drug Abuse.

25. Fardy, P.S., White, R.E.C., Clark, L.T., Amodio, G., Hursler, M.H., McDermott, K.J., and Magel, J.R. 1995. Health promotion in minority adolescents: A Healthy People 2000 pilot study. *Journal of Cardiopulmonary Rehabilitation* 15:65-72.

26. Stein, K.F. 1994. Complexity of the self-schema and responses to disconfirming feedback. *Cognitive Therapy and Research* 18:161-178.

27. Vega, W.A., Sallis, J.F., Patterson, R.L., Rupp, J.W., Atkins, C.J., and Nader, P.R. 1987. Assessing knowledge of cardiovascular health-related diet and exercise behaviors in Anglo- and Mexican-Americans. *Preventive Medicine* 16:696-709.

28. Moberg, D.P., and Piper, D.L. 1990. An outcome evaluation of Project Model Health: A middle school health promotion program. *Health Education Quarterly* 17:37-51.

29. Garcia, A.W., Pender, N.J., Antonakos, C.L., and Ronis, D.L. 1998. Changes in physical activity beliefs and behaviors of boys and girls across the transition to junior high school. *Journal of Adolescent Health* 22:394-402.

30. Epstein, L.H., Valoski, A., Wing, R.R., and McCurley, J. 1994. Ten-year outcomes of behavioral family-based treatment for childhood obesity. *Health Psychology* 13:373-383.

31. Campbell, M.A., and Rapee, R.M. 1994. The nature of feared outcome representations in children. *Journal of Abnormal Child Psychology* 22:99-111.

32. McCubbin, H.I., Needle, R.H., and Wilson, M. 1985. Adolescent health risk behaviors: Family stress and adolescent coping as critical factors. *Family Relations* 34:51-62.

33. Norbeck, J. 1984. Modification of recent life event questionnaires for use with female respondents. *Research in Nursing & Health* 7:61-71.

34. Norbeck, J. 1981. The development of an instrument to measure social support. *Nursing Research* 30:264-269.

35. Colley, A., Griffiths D., Hugh, M., Landers, K., and Jaggli, N. 1996. Childhood play and adolescent leisure preferences: Associations with gender typing and the presence of siblings. *Sex Roles* 35:233-245.

36. Harris, A.C. 1994. Ethnicity as a determinant of sex role identity: A replication study of items selection for the Bern Sex Role Inventory. *Sex Roles* 31:241-273.

37. Levit, D.B. 1991. Gender differences in ego defenses in adolescence: Sex roles as one way to understand the differences. *Journal of Personality and Social Psychology* 61:992-999.

38. Covey, L.A., and Feitz, D.L. 1991. Physical activity and adolescent female psychological development. *Journal of Youth and Adolescence* 20:463-474.

39. Blanchard-Fields, F., Sulsky, L., and Robinson-Whelen, S. 1991. Moderating effects of age and context on the relationship between gender, sex role differences and coping. *Sex Roles* 25:645-660.

40. Adleman, H.S., Smith, D.C., Nelson, P., Taylor, L., and Phares, V. 1985. An instrument to assess life satisfaction among children and adolescents with psychoeducational problems. Manuscript submitted for publication.

41. Marshall, W.A., and Tanner, J.M. 1969. Variations in pattern of pubertal changes in girls. *Archives of Disease in Childhood* 44:291-303.

42. Harter, S. 1988. Self-Perception Profile for Adolescents. Unpublished paper. University of Denver. Reference: Kupermine, G.P., Blatt, S.J., and Leadbeater, B.J. 1997. Relatedness, self-definition, and early adolescent adjustment. *Cognitive Therapy and Research* 21:301-320.

43. Hagborg, W.J. 1993. Gender differences on Harter's self-perception profile for adolescents. *Journal of Social Behavior and Personality* 8:141-148.

44. Campbell, M.A., and McGrath, P.J. 1997. Use of medication by adolescents for the management of menstrual dis-comfort. *Archives of Pediatrics and Adolescent Medicine* 151:905-913.

45. Havens, B., and Swenson, I. 1986. Menstrual perceptions and preparation among female adolescents. *Journal of Obstetric, Gynecologic, and Neonatal Nursing* 15:406-411.

46. Janes, B.A., and Morse, J.M. 1990. Adolescent girls' perceptions of and preparation for menarche. *Canadian Journal of Nursing Research* 22:47-59.

47. Whitehead, W.E., Busch, C.M., Heller, B.R., and Costa, P.T. 1986. Social learning influences on menstrual symptoms and illness behavior. *Health Psychology* 5:13-23.

48. Rippon, C., Nash, J., Myburgh, K.H., and Noakes, T.D. 1988. Abnormal Eating Attitude scores predict menstrual dysfunction in lean females. *International Journal of Eating Disorders* 7:617-624.

49. Garner, D.M., Olmsted, M.P., and Polivy, J. 1983. Development and validation of a multidimensional Eating Disorder Inventory for anorexia nervosa and bulimia. *International Journal of Eating Disorders* 2:15-34.

50. Mellin, L.M. 1986. *Youth Evaluation Scale (YES): A biopsychosocial assessment instrument for adolescent weight problems*. Balboa Pub., 11 Library Place, Larkspur, CA 94960.

51. American Alliance for Health, Physical Education, Recreation and Dance. 1980. *AAHPERD Health Related Physical Fitness Test Manual*. Reston, VA: AAHPERD.

52. American College of Sports Medicine. 1995. *Guidelines for exercise testing and prescription,* 5th ed. Philadelphia: Lea & Febiger.

53. Bar-Or, O. 1983. *Pediatric sports medicine for the practitioner: From physiologic principles to clinical applications*. NY: Springer-Verlag.

54. Aaron, D.J., and LaPorte, R.E. 1997. Physical activity, adolescence, and health: An epidemiological perspective. *Exercise in Sport Science Review* 25:391-405.

55. McGraw, S.A., Stone, E.J., Osganian, S.K., Elder, J.P., Perry, C.L., Johnson, C.C., Parcel, G.S., Webber, L.S., and Luepker, R.V. 1994. Design of process evaluation with the Child and Adolescent Trial for Cardiovascular Health (CATCH). *Health Education Quarterly* (Suppl 2):S5-S26.

56. Liederbach, M. 1997. Screening for functional capacity in dancers: Designing standardized, dance-specific injury prevention screening tools. *Journal of Dance Medicine & Science* 1(3):93-106.

57. Poggini, L., Lossasso, S., and Iannone, S. 1999. Injuries during the dancer's growth spurt: Etiology, prevention, and treatment. *Journal of Dance Medicine & Science* 3(2):75-79.

58. Blair, S.N. 1984. How to assess exercise habits and physical fitness. In J.D. Matarazzo, et al. (eds.), *Behavioral health: A handbook of health enhancement and disease prevention*. NY: Wiley.

59. Blair, S.N., Haskell, W.L., Ho, P., Paffenbarger, R.S., Vranizan, K.M., Farquahr, J.W., and Wood, P.D. 1985. Assessment of habitual physical activity by a seven-day recall in a community survey and controlled experiments. *American Journal of Epidemiology* 122:794-804.

60. Janz, K.F., Golden, J., Hansen, J., and Mahoney, L. 1992. Heart rate monitoring of physical activity in children and adolescents. *Pediatrics* 89:256-261.

61. Garcia, A.W., George, T.R., Coviak, C., Antonakos, C., and Pender, N.J. 1997. Development of the child/adolescent activity log: A comprehensive and feasible measure of leisure-time physical activity. *International Journal of Behavioral Medicine* 4:324-339.

62. Godin, G., and Shephard, R.J. 1985. A simple method to assess exercise behavior in the community. *Canadian Journal of Applied Sport Sciences* 10(3):141-146.

63. Godin, G., Jobin, J., and Bouillon, J. 1986. Assessment of leisure time exercise behavior by self-report: A concurrent validity study. *Canadian Journal of Public Health* 77:359-362.

64. Sallis, J.F., Buono, M.J., Roby, J.J., Micale, F.G., and Nelson, J.A. 1993. Seven-day recall and other physical activity self-reports in children and adolescents. *Medicine and Science in Sports and Exercise* 25(1):99-108.

65. Aaron, D.J., Kriska, A.M., Dearwater, S.R., Anderson, R.L., Olsen, T.L., Cauley, J.A., and LaPorte, R.E. 1993. The epidemiology of leisure physical activity in an adolescent population. *Medicine and Science in Sports and Exercise* 25(7):847-853.

66. Aaron, D.J., Kriska, A.M., Dearwater, S.R., Cauley, J.A., Metz, K.F., and LaPorte, R.E. 1995. Reproducibility and validity of an epidemiologic questionnaire to assess past year physical activity in adolescents. *American Journal of Epidemiology* 142(2):191-201.

67. Bukowski, W.M., Gauze, C., Hoza, B., and Newcomb, A.F. 1993. Differences and consistency between same-sex and other-sex peer relationships during early adolescence. *Developmental Psychology* 29:255-263.

68. Gardner, M.F. Test of visual-motor skills. Psychological and Educational Publications, PO Box 520, Hydesville, CA 95547-0520.

69. Maehr, M.L., and Haas, H.I. 1976. Physical self test. In O.G. Johnson (ed.), *Tests and measurements in child development: Handbook II* (vol. 2). San Francisco, CA: Jossey-Bass.

70. McAuley, E., and Courneya, K.S. 1994. The subjective exercise experience scale (SEES): Development and preliminary validation. *Journal of Sport and Exercise Psychology* 10:163-177.

71. Botuck, S., and Turkewitz, G. 1990. Intersensory functioning: Auditory-visual pattern equivalence in younger and older children. *Developmental Psychology* 26:115-120.

72. Garcia, A.W., Broda, M.A.N., Frenn, M., Coviak, C., Pender, N.J., and Ronis, D.L. 1995. Gender and developmental differences in exercise beliefs among youth and prediction of their exercise behavior. *Journal of School Health* 65(6):213-219.

73. In the author's conversations with health care workers and fitness instructors who serve the Hawaiian population, these terms were identified as part of the culture of helping that is specific to this ethnic group, and which girls learn primarily in the home. Hawaii Department of Health, Physical Activity Promotion Project Training Sessions, Honolulu, HI, November, 2000.

74. Godin, G., and Shephard, R.J. 1985. A simple method to assess exercise behavior in the community. *Canadian Journal of Applied Sport Sciences* 10:141-146.

75. National Dairy Council. 1994. *Food model comparison cards.* Rosemont, IL 60018-5616.

76. Hutchinson, A. 1970. *Labunotation.* NY: Theatre Arts Books.

77. Laban, R., and Lawrence, F.L. 1947. *Effort.* London: Macdonald & Evans.

78. Laban, R. 1984. *A vision of dynamic space.* Compiled by Lisa Ullman. London: Falmer Press.

PART II

PREGNANCY

On the biological level, life has only one purpose: to reproduce. All the rest of the accoutrements of living are measures for achieving survival or comfort. From this perspective, the processes of gestation, birth, and lactation take on a great significance. One promising aspect of the growing visibility of women in the marketplace of policy is the increasing focus on childbirth and parenting, both as underpinnings of a healthy society and as productive work worthy of valuation.

Bearing children is an event that can happen over several decades of women's biological existence. In some cultures and settings, girls become pregnant while still in adolescence. With the rise of affluence and women's education, pregnancy tends to become more rare and occurs later in the female life cycle. Whenever it occurs, it is a major—if not *the* major—identity-shaping moment in a woman's life.

Although the prenatal (or antepartum) and postpartum periods are often lumped together, they are, in fact, two very distinct and separate phases of the life cycle. Growing a life within your body naturally causes an inward, reflective focus. This is a wonderful time for women to learn mind/body techniques because there is already an interest in internal sensations and cues. It is also a time of preparation. Some women like to "nest," especially toward the end of their pregnancy. On the other hand, the postpartum period is marked by an outward turn of focus as the baby's needs pull the mother's attention outside herself. An adequate preparation for the endurance events of birth and parenting includes physical conditioning. However, the needs and concerns of exercising pregnant and postpartum women are best addressed as distinct phases in the female life cycle.

This part of the text begins with a chapter that outlines the development of the prenatal fitness field and reviews research that has influenced safety guidelines and screening procedures. The chapter then addresses maternal/fetal anatomy and physiology and how these affect exercise protocols and outcomes. Chapter 6 reviews research findings on the interactions of exercise and pregnancy. This is followed by a chapter that discusses goals and priorities for prenatal fitness programs, and then a chapter that considers how to design and evaluate effective programs for the pregnant population.

CHAPTER 5

UNDERSTANDING PREGNANCY

This chapter examines the close relationship between pregnancy and exercise—both of which the female body perceives as work. We start with the development of the prenatal fitness field, looking at early pioneers and research findings that led to some of the first guidelines and protocols. The chapter then reviews basic aspects of maternal/fetal physiology and physical fitness that are critical to understanding the interactions of pregnancy and exercise, the topic of the next chapter.

The prenatal fitness field, like most areas of inquiry and practice, grows out of preexisting fields. In this sense, it owes its existence to a unique fusion of insights and efforts on the part of creative instructors who followed intuition to develop imaginative prenatal programs combining education, support, and physical activity; dedicated pregnant athletes who trusted their mind/body to give them signs they were pushing too hard; and researchers who attached wires to everything they could to find out just what was happening when pregnant women did what we've always done, worked.

DEVELOPMENT OF THE PRENATAL FITNESS FIELD

The current *fitness industry* can trace its immediate roots to the early 1970s. Although there are also older precedents, it was research on cardiovascular fitness (stimulated by the work of Cooper in 1968 [1]) and stress reduction (given impetus by Benson in 1974 [2]) that began to build the growing list of health benefits from strenu-

ous activity and mind/body relaxation techniques, and that gave legitimacy to the concept of charging money for access to exercise. One of the first aspects of women's health to receive major research attention was prenatal exercise, although interactions of exercise and women's health from the onset of menses through old age have been documented [3-5]. But, even before the fitness revolution, pioneers were working on the question of how exercise might improve the outcome of labor and birth for women in an age when it was no longer necessary to do physical work for survival purposes.

Pioneers in Prenatal Exercise Programming

As the prenatal exercise field began to develop, three key areas were being addressed. Over time, knowledge in these areas has converged to become an essential component of women's health and fitness. These three areas are the somatic arts, recreational physical activity, and childbirth education. In each area, practitioners have been addressing issues of exertion during pregnancy, as well as its impact on the body, the baby, the birth, and parenting.

The Somatic Arts

The somatic arts include relaxation techniques, body/mind disciplines, physical therapy, and dance/movement therapy. These methods rely on a combination of physical and mental education (and sometimes emotional and spiritual awakening) to effect their common objective: release tensions or imbalances that impede functional movement and personal development. By observing the childbearing process, practitioners in these areas have uncovered particular motions and attitudes that aid in reducing discomforts and improving outcomes. With both ancient roots (e.g., yoga, tai chi, meditation) and modern roots (e.g., physical therapy, Alexander, Feldenkrais, ideokinesis, Pilates), these areas have contributed substantially to the ability to perceive exertion and to design special strength and relaxation exercises that assist women in coping with the rigors of pregnancy, birth, and nurturing. The 1960s and 1970s saw many practitioners—often collectively referred to as bodywork professionals—begin work on these issues.

Recreational Physical Activity

When Cooper published his work, he codified one of the great truths about the human animal: we are equipped to endure. Employing inborn adaptive conditioning mechanisms, we humans can teach our bodies to put up with tremendous physiological stresses. The development of technology helped Cooper and others to examine cardiovascular conditioning and pushed open the edges of endurance training. It also permitted researchers to peer into the mysteries of gestation. While a cadre of young, fertile women entered the recreational fitness arena, the ranks of elite competitive female athletes choosing to train throughout their pregnancies began to grow. Interested researchers began asking questions: What happens when pregnant women exercise or participate in sport? What is safe? And, what do we study to decide what is safe? Some early studies, particularly in animals, produced theoretical concerns about possible adverse effects of intense cardiovascular training. When these theoretical negative consequences did not materialize in recreational and competitive exercisers, and improved technology and more subtle analysis revealed feto-protective mechanisms at work, the obstetrical community concluded that guidelines varied greatly from individual to individual depending on exercise history and genetic potential—and that women should pay attention to fatigue as an indicator that they have reached their limit.

On the practical side, one of the first exercise proponents to develop a methodology was Helen Heardman. She is credited with designing a program of calisthenics, including squatting (as in *birth squat* rather than *fitness squat*), alignment work, and abdominal and pelvic floor toning, in 1951 [6]. Around the time that Cooper was working on aerobics, childbirth educator Elizabeth Bing (*Six Practical Lessons to an Easier Childbirth* [7]) was likening birth to a 12-mile hike, in which stamina and muscle tone would play a critical part. Bing (*Moving Through Pregnancy,* 1969 [8]) and physical therapist Elizabeth Noble (*Essential Exercises for the Childbearing Year,* 4th ed., 1995 [9]) were among the first to write about how particular exercises could benefit the preparation for childbirth, although these books offered little cardiovascular work other than walking. Carol Difler (*Your Baby Your Body,* 1977 [10]) proposed combining the known calisthenics and bodywork exercises with aerobic conditioning such as jogging, swimming, running, or dancing. Along similar lines, but beginning from a yoga base and later adding cardiovascular fitness, the late Sylvia Klein Olkin developed her *Positive Pregnancy Fitness* [11]. *Dancing Thru Pregnancy®*, designed by Ann Cowlin [12], and *Bellies Up!* by Barbara Holstein [13] are dance/fitness programs created in the late 1970s that teach women to increase their range of motion and aerobic component by using the dance technique of *centering* to help evaluate perceived exertion and develop an internal locus of control for safe, balanced, relaxed movements. In the late 1970s, running and swimming also began to be employed by increasing numbers of women as fitness methods. By the early 1980s, a number of exercise programs were emerging that included increasing emphasis on fitness during pregnancy and the postpartum period. The work of Rhulena White and such programs as Susan Regnier's *You & Me, Baby©* for the YMCA, Bonnie Berk's *Motherwell®*, and Susan Bullen-Lawler's *Moms on the Move™* emerged to swell the ranks of those promoting pre/postnatal health and fitness. Since that time, increasing numbers of prenatal programs for beginning exercisers, as well as intermediate and advanced, have become available in the United States and abroad.

Childbirth Education

Beginning in the 1940s, a number of preparation-for-childbirth systems of educating both women and their partners about the birth process were introduced into the United States. Grantley Dick-Read (*Natural Childbirth,* 1933 [14]; *Childbirth Without Fear,* 1944 [15]), an English obstetrician, had put forth the theory that fear of birth causes a physical tension resulting in restriction of blood flow to the uterine muscles that in turn causes pain and leads to more fear, and that one could interrupt this fear-tension-pain cycle by teaching the mother about childbirth and by physical conditioning in relaxation and deep abdominal breathing. He also introduced the practice of holding one's breath (Valsalva maneuver) during the pushing stage of labor. Fernand Lamaze (*Painless Childbirth,* 1972 [16]), a French obstetrician, based his highly structured method of controlled neuromuscular relaxation on the Pavlovian stimulus-response theory after observing Russian women in labor in the 1950s. A dissociative mental focus and patterned breathing technique are also central to his method. A Denver-based obstetrician, Robert Bradley (*Husband-Coached Childbirth,* 1970 [17]), introduced his method in the 1950s. He emphasized the husband or support person as a key figure in helping the woman go through labor and birth with as little intervention as possible.

The first woman theorist to have a profound impact on theory in the childbirth education field was Sheila Kitzinger (*The Complete Book of Pregnancy and Childbirth,* 1989 [18]), an English social anthropologist and childbirth educator who was influenced by Dick-Read. Her philosophy centers on pregnancy and birth as key aspects of a woman's psychosexual identity and encourages each woman to release into the flow of sensations, tactile cues, and imagery within the body that life experience produces. Although she describes techniques to achieve the openness needed to release a baby from the body, she focuses more on creating an environment that will permit a woman to tap into her own female sexual/birthing rhythms than on any structured methodology. In so doing, she counters Dick-Read's concept of holding the breath and straining during the pushing stage—which she considers to be based on a male sexual rhythm.

Convergence of Professions

These three areas have been steadily converging. With cardiovascular conditioning well established as safe and effective for producing beneficial outcomes for pregnancy and birth when appropriate, exercise scientists are beginning to investigate questions of pregnancy-specific strength training, proprioception in pregnancy, and relaxation for labor. Meanwhile, somatic practitioners and birth educators are expanding their work to include more vigorous activities. Whereas the first childbirth educators were often nurses, increasing numbers of fitness instructors, physical therapists, and movement educators are becoming certified birth educators and doulas (women who provide support and assistance to the birthing mother). Penny Simkin [19], a physical therapist instrumental in organizing doulas into a profession, has also been active in delineating movements that promote labor progress and relieve common discomforts.

Early Research Findings

Research concerning exercise and pregnancy has focused primarily on two areas. One is the interaction of pregnancy-induced maternal adaptations and standard measurable responses to exertion. The second area is fetal response to exertion, including acute responses and birth outcome. As is frequently the case with scientific investigation, research in this field has produced an interesting history of inquiry, with early findings sometimes misleading, sometimes divergent, but always challenging. During the course of research in this field, advances in medical technology have helped enlarge our understanding of what happens when a pregnant body meets physical activity.

An in-depth discussion of the interactions of pregnancy and exercise as we currently understand them appears in chapter 6, but it is useful to point out historically significant findings here. This information forms the foundation for the first pregnancy exercise guidelines issued in the mid-1980s, and reviewing it provides insight into continuing controversies, such as whether or not it is safe to do exercise in the supine position in the second and third trimesters and how the fetus responds to maternal exertion.

The 1940s through the early 1980s produced many findings regarding maternal cardiovascular, respiratory, and metabolic adaptations of pregnancy and the effects of physical work on pregnancy [20-41]. Important findings include those of McLennan in 1943 [20], Veal and Hussey in 1947 [22], and Wright and Osborn in 1950 [23] concerning lower-extremity venous pressure in the supine and standing positions, which point to theoretical concerns about exercise in these positions. In 1960, Ihrman [26] first noted the similarity between circulatory adjustments of pregnancy and those occurring during physical training. The increased ventilatory response of pregnancy, first noted by Widlund in 1945 [21] (and later by Hytten and Leitch in 1971 [29]; Knuttgen and Emerson in 1974 [32]; Pernoll, Metcalfe, Schlenker et al. in 1975 [36]; and Edwards et al. in 1981 [39]) is important to our understanding of feto-protective mechanisms associated with exertion. Hytten and Leitch's 1971 textbook [29], describing the physiology of pregnancy, first brings together information concerning increases in blood volume and composition, shifts in cardiac output and stroke volume, and changes in blood pressure and oxygen consumption. Conflicting findings during this research period concerning maternal tolerance of exercise and the level of fitness attainable by pregnant women reflect inconsistency both in the use of the term *exercise* and in the varying protocols for measurement employed, as well as the small sample sizes in many studies. In the early 1980s, Artal [40] and Clapp [41] began to track the energy cost of vigorous exercise in pregnancy into the metabolic consequences during pregnancy and offspring outcomes.

Finding clues to fetal outcome became an increasingly popular topic as research proliferated in the 1970s and early 1980s. One of the first mechanisms perceived as a possible connection between maternal adaptations and the well-being of the fetus was the drop in uterine blood flow during maternal exertion. Although intuition suggests that decreased uterine blood flow might result in intrauterine growth restriction (IUGR), it appeared from this early research that there are fetal protections at work, including a shift in the distribution of nutrients and the delivery of oxygen. During this research period, the work of Clapp and others—although predominantly done in animals—gave us insight into three important features: first, nutrients appear to move to the area of greatest tissue demand, and the fetus is very demanding; second, when the fetus is already compromised, maternal exertion is detrimental to the fetus; and, third, reduction in uterine blood flow is related to maternal exertion intensity [42-55].

Intrauterine growth restriction is one sign of a compromised fetus and, if not corrected, leads to low birth weight. If the energy demands of maternal exercise, decreased uterine blood flow, or damage to the placenta result in low birth weight, they are causes of poor birth outcomes. During this research period, findings concerning birth weight and maternal exercise produced conflicting results [56-64]. Inconsistent methodologies and the variety of animals and humans tested raised questions about dose effect and differences between animal and human physiology. Damage to the placenta, leading to uteroplacental insufficiency, was still a question in relation to maternal exercise in 1984. Clapp's 1981 study [62] concerning growth restriction with repetitive placental damage in sheep illustrates the importance of screening for uteroplacental insufficiency with women who wish to exercise. In addition, questions of thermoregulation during maternal exercise were still unanswered at this time. Results of some of the animal studies raised questions about the possibility of neural tube defects due to rising core body temperature.

One sign that the fetus is compromised or is experiencing distress is deviation from the normal fetal heart rate pattern, a range of 120 to 160 beats per minute with variability. Symptoms include fetal bradycardia (<120), tachycardia (>160), lack of variability, and slow return or failure to return to a baseline reading following a change. Early findings concerning fetal heart rate and maternal exercise were influenced by the fact that a number of the studies looked at small groups and included women with serious medical conditions [65-74]. Limits in the technology employed were discovered later to have created some false impressions of fetal distress. Other factors that may influence fetal heart rate, such as stress hormones associated with maternal exercise or the waking state of the fetus, may also color results. Because of the broad range of results, by 1984 there was still no clear signal as to whether or not maternal exercise in healthy women is safe for the fetus, even at the low intensities involved in most of these studies.

Two other issues remained unresolved in 1984. One was the question of who gets the available carbohydrates first—the woman (i.e., her exercising muscles) or the fetus. Clearly, for safety's sake, it made sense that keeping intensities low would allow the available fuel to go farther. The second issue was the interaction of changes in the connective tissue and center of gravity with the biomechanical stresses of exercise.

Development of Safety Guidelines

Such was the state of affairs in 1985 when the American College of Obstetricians and Gynecologists (ACOG) issued its first guidelines concerning exercise in pregnancy and the postnatal period [75]. Among the features of these guidelines for pregnancy were the following: 140 beats per minute: maximal maternal heart rate; limiting "strenuous" exercise to 15 minutes; no exercise in the supine position after four months of gestation; and 38° C maternal core temperature maximum. Among the features for both pregnancy and the postpartum period were regular exercise (at least three times per week) rather than binge activity; no competitive activities; no ballistics, jumping, or quick changes of direction; no deep flexion or extension; heart rate measurement at peak of activity; and very low beginning intensities for sedentary women. The guidelines also included information on the importance of nutrition and hydration.

Controversial Guidelines

Most of these and the other guidelines seemed logical enough, but several items became controversial, and—despite changes in the 1994 ACOG guidelines [76]—have continued to be controversial. The 140 beats per minute and 15 minutes of vigorous activity were questioned by individual athletes and aerobics instructors because they were so very conservative compared with what many people were actually doing in their workout routines. Fortunately, research has emerged to provide clear evidence that *in the absence of limiting medical conditions,* there are many benefits for both pregnant and postpartum women who exercise at levels appropriate to their prior exercise history and personal preferences (even if these levels are in excess of ACOG's original guidelines), without detriment to the fetus. In addition, emerging research information indicates that benefits also accrue for those with little or no exercise history who participate in carefully monitored exercise programs. The 1994 ACOG guidelines were more liberal, focusing on individual variations for cardiovascular conditioning. Unfortunately, one still hears the 140 beats per minute stricture from those who are less informed.

Another controversial item was the restriction on supine exercise. Although theoretical concerns made it apparent that the supine position might be more dangerous than standing on the feet for long periods of time, adverse outcomes were not associated with supine position exercise, but were with jobs that required many hours of standing up. To athletes and instructors who had not seen adverse outcomes from abdominal exercises in the supine position for a few minutes in the course of a workout, it seemed mysterious that this activity would be restricted when there was no mention of getting nurses, waitresses, and retail clerks off their feet! This controversy remains today, as ACOG continues to advise that no exercise should be done in the supine position after the first trimester.

The third controversy from the 1985 guidelines was the stricture against deep flexion and extension. Most affected by this were midwives, childbirth educators, and exercise instructors who taught birth squats as a preparation for labor and as a potential delivery position for birth. Fortunately, after nearly a decade of justifying this movement to institutions and businesses that required their facilities to follow the ACOG guidelines, those working with women preparing for birth were relieved to find that the 1994 guidelines removed this stricture as well.

Contraindications

The following absolute contraindications for exercise were given in ACOG's 1985 guidelines: ruptured membranes, premature labor, a history of three or more spontaneous abortions, diagnosed multiple gestation, incompetent cervix, bleeding or diagnosed placenta previa, and diagnosed cardiac disease [75]. The 1994 guidelines added or adjusted contraindications to include pregnancy-induced hypertension (PIH), preterm rupture of membranes (PROM), preterm labor during the prior or present pregnancy, incompetent cervix, persistent second- or third-trimester bleeding, and IUGR [76].

Refining the Guidelines

In 1987, Melpomene Institute in Minnesota published guidelines on selecting a prenatal exercise program [77]. Although the authors of the guidelines made note of ACOG's 140 beats per minute recommendation, they did not issue heart rate or duration limits but rather focused on the quality of the program, including the instructor's qualifications and sensitivity. They suggested consulting the primary care provider and obtaining medical permission. Program guidelines included proper warm-ups and cool-downs; combining cardiovascular work, strength work, and relaxation; and health education. Also in 1987, the International Dance Exercise Association included information on exercise in pregnancy in its teacher preparation materials, based largely on the ACOG guidelines.

In the mid-1980s, Dancing Thru Pregnancy began work on creating forms for medical screening and for evaluating a woman's exercise history and nutritional status in preparation for entering a prenatal exercise program or receiving an exercise prescription. The forms and methods that evolved are included in chapter 8 of this text. In 1983, DTP, Inc. began its educational seminars to prepare instructors.

In 1988, a dozen leaders in the field formed the Perinatal Health and Fitness Network (PHFN) as an informal communication system to share information and knowledge about research findings, exercise methods, safety guidelines, and benefits for this special population. Under the leadership of Cowlin, Holstein, Olkin, Berk, Jacqueline White, MaryAnn Brundage, Geri Flynn, and others, the group worked to put research findings and practical experience into the hands of as many fitness and movement specialists, childbirth educators, nurses, midwives, and physicians as possible. Recognizing the individual nature of exercise prescription for this population, PHFN strove not to set up rules but to educate instructors, trainers, and health care providers about key issues. By 1993, professional fitness, childbirth education, and medical organizations had begun to include pre/postnatal fitness in their discussions of a healthy childbearing experience. Its goal accomplished, PHFN disbanded in 1995.

Research since 1985 has made it clear that, in the absence of medical problems, moderate amounts of vigorous-intensity exercise, even though we do not recommend it, continued into pregnancy or begun in the first half of pregnancy has benefits for mothers and their offspring. The 1994 ACOG guidelines, though still considered conservative, provide a baseline for safety by advising pregnant women to seek approval of their health care provider; to exercise regularly and in line with their pre-pregnancy fitness level; to avoid discomfort in movement; and not to engage in activity when labor signs appear, when fatigued, or when unusual conditions such as bleeding occur.

Since the late 1970s, prenatal exercise has moved from a subject of fringe awareness to a central theme in women's health. As a research topic concerning female function, exercise in pregnancy may be the most complex physiological model for study. Almost all women are pregnant women at some point in their lives; and because women are slightly more than half the population, a working model of healthy and fit pregnant women is a large piece of the public health model of a physically active population.

Much remains to be discovered through research about the dose effect of exercise in pregnancy, but a basic understanding of the beneficial physiological interactions of exercise and pregnancy has been established (detailed discussion is included in chapter 6). The benefits of this work will carry far into the future as improvements are made not only in the lives of pregnant and postpartum women, but also in the lives of their children, because these women have been encouraged to observe, interact with, and enjoy their babies. And many of these women will suffer less in midlife. Their mothers too often faced incontinence or uterine prolapse because they were not taught anatomy of the female pelvis or the fact that the pelvic floor is a muscle group. And as knowledge increases, trauma to the pelvis becomes more preventable and manageable. Emotional support for women in the childbearing years is also a critical service, leading to reductions in depression and alienation among new mothers. Programs for these women are growing, and with them a greater standard of care for women.

PREGNANCY-RELATED ANATOMY

For a health and fitness program to have a positive effect on the pregnancy, birth outcome, and recovery of pre/

postnatal clients, the designer of the program must understand the anatomical features and physiological functions of the female body pertaining to pregnancy. Without a clear concept of how a woman's body is constructed, how it reacts in a normal pregnancy, and how it is affected by physical activity, it is impossible to design an effective program.

The Pelvis

With the exception of the breasts, female sexual organs are encased in the *pelvis,* the bony structure surrounding the center of gravity. The word *pelvis* comes from the Latin word for bowl—an apt identifier. Viewing the female pelvis (see figure 5.1), it is easy to see how the concept of the pelvis as a bowl comes about. The major bones of the pelvis are the *iliacus,* the *ischium,* and the *pubis.* Each bone is present on both the left and right sides, and during infancy these bones grow together via suture joints at their junctures and within the *acetabulum*

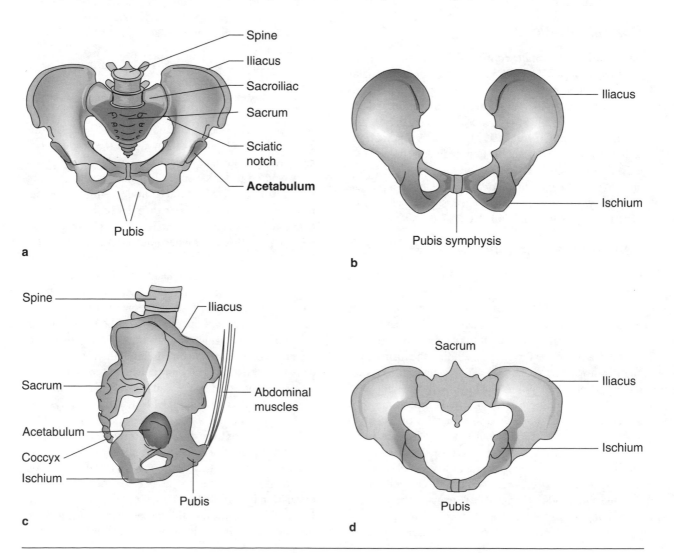

Figure 5.1   Views of the pelvis: *(a)* anterior, *(b)* posterior, *(c)* right lateral, *(d)* superior.

or socket of the *iliofemoral joint* (the femur/pelvis ball-and-socket joint) .

Sacrum

The *sacrum,* or next-to-last section of the spine, fits down into the space created at the back of the pelvis between the left and right iliacus bones. The bones of the pelvis, the sacrum, and the abdominal muscles form a bowl surrounding the viscera.

The many-faceted, three-dimensional right and left *sacroiliac joints* (SI joints) are often the source of discomfort during pregnancy and the postpartum period. Normally held fairly rigid by a complex of ligaments and tendons, during pregnancy these joints are loose because the connective tissues become soft and consequently allow a large and often unstable range of motion. The joints can slip and become stuck, causing stiffness, misalignment, and discomfort.

Sciatic Nerve

The *sciatic nerve* (figure 5.2) can also contribute to discomfort in this area. This large, major nerve plexus exits the spine through several of the intervertebral spaces at and above the sacral table (top of the sacrum), passes along the front of the SI joint and exits the pelvis under the sciatic notch. It can become impinged in the SI joint or under the *piriformis muscle* that runs from the sacrum over the nerve, and then to the greater trochanter on the lateral aspect of the femur. The forward shift of gravity, especially in the later stages of pregnancy, causes the sacrum to be pulled forward, contributing to the instability of the SI joint and causing the piriformis muscle to contract in response to being stretched by the forward momentum of the sacrum.

Pelvic Floor Muscles

The *pelvic floor muscles* (shown in figure 5.3) are located between the pubic bone and the coccyx and are bounded on the sides by the *ischial tuberosities* (popularly called the *sitsbones*). The term for this area is the *perineum.* Embedded within these muscles are the outlets for the *urethra,* the *vagina,* and the *anus.* The *perineal body* is the tissue between the opening of the vagina and

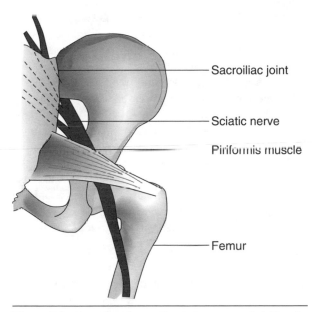

Figure 5.2 Posterior view with sciatic nerve and piriformis muscle.

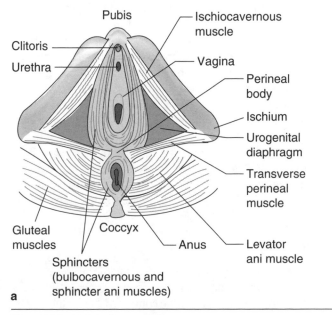

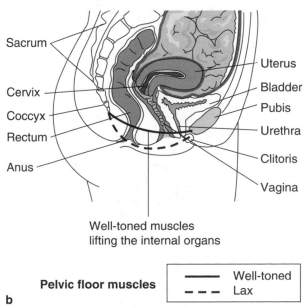

Figure 5.3 Pelvic floor muscles.

anus, created by the intersection of the two *sphincter muscles,* the first of which surrounds the vagina and urethra, and the second of which surrounds the anus. These two muscles are responsible for closing the outlets by contracting, and opening the outlets by relaxing.

Other muscles in the pelvic floor include the *ischiocavernous, transverse perineal, urogenital diaphragm,* and *levator ani muscles.* When contracted, the ischiocavernous and transverse perineal muscles close the space between the pubis and sitsbones, and the diaphragm and levator muscles close and lift the pelvic floor. Collectively the pelvic floor muscles are called the pubococcygeal muscles; and their actions—squeezing the outlets, closing and lifting the pelvic floor, and then releasing these muscles—are known as the *Kegel exercises* and are vital to pelvic floor fitness.

The functions of the pelvic floor muscles include maintenance of alignment and integrity of the internal viscera, control of urine flow, sexual enhancement, and elimination of waste from the rectum. Some of the problems associated with a weak pelvic floor include prolapse of internal organs due to lack of support, limited sexual pleasure during intercourse, stress incontinence (uncontrollable leakage of urine especially during exercise or coughing or sneezing), and delayed recovery of tissue in the case of an episiotomy.

Internal Organs of the Abdomen

Internal organs (refer to figure 5.4) include the *bladder* (located between the pubic bone and uterus), the *vagina* (or *birth canal*), and the *uterus,* the hollow bag of invol-

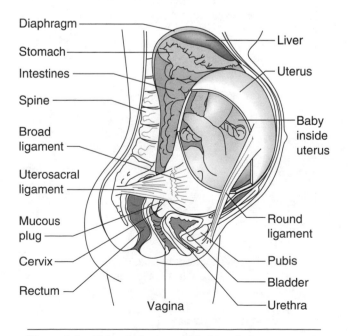

Diaphragm
Stomach
Intestines
Spine
Broad ligament
Uterosacral ligament
Mucous plug
Cervix
Rectum
Vagina
Liver
Uterus
Baby inside uterus
Round ligament
Pubis
Bladder
Urethra

Figure 5.4 Abdominal organs, right lateral view.

untary muscle located above the bladder between the pubic bone and rectum and normally having an anterior tilt. The uterus is held in place by the *uterine ligaments.* The bottom of the uterus, or the *cervix,* is the opening through which the baby emerges into the vagina during labor and birth.

Uterine Ligaments

Uterine ligaments that hold the uterus in place are shown in figure 5.4. These ligaments undergo prolonged stretching during pregnancy. The *round ligaments* attach the uterus to the pubic bone and help maintain the uterus in the midline. During periods of rapid uterine growth, often in the fifth or sixth month, the round ligament is the source of discomfort as it is stretched. The sensation of sharp pain or a dull ache is common, and to relieve the discomfort it is helpful to bend into the pain at the iliofemoral joint so that the space between the ligament attachments is shortened. The *uterosacral* or *broad ligaments* connect the uterus to the sacrum and are often involved in backaches during pregnancy because of stress in the low back resulting from weak abdominals, poor posture, and weight of the abdomen. They can also cause discomfort during labor in the case of a posterior presentation of the baby (i.e., when the posterior aspect of the baby's spine is pressing against the mother's sacrum).

Uterus

In the nonpregnant state the uterus weighs approximately 70 grams or slightly more than 2 ounces, is about the size of a pear, and has a cavity with capacity of approximately 10 milliliters or 2 teaspoons. In pregnancy the uterus grows to a weight of about 1100 grams or 39 ounces and has a cavity capacity of approximately 1.5 to 2.5 gallons. It enlarges through the stretching of muscle fiber until it is about the size of a watermelon and has an increased number and size of blood vessels and nerves.

After the first trimester, the uterus begins to prepare for labor and delivery by contracting involuntarily and sporadically. These contractions are called *Braxton-Hicks contractions* and are irregular, without the increasing length, frequency, or intensity associated with labor. They are usually painless.

The *fundus* is the upper one-third of the uterus. Fundal height is used as an indicator of gestational age and is measured from the pubic bone to the top of the uterus. In labor, the lower part of the uterus contracts toward the fundus.

Cervix

The *cervix* is the cylindrical opening of the uterus, leading into the birth canal. During pregnancy it is a long corridor with a *mucous plug* composed of tiny blood vessels and mucus that serves as a barrier against infection. At some point leading up to labor or in its early phases, this plug loosens and falls out in sections or as a whole.

In the early phase of the first stage of labor, the cervix softens and thins, in a process known as *effacement*. This process can take several days and may or may not occur before the onset of regular contractions. The cervix then opens slowly, in a process that is termed *dilation* (or *dilatation*). This part of labor generally requires several hours. The mechanisms that cause these actions are the *labor contractions* of the uterine muscle fibers, mediated by the hormone *oxytocin,* produced in the maternal posterior pituitary gland. Labor is probably initiated in response to a signal released from the baby's paraventricular nucleus in the basal ganglia of its brain [78-81].

In order for labor to be effective, uterine contractions must be strong enough to cause effacement and dilation. A number of factors can influence the strength of contractions, including how hard the baby is pressing on the cervix; the position and size of the baby; and the responses of the mother's sympathetic nervous system to genetics, environment, emotional factors, nourishment, and hydration.

Other Reproductive Organs

Other glands and organs within the abdomen include the *ovaries,* which produce the *ovum* or *egg,* and the hormones *estrogen, progesterone,* and *relaxin.* Relaxin is responsible for softening the connective tissue within joints, muscles, and vascular vessels. The *fallopian tubes* are the ducts that lead from the ovaries to the uterus and carry the ovum (which may be fertilized during its journey through the fallopian tube or shortly after its arrival in the uterus) toward the *endometrium* or uterine lining. The *embryo*—or developing fertilized egg—will attach itself to the lining. The entire process of release of the ovum by the ovary, its journey to the uterus, fertilization, and *implantation* in the lining transpires in about one to two weeks.

The Placenta

The *placenta* (figure 5.5) develops as the embryo implants in the uterine lining. Within a few days of implantation, a primitive placental circulation is established, with further development occurring around the eighth week. The placenta, or interface of maternal and fetal circulations, includes the fetal placenta *(villous chorion)* and maternal placenta *(decidua basalis).* Inflowing maternal arterial blood is spurting into the *intervillous space,* pushing venous blood out into the endometrial veins of the decidua basalis. Substrate exchanges (molecular structures, including nutritional components, gases, and toxins) between maternal and fetal blood occur across a permeable barrier or membrane as the maternal blood flows around the villi—the fingerlike projections of the fetal vasculature.

The placenta has three functions: (1) metabolism; (2) transport or exchange; and (3) synthesis, production, and secretion of protein and steroid hormones. In early pregnancy the placenta synthesizes glycogen. This function declines as the fetal liver develops. The placenta is also involved in the synthesis of cholesterol and fatty

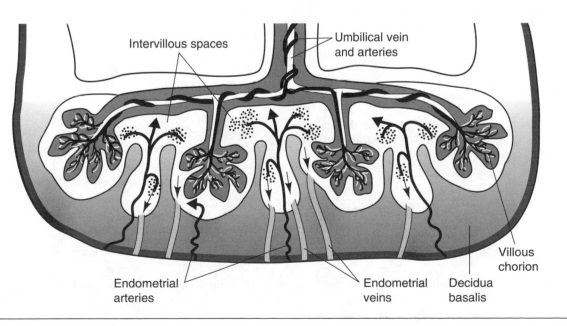

Figure 5.5 Placental circulation.

acids that provide energy. While maternal nutrients pass to the fetus through the placenta, so do many drugs, including caffeine, alcohol, nicotine, and carbon monoxide, as well as antibiotics, antihistamines, sedatives, analgesics, narcotics, and anesthetics. Man-made and naturally occurring substances such as plant toxins can be responsible for fetal defects. The fetal liver is immature and cannot metabolize substances as quickly as the adult liver does.

Placental function is highly dependent on maternal circulation. Such factors as blood pressure, maternal position, blood volume, and uterine contractions affect delivery of nutrients to the fetus and the removal of waste.

Nutrient Transfer Across the Placental Membrane

Simple *diffusion* accounts for transfer of oxygen (O_2), electrolytes, water, and drugs from mother to fetus and of carbon dioxide (CO_2) from fetus to mother. Glucose is transferred by facilitated diffusion. More active transport delivers vitamins, minerals, proteins, and other complex structures, including infections.

The direction of substrate diffusion is regulated by such factors as internal temperature, pH (acidity), and pressure gradients. A high concentration of gas within a fluid on one side of a barrier creates a pressure difference when concentration is less on the other side, facilitating the flow of gas from the side with greater concentration to the side with lesser concentration.

Concentration is determined by pressure and solubility. CO_2 is very soluble in water, and O_2 is not. In addition, CO_2 is easy for tissues to unload, and O_2 is difficult for tissues to take up. The exchange process is assisted by a greater concentration of *hemoglobin* (the specific oxygen-binding protein) in the fetal blood. While pressure gradients favor the flow of oxygen to the fetus and carbon dioxide to the mother, the higher concentration of hemoglobin in the fetal blood is necessary to help unload oxygen at the high internal temperatures associated with pregnancy and the fetus. In the process of creating additional blood, the mother's system produces a higher percentage of *plasma* (the fluid portion of the blood) than *red blood cells* or *RBCs* (hemoglobin-carrying cells), thereby having the effect of lowering the *hematocrit* (or percentage of RBCs in the total blood volume). In addition, fetal hemoglobin can carry 20% to 30% more oxygen than maternal hemoglobin, further facilitating the flow of oxygen to the fetus.

Net diffusion is also pH sensitive (the Bohr effect). As the pH lowers—that is, as the blood becomes more acidic—the hemoglobin-oxygen bond is weakened, further enabling the mother's blood to give up oxygen to the fetus. When PO_2 (or the pressure gradient) is higher, the Bohr effect is lessened.

Importance of Blood Volume

During pregnancy, blood volume increases by about 40%; the majority of the increase is in plasma. This increased volume is necessary to maintain a healthy placenta and thus facilitate fetal growth. The increase in plasma results in a normal reduction in the percentage of RBCs in the maternal blood. This can cause a state termed *physiologic anemia,* which is not true anemia because the absolute level of hemoglobin is adequate. It is possible that this reduction is part of nature's provision to ensure adequate calcium uptake. Because iron interferes with calcium uptake, a reduction in the percentage of RBCs means that iron, though necessary to the oxygen-binding process, will not be present to a degree that inhibits fetal skeletal development.

Fluids and proteins are important in the diet of the pregnant woman because they are needed to make this plasma. *Albumin* (the specific osmotic amino acid that draws fluid from the cells and into the blood) is required and is produced by the liver. Eggs are an excellent dietary source of albumin. Some researchers believe that toxemia—a disease of pregnancy—is caused or affected by insufficient protein in the diet [82]. Adequate protein for the average woman is 70 to 90 grams per day for a single baby, or 30 grams per day per baby beyond her other protein requirements. Adequate water is 2 quarts per day, except in high altitudes, where requirements may be double that amount.

Umbilical Cord

The *umbilical cord*—the conduit between the placenta and fetus—contains one vein and two arteries. The average length is 53 centimeters or 21 inches. The cord is spiral and is covered with a substance called Wharton's jelly that prevents kinking, compression, and interference with fetal circulation. The jelly has a high water content and contains prostaglandins that cause the umbilical cord to shrink quickly and its blood vessels to vasoconstrict following birth.

Embryo

Embryo refers to the organism between fertilization and about eight weeks. This is a critical period marked by rapid cell division and the differentiation of major organs. During this early period of development, the embryo's systems are extremely vulnerable to environmental agents such as drugs, viruses, radiation, or infection.

Fetus

Fetus is the term used after eight weeks, when skeletal formation begins. Although somewhat less vulnerable, the fetus is still susceptible to *teratogens,* or agents that can cause defects, especially to the brain.

The Amniotic Sac and Fluid

In the course of placental development, *membranes* (an *amniotic sac*) that encase the *amniotic fluid* and the fetus are created. The membrane or sac acts as a protective barrier against infection as well as housing the amniotic fluid in which the fetus is immersed. The fluid, or fetal urinary output, is clear, slightly yellow, and odorless. It protects the fetus from impact trauma, allows freedom of movement, facilitates growth and development of the musculoskeletal system, maintains a relatively constant fetal body temperature, is the source of oral fluids for the fetus, and aids in the development of the respiratory system.

Rupture of Membranes

The rupture of the membranes normally occurs at the end of the first stage of labor. Rupture prior to labor is termed *premature rupture of the membranes* (PROM). A premature rupture can be caused by infection, and when it occurs prior to term it is an absolute contraindication for exercise. This is a serious situation that requires immediate attention from the health care provider. Sometimes women will begin spontaneous labor following a rupture. The rupture of membranes and loss of amniotic fluid is popularly called *breaking the bag of waters.*

PHYSIOLOGICAL CHANGES IN PREGNANCY

Dramatic changes occur in the female body during pregnancy. In order to make a baby, the body must adjust many systems. The five major physiologic systems affected by pregnancy are the cardiovasculature, thermoregulation, metabolism, respiration, and biomechanics. More than 30 changes in these systems affect the mother's body and, in turn, its response to exercise. Readers wishing a more extensive discussion of the physiological changes in pregnancy are referred to the most recent editions of *Varney's Midwifery, Williams Obstetrics,* or *Guyton and Hall's Physiology of Human Disease.*

Cardiovasculature System

The cardiovascular system includes the heart, blood, arteries, and veins. It delivers oxygen and nutrients to all parts of the body. It works not just for the pregnant woman, but also delivers nutrients to the growing baby through the placenta. To accommodate the additional circulatory demands, blood volume increases by approximately 40%, as noted earlier. The mother's heart becomes more efficient at pumping blood. Cardiac (heart) output, stroke volume, and end-diastolic volume increase, so the heart pumps more blood, but not 40% more. In order to pump the extra blood, resting pulse increases by as much as 8 beats per minute in the first trimester and 15 beats per minute by the third trimester. Cardiac reserve (blood left in the heart on each stroke) decreases.

Blood plasma increases, and the percentage of RBCs (which hold oxygen) decreases. As a result, hematocrit (percentage of oxygen in the blood) decreases due to pregnancy, but is higher in women who participate in vigorous exercise. The blood pressure normally decreases; but in PIH (pregnancy-induced hypertension, or high blood pressure), blood pressure increases and exercise must stop, though relaxation activities should continue. The blood supply to the uterus during continuous, vigorous exercise decreases 50% in recreational activity and 70% in competitive athletic events. Although there are theoretical concerns due to this diversion of uterine blood flow, there appear not to be adverse effects on the fetus in fit women as long as there are no medical problems.

Thermoregulatory System

The thermoregulatory system regulates body temperature. After the first trimester, a pregnant woman's body temperature tends to be slightly higher than a nonpregnant woman's. She perspires more rapidly; this helps her body cool more efficiently. However, if her temperature rises above 100.5° to 101° F (38° C), this could be a fever related to illness, and the woman should see her health care provider. Basal metabolic rate probably declines in early pregnancy, but it then increases steadily during the remainder of the pregnancy, affecting internal (core) temperature. Core temperature at rest increases, but during the first few minutes of vigorous exercise it decreases because pregnant women are more efficient at cooling; after that it increases steadily. An upper limit of 100.5° to 101° F should also be observed during exercise. In fit women, core temperature following exercise at low to moderate intensity appears to decline slightly, according to ACOG; the decline is probably related to the ability of fit individuals to better regulate internal temperature as well as the increased capacity for cooling in fit pregnant women. A less fit pregnant woman will experience slower and less cooling than the fit pregnant woman will.

Metabolic System

The metabolic system includes energy production. We measure how much energy we use by how many calories we burn. High metabolism burns more calories. When a person exercises, her metabolic rate increases and she uses more calories. A pregnant woman's metabolic rate also increases to provide more energy for the baby. The extra energy required for pregnancy is only about 300 calories per day. Carbohydrate utilization during exercise increases as weight increases. Protein and fluid requirements, as already noted, increase in order to make additional blood to nourish the placenta, fetus, and mother. It is essential to emphasize the importance of adequate protein and fluids.

Metabolism also involves hormone production, which alters in pregnancy as well. Major changes include increases in insulin production (the body seeks to store energy more frequently). In some women this may lead to insulin resistance and fatigue and eventually cause gestational diabetes, or too little insulin. Because insulin is released more often in normal pregnancy, the amount of time during which glucose (sugar that provides energy) remains in the blood decreases, and the body needs energy (food) in small doses more often.

The level of estrogen increases, which helps with fetal growth and uses energy. Progesterone increases, which helps the uterus nurture the placenta, affects thermoregulation, and contributes to relaxation of vasculature and lowering of blood pressure in normal pregnancy. Relaxin increases, causing connective tissue to soften and affecting range of movement.

Respiratory System

Pregnancy also affects the respiratory system. In the first trimester, increases in progesterone levels as the placenta takes over the production of ovarian hormones make the body more sensitive to CO_2, and may make the woman feel short of breath and cause her to hyperventilate. In the third trimester, the uterus pushes up on the diaphragm, causing the woman to feel short of breath again. She has enough oxygen; she just needs to take a deep breath to ease the sensation. As the abdomen grows, the respiratory capacity increases; to take advantage of this, women can inhale as they do a side bend and exhale when they return to upright. This helps develop breathing in the back lobes of the lungs and uses intercostal muscles.

Because of pressure changes, the increased workload of breathing exertion, and the amount of oxygen going to the fetus, less oxygen is available for aerobic exercise as the pregnancy progresses, except in very fit women. Carbon dioxide sensitivity is increased by increasing levels of progesterone around 8 to 12 weeks. According to ACOG, physiologic dead space remains unchanged, but these findings are based primarily on non-weight-bearing activities. There is increased risk of lactic acidosis

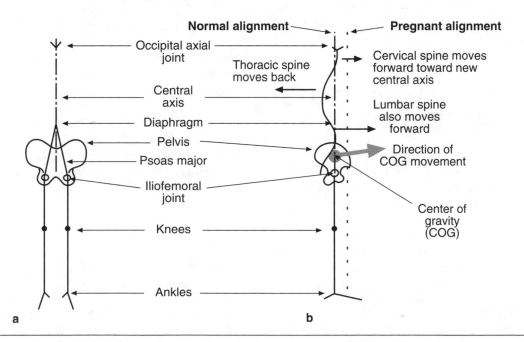

Figure 5.6 Central axis: *(a)* frontal view, *(b)* lateral view, showing both normal alignment and pregnant alignment. In normal alignment, half of the body's weight falls behind the ankle and half falls in front; but, in pregnancy all the weight falls forward.

(muscle fatigue and soreness) when women maintain high intensity for long periods in the last few weeks of pregnancy, except when they have maintained a high level of fitness.

Biomechanical System

The biomechanics system includes the bones, muscles, and nerves and governs how they work together to make the body move. Two major changes have a tremendous effect on biomechanics: one is the shift in the center of gravity (COG), and the other is the increase in relaxin and other hormones that cause loosening of connective tissue. The postural shift that accompanies the baby's growth during the second half of pregnancy is significant because of the redistribution of weights as the COG moves forward and slightly up. In the nonpregnant female population, the COG lies in the pelvis at a point just anterior to the second sacral segment. It is a dynamic balance point. The vertical extension of the COG is the *central axis* (see figure 5.6), also called the *gravity line* or *plumb line.*

The growing uterus shifts the COG and central axis forward, changing the alignment of bones, muscles, and supporting structures and also the way the brain processes what is normal posture and movement. The slight upward direction of the COG tends to destabilize the upright body. This creates alterations in posture and balance during standing, including increased flexion in the hip sockets. The back of the waist curves in (increased lumbar lordosis); the top of the pelvis tilts forward (increased anterior pelvic tilt); and the outward curve in the thoracic spine (kyphosis) increases, as does the inward curve in the cervical spine. The head may shift forward as well.

These changes put stress on joints and muscles. Changes in joint movement occur because of changes in weight distribution (there is more weight on one side of a joint than the other, where before there was balance). The increased lumbar and cervical curves place a greater load on the posterior aspect of the bodies of the vertebra in those regions, and changes in the thoracic curve place a greater load on the anterior aspect of the vertebral bodies in that region. And while the core of the body is dramatically affected, alterations in the angles of peripheral joints occur as well.

The balance of muscle strength around the joints is affected to accommodate the new weight distribution. Among the effects are shortening and tightening of low back and iliopsoas (hip flexors) muscles, shortening of thoracic spinal flexors and pectoral muscles, overstretching and weakening of gluteals and hamstrings, overstretching and weakening of abdominals and pelvic floor, and overstretching and weakening of upper back muscles. In addition, the quadriceps and calf muscles require additional strength to carry the added weight. Because mechanical advantage is decreased, postural and mobility muscles must use increased energy to maintain balance against gravity and produce movement.

Hormone changes affect the looseness of ligaments and tendons, making the joints more mobile. Although this helps with the birth of the baby, it can also stress joints and muscles and contribute to joint laxity. Other problems that derive from these changes in bony alignment include erosion (grinding) of joint surfaces, abnormal compression and shearing forces on discs and facets of the spine, and decreased joint spaces leading to nerve or blood vessel entrapment (causes numbness or poor circulation). There can be more structural discomfort, such as low back pain, sciatica, or carpal tunnel syndrome. Meanwhile, the nervous system adapts to the new abnormal alignment. Changes in joints to keep the head and body upright against gravity, as just described, contribute to an alteration in the brain's configuration of alignment. This occurs slowly over the nine months of pregnancy. Following birth, however, the physical change of weights occurs quite suddenly, while the brain requires retraining over time.

Figure 5.6 helps demonstrate how these changes affect the pregnant body. For example, the figure shows how, as the weight shifts forward, it is carried more by the arch of the foot during pregnancy than by the ankle, which in the nonpregnant body normally distributes the weight evenly forward and back. This, coupled with softening ligaments, often leads to foot discomfort and enlarged feet.

CHARACTERISTICS OF PREGNANCY BY TRIMESTERS

The average pregnancy comes to full *term* at 280 days, the equivalent of 10 lunar months of 28 days each or 40 weeks. This is equal to approximately nine calendar months, or three *trimesters* of about three months each. The range of term delivery is considered to be between 38 weeks (266 days) and 42 weeks (294 days). To calculate the *due date,* one starts from the first day of the last menstrual period, adds seven days, and counts back three months. However, *gestational age* is also figured by fundal growth and often via ultrasound.

First Trimester

The first 13 weeks, or approximately three months, is often characterized by fatigue. The mother's body is working to establish a supportive vasculature and is producing insulin more frequently; both these processes contribute to the sensation of fatigue. Nausea, resulting from changes in insulin production and the body's response to environmental toxins, may also occur. Resting, eating small meals every 2 or 3 hours, eating adequate protein, and drinking plenty of water help with fatigue and nausea.

Embryo/Fetus

- The embryo/fetus grows from 1/4 inch to 3 inches.
- Weight increases to about 1/2 to 1 ounce.
- The heart is beating by the third week.
- The heart, circulatory system, and brain show the most development.
- The digestive system, nerves, lungs, liver, kidneys, and reproductive organs begin development.
- External genitalia show a definite sex by the third month.
- Facial features are present.
- Calcified bones begin to replace cartilage.
- Buds for arms and legs differentiate into hands, fingers, feet, toes, nails.
- Spontaneous movement begins but is not yet felt by mother.

Mother

- The mother has missed a period.
- She may have emotional reactions and may be ambivalent.
- Breasts swell and become tender as a result of increased estrogen and progesterone.
- She experiences urinary frequency.
- She experiences nausea and fatigue due to changing hormone levels and insulin and glucose levels.
- Vaginal secretions are increased.
- Perspiration and salivation are increased.
- There are changes in skin, hair, sense of taste, and sense of smell, as well as food cravings.
- The breasts may secrete colostrum.
- The waistline thickens.

Second Trimester

Weeks 14 to 27 are often accompanied by increased energy and a feeling of well-being. By the mid or later weeks, changes in biomechanics have become significant because of the increasing size of the uterus and resulting displacement of normal body alignments.

Fetus

- The fetus grows to 12 to 14 inches.
- Weight increases to 1 1/4 to 1 1/2 pounds.
- Thyroid and liver begin to function.
- The skeleton is visible on X-ray.
- Hair and lanugo (downy hair covering body) are forming.
- Facial features are well formed; eyebrows and lashes are present.
- The fetus sucks, swallows, grimaces, develops grip, and moves away from stimuli.
- Skin is wrinkled, but fat is slowly filling it in.
- Buds for permanent teeth develop.
- Rapid growth begins.

Mother

- Nausea and urinary frequency generally improve.
- Blood volume increases greatly (there may be bleeding from gums, and a flush or "glow").
- Pigmentation changes. Linea negra (dark center line along the abdomen) appears, and nipples may enlarge and darken.
- Heartburn, indigestion, or constipation may occur as a consequence of sluggish gastrointestinal mobility and crowding by uterus.
- She may experience round ligament discomfort in the lower abdomen, above either or both hip sockets.
- She feels fetal movement.
- She may experience leg cramps.
- She may feel Braxton-Hicks contractions.

Third Trimester

The final weeks (approximately 28 to 40) can be characterized by a sense of sluggishness, especially as term approaches. Alternating activity, eating, and rest often proves a useful rhythm for remaining productive.

Fetus

- The fetus grows to 18 to 22 inches.
- Weight increases to 7 to 8 pounds.
- The fetus begins to store subcutaneous fat.
- Lanugo is shed near term.
- The fetus has fingerprints.
- Internal organs and bones are developed.
- Movement is energetic but may decrease during the last month because of lack of room.
- The fetus has periods of wakefulness and sleep.

Mother

- Discomforts may increase, especially backaches.
- She is susceptible to *varicosities* due to relaxation of smooth walls of veins; pressure on pelvic vessels reducing venous return; and increased blood volume distending vessels in pelvis, perineal region, and lower extremities.
- Emotions may be fluid; she may have fears and may dream a lot.
- Breathing may be difficult because the uterus is displacing diaphragm upward.
- There may be swelling or *edema* due to reduced venous return.
- She experiences urinary frequency.
- She can eat only small amounts at one time.

COMMON DISCOMFORTS OF PREGNANCY AND NONINVASIVE COMFORT MEASURES

The list of possible discomforts and problems of pregnancy is very long—too long to recite to clients. It is impossible to know which (if any) potential problems may arise for a given individual, and it is not the role of the fitness specialist to make diagnoses of what may well be medical conditions. On the other hand, some common discomforts are seen with great frequency, can be alleviated by simple and noninvasive methods, and are within the province of the fitness specialist.

Nausea and Vomiting

Eating often in small amounts prevents extremes in blood sugar levels, which can prompt nausea. Eating late at night and first thing in the morning also helps prevent blood sugar swings. Women must be sure to consume adequate protein (70-90 grams per day, or an additional 30 grams per baby per day above her nonpregnant needs). For first-trimester nausea, some women find these effective: sports drinks, wristbands for seasickness, ginger ale, or ginger tea. Avoiding foods that seem noxious, especially in the first trimester, is a common means of preventing nausea. A prenatal vitamin—prescribed by the health care provider—helps ensure adequate micronutrients. However, the woman needs to be sure to take these with food and, if helpful, to cut the vitamins into smaller sections and take them several times during the day. In extreme cases (*hyperemesis gravidarum*), her care provider will prescribe appropriate drugs.

Tiredness

Women can take several steps to decrease tiredness. Resting on the side to maximize blood flow helps reduce the amount of metabolic waste remaining in the muscles. Eating small meals of protein and complex carbohydrates often over the course of the entire day helps ensure a steady blood sugar level. Women should be encouraged to drink at least 2 quarts of water a day. They should be sure to get extra sleep if they need it, especially in the first trimester when the body is working hard to establish its new cardiovasculature and metabolic status. Regular exercise is helpful. They should get checked for anemia.

Tender Breasts

For tenderness of the breasts, it helps to wear good support. Sometimes ice is helpful. The breasts may grow by a pound or two by the end of pregnancy in preparation for lactation, and most women are likely to need a new, larger, supportive bra.

Groin Spasms or Round Ligament Pain

If a woman experiences a sharp pain or dull ache in the region of the hip socket, it may well be round ligament spasms, which occur commonly in midpregnancy when the uterus begins to grow more rapidly. The round ligament has to stretch extensively to accommodate this growth. In the process, the ligament is pulled. This can cause pain, as can spasms in the uterus near the attachment of the ligaments. Bending into the pain (flexing the iliofemoral joint) brings the ends of the round ligament closer together, reducing the pull on them.

Constipation, Gas, Hemorrhoids

For constipation, women need to make sure that fluids and fiber are adequate. Someone who is taking iron for anemia should cut the pill up into more than one piece and consume it during the course of several meals. She should take the pill with orange juice or another source of vitamin C to improve absorption. For gas, she should try the deeply folded position (see special exercises in chapter 8); this opens the bowels. For hemorrhoids, witch hazel is commonly used; sometimes ice is also helpful, and Kegel exercises are effective.

Backache

Resting on the side with a pillow between the legs is the common method of resting the back. In addition, a woman can simultaneously hold a pillow between the arms, place more than one pillow under the head, and place a pillow under the abdomen, as this stabilizes the entire spine. Women should be told to get up slowly, stabilizing the SI joint. In case of SI joint slippage or a sensation of impingement on one side of the low back, a woman should see a physical therapist or other professional bodywork specialist.

Sciatic Nerve/Piriformis Muscle Syndrome or Severe Sciatica

For mild sciatica, resting on the side, with the iliofemoral joint slightly flexed, is effective. There are also special exercises in chapter 8 for this problem. In the case of severe sciatica, women should refrain from exercise and consult their care provider.

Carpal Tunnel Syndrome

There can be several causes and solutions to carpal tunnel syndrome. For some women it works well to wear a splint, particularly at night, to immobilize the joint. For others, holding the thumb and little finger together with a slightly flexed and relaxed wrist creates more space for the nerves and circulation in the wrist tunnel. Carpal tunnel syndrome may be partially caused by pressure of increased breast tissue on nerves that go to the hands, so a woman with this problem should try stretching the chest/shoulder area (see special exercises in chapter 8).

Headache

If a woman complains of recurring headaches, she should report them to her care provider. She may simply need to rest in a dark room or eat and drink more often. However, severe headaches can be a sign of hypertension and should receive medical attention.

Hypertension or Anxiety

High blood pressure may be a sign of PIH or toxemia and requires medical attention. A slightly elevated reading and anxious feeling may simply require attention to stress management, including relaxation.

Edema

To help lessen edema, women should drink fluids and use salt to taste, unless otherwise directed by their care provider. If the onset of edema is sudden, or if it appears in the face and hands, they should check immediately with their care provider. Resting on the side and avoiding hot, humid locations are also standard means of averting problems. However, sudden edema is a possible sign of PIH and should be assessed by a health care provider.

Dizziness

If a woman is dizzy or light-headed, she must get off her feet and rest on her side. She may need food or fluids. If dizziness does not immediately abate with rest or fluids, she needs to see her health care provider. Dizziness or "seeing stars" can be other signs of PIH.

Abdominal Cramps

If a woman reports that she is having regular cramps or contraction-like sensations, she should drink at least four 8-ounce glasses of water, void her bladder, and rest on her left side; if the sensations do not subside within 10 minutes, she must contact her care provider.

Leg Cramps

Leg cramps are often caused by blood pooling in the lower legs. To alleviate cramps, women should get off their feet and lie on their side. If leg cramps occur at night, flexing the ankles is effective; ice on the calf muscles before bed can be helpful. Although leg cramps may signal inadequate calcium and potassium or excessive phosphorus, they are most commonly a problem of circulation. It is important for women to make sure that the cool-down of aerobic or cardiovascular activity includes adequate movement that drives blood back from the extremities toward the abdomen.

Varicosities

If varicosities occur in the legs or perineum, women can use support stockings or a prenatal support "girdle." Ice can also relieve discomfort. Resting on the side several times during the day helps maximize blood flow.

Insomnia

At the end of pregnancy, insomnia is not uncommon. Many women are physically uncomfortable and have dreams or obsessive thoughts. Relaxation or stress reduction techniques are helpful. Some women find that chamomile tea or milk products before bed help them sleep. If a woman is experiencing diaphragm pressure, she can sleep propped up with pillows. Stretching the arms overhead and breathing slowly and deeply also helps. If she is distraught, she should be referred to a mental health professional.

MODIFYING EXERCISE PROTOCOLS FOR PREGNANCY

The changes that occur during pregnancy require modification of exercise programs. Alterations due to pregnancy relate to our assessment of exercise intensity; prevention of low blood pressure due to position; avoidance of fatigue; the inclusion of slow, deep breathing in all phases of activity; and biomechanical adjustments—all of which are briefly discussed in the following pages. Also, the nature of pregnancy and birth—a major identity-building experience for women—requires special psychosocial elements in programming. These are covered in chapters 7 and 8, where we discuss goals and priorities and program design.

Assessing Exercise Intensity

Outside of the laboratory, we normally measure heart rate to determine how hard a person is working during vigorous exercise. In pregnancy, because of the changes in the cardiovasculature mentioned earlier, the heart rate is not always a good indicator of how hard someone is working, so we use rate of perceived exertion (RPE), especially in the second and third trimesters. However, it is useful to measure heart rate via a conservative method in the first trimester and postpartum to determine the target heart rate range for cardiovascular conditioning, or aerobic fitness at a moderate intensity, as recommended by ACOG.

Heart Rate Formula

For a healthy woman, the simplest, safest formula for determining the target heart rate uses a percentage of the age-predicted maximal heart rate. In this formula, you subtract the mother's age from 225 to get the maximal heart rate, then multiply by 60% to find the bottom of the range and by 80% to find the top of the range. This will give you a conservative range of heart rates (measured in beats per minute, or bpm) for effective cardiovascular conditioning. Table 5.1 gives some examples of this system.

Rate of Perceived Exertion

The scale most often used to determine how hard a person is working based on her subjective sense is the Borg scale or the rate of perceived exertion (RPE). This and other subjective scales for rating exertion can be found in exercise physiology texts. Some exercisers prefer to use words to express the perceived exertion, and others prefer numbers. *Somewhat hard* to *hard* is a safe, moderate range that is effective for cardiovascular conditioning. If exercisers report they are working at a level of 12 to 16 on a scale from 6 to 20, they are in this range.

In practice, subjective methods of assessing how hard a pregnant woman is working are generally more useful than the heart rate range. Women who are working at an effective intensity will be working at a *somewhat hard* to *hard* level, and should be encouraged to work in this range if they want their exercise routine to help in reducing discomforts, promoting placental proliferation, and improving or maintaining aerobic fitness in preparation for labor. The instructor must be aware, however, that if a woman has had a sleepless night, is still experiencing nausea, or has recently had a procedure such as a sugar test, she may be more comfortable working at a *fairly light* level, around 10 or 11.

Some women prefer to work at the higher subjective level of *very hard*. When the instructor or trainer finds this to be the case, she should insist that the client provide

Table 5.1 Conservative Heart Rate Range for Aerobic Exercise in Pregnancy

	225 bpm	225 bpm
Minus age:	−20	−30
MHR	205	195
MHR × 60% =	123 bpm	117 bpm
MHR × 80% =	164 bpm	156 bpm

For a 20-year-old, the range would be 123 to 164 beats per minute. For a 30-year-old, the range would be 117 to 156 beats per minute. Figuring target heart rates in this way produces a safe, effective range for most average, healthy women. MHR = Maximum heart rate.

her with written instructions from the health care provider stating it is acceptable for this woman to work in the range above 16, or *very hard.*

Preventing Orthostatic Hypotensive Syndromes

Orthostatic hypotensive syndrome refers to very low blood pressure due to body position, which is a concern. Lying in the supine position (on the back) after the first trimester is not advised, according to ACOG, because it can cause this situation. Standing still for long periods of time may also lead to the problem. Therefore, in the second and third trimesters, exercises normally done on the back should be done on the side, seated, or on hands and knees. And the time frame for weight-bearing aerobic sessions should be from 20 minutes to a maximum of 45 minutes.

Avoiding Exercise When Fatigued

During pregnancy, less glucose (blood sugar) is available for exercise. Women should stop when fatigued, rather than push through. Sometimes a small carbohydrate snack and water or juice will provide enough sugar to allow continuing. But attention to adequate protein in the overall diet is important in maintaining energy over the long term.

Including Slow, Deep Breathing During All Phases of Exercise

The hormone progesterone makes the body more sensitive to CO_2, so pregnant women have a tendency to hyperventilate. Women should breathe slowly and deeply and should slow down for a moment, if needed. In later pregnancy, the uterus pushes up on the diaphragm, increasing tidal volume (how much air goes in and out) and possibly decreasing tidal reserve (reserve air); this can also lead to feelings of breathlessness. A woman should use intercostal breathing and breathe into the back lobes of the lungs—by inhaling when she does a side bend and exhaling when she returns to upright.

It is also helpful to use slow, deep breathing during aerobic or cardiovascular conditioning activities. For one thing, this more closely approximates the difficulties a woman encounters in active labor than any other method of breathing to stay focused during labor. It also helps the woman learn to remain calm and relaxed during challenging activity. In addition, inhaling and exhaling during strength and flexibility exercises are important to

preventing undesirable intra-abdominal pressure during pregnancy.

Making Biomechanical Adjustments

Major changes in body alignment during pregnancy are due to two major factors: (1) the shift in the COG forward and slightly up and (2) hormonal changes that soften connective tissue. As a result, a pregnant woman's body has more potential for damage from the effects of gravity than when she is not pregnant.

Using Low-Impact Movements and Modifying Exercises to Prevent Injury

The impact of ground forces varies from person to person, so some pregnant women tolerate running, step aerobics, and so on; but many don't. Kegels and squatting may help prevent pelvic floor trauma. Strong abdominals and pelvic tilts help relieve low back pain and maintain more normal alignment.

Because of the decreased mechanical advantage, muscles must use increased energy to maintain balance against gravity and produce movement. The particulars have been already described (in the section "Physiological Changes in Pregnancy").

To counteract these effects, the strengthening parts of a prenatal program should emphasize the following:

- Strengthening the gluteals, hamstrings, and quadriceps for hip and leg strength
- Strengthening the abdominals and pelvic floor
- Strengthening the upper back

In addition, the following should be emphasized during the stretching parts of the program:

- Stretching the low back and hip flexors
- Stretching the chest
- Lengthening the spine

Increased production of estrogen, progesterone, relaxin, and elastin results in the loosening of connective tissue structures. This has a detrimental effect on stability and alignment of joints and muscles. Crelin [83] demonstrated that during pregnancy the collagen in connective tissue in the symphysis pubis of the rat realigned from a strong criss-cross pattern to a weaker linear pattern, resulting in joint instability. Increasing ligament laxity and softening of connective tissue, such as the symphysis pubis, linea alba, and suture joints in the pelvis, contribute to the potential for injury caused by prolonged overstretching or sudden, forceful abnormal movement.

Connective tissue has both elastic and plastic characteristics. Its elastic quality contributes to its ability to provide flexibility and an extended range of motion at the joint. However, when stretching becomes extreme for a prolonged period of time or when there is a sudden forceful movement beyond a safe range, there is a plastic effect; that is, the connective tissue becomes permanently stretched, resulting in long-term instability.

Ligaments are also pain-producing structures and thus play a part in the increasing discomfort associated with biomechanical problems. The pathogenesis of injury due to the biomechanic difficulties of pregnancy is described in figure 5.8. It is important to note that Vullo et al. [84] found lower-extremity pain more common in pregnant and postpartum women than in nulliparas (women who have not carried a baby to a viable birth stage), with timing of onset frequently in mid to late pregnancy, suggesting that biomechanics rather than hormones is the primary cause of pain.

Importance of Normal Alignment

The importance of normal alignment is in providing a stable base for normal movement. Normal movement permits the safety and efficiency associated with healthy biomechanics. The joint stability, balance, efficiency, and relief from fatigue that result from healthy biomechanics are helpful in preventing damage to the pregnant or postpartum body.

It is important to note that during pregnancy, some degree of change in the alignment of the pelvis and spine is necessary to bring the weights and forces into balance around the central axis, resulting in some level of abnormal movement and potential for injury. The degree to which the change is necessary depends on the individual body and the stage of pregnancy. Special exercises designed to minimize the adverse effects of abnormal alignment and to alleviate symptoms associated with common biomechanical problems are discussed in chapter 8.

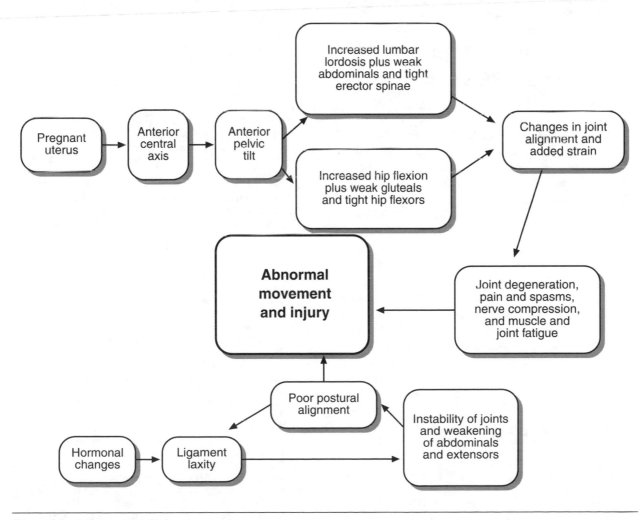

Figure 5.8 Pathogenesis of injury in pregnancy.

Because they are the central structures in the female body, the spine and pelvis are the most critical areas in which to work to achieve near-normal alignment. Proper alignment of the pelvis and spine can be achieved through a combination of postural education, awareness, and correction, along with exercises to strengthen weak muscles and exercises to stretch tight muscles. Imagery and constructive rest—essentially "passive" from an effort standpoint—are among the most effective means of establishing healthy alignment (for an explanation of constructive rest, see chapter 11) [85].

Biomechanical problems associated with the prenatal and postpartum periods represent great challenges to the skills of the health and fitness professional. During pregnancy a woman's body is changing by opening, expanding its function, and growing in an outward direction, while her psyche is often focused on inner dynamics—both the new life stirring inside her and her own evolving identity. In the months following birth, these two processes reverse—her body dynamic shifts inward to closing and healing, while her psychological dynamic moves outward, focusing on the new baby.

REVIEW OF THE PRENATAL FITNESS FIELD

The prenatal fitness field has developed since the 1940s out of the combined concerns of athletic women, birth educators, practitioners of body therapies, and medical researchers spurred by the technological advances that allowed us to see into the womb. Early findings led to the eventual discovery of feto-protective mechanisms at work during exertion in pregnancy. Many of the theoretical concerns about physical activity in pregnancy have not materialized in humans. Consequently, guidelines for prenatal exercise focus on individual tolerances, prior fitness training, and proper medical screening. Fitness professionals working with this population need an understanding of the fundamental anatomical and physiological adaptations of pregnancy and the basic modifications of exercise protocols that are appropriate for pregnant women. A detailed discussion of the interactions of pregnancy and exercise follows in chapter 6.

REFERENCES

1. Cooper, K.A. 1968. *Aerobics*. NY: Evans & Co.
2. Benson, H., Beary, J.F., and Carol, M.P. 1974. The relaxation response. *Psychiatry* 37:37-46.
3. Moison, J., Meyer, F., and Gringras, S. 1991. Leisure physical activity and age at menarche. *Medicine and Science in Sports and Exercise* 23(10):1170-1175.
4. Pivarnik, J.M., Lee, W., and Miller, J.F. 1991. Physiological and perceptual responses to cycle and treadmill exercise during pregnancy. *Medicine and Science in Sports and Exercise* 23 (4): 470-475.
5. Nelson, M.E., Fiatarone, M.A., Morganti, C.M., Trice, I., Greenberg, R.A., and Evans, W.J. 1994. Effects of high-intensity strength training on multiple risk factors for osteoporotic fractures. *Journal of the American Medical Association* 272(24):1909-1914.
6. Blankfield, A. 1967. Is exercise necessary for the obstetrical patient? *Medical Journal of Australia* 1(4):163-165.
7. Bing, E. 1967. *Six practical lessons to an easier childbirth.* NY: Bantam.
8. Bing, E. 1969. *Moving through pregnancy.* NY: Bantam.
9. Noble, E. 1995. (1st ed. 1976) *Essential exercises for the child-bearing year,* 4th ed. Harwich, MA: New Life Images.
10. Difler, C. 1977. *Your baby your body—physical fitness in pregnancy.* NY: Crown.
11. Olkin, S.K. 1987. *Positive pregnancy fitness.* Garden City Park, NY: Avery.
12. Cowlin, A.F. 1981, 1992, 1996. *Dancing Thru Pregnancy instructor's guide.* Branford, CT: DTP, Inc.
13. Holstein, B.B. 1988. *Shaping up for a healthy pregnancy.* Champaign, IL: Life Enhancement Publications.
14. Dick-Read, G. 1933. *Natural childbirth.* NY: Harper & Row.
15. Dick-Read, G. 1944. *Childbirth without fear.* NY: Harper & Row.
16. Lamaze, F. 1972. *Painless childbirth.* NY: Pocket Books.
17. Bradley, R.A. 1970. *Husband-coached childbirth,* rev. ed. NY: Harper & Row.
18. Kitzinger, S. 1989. *The complete book of pregnancy and childbirth.* NY: Alfred A. Knopf.
19. Simkin, P. 1995. *Comfort measures for childbirth with Penny Simkin, P.T.* Video Tape. Seattle: Penny Simkin, Inc. 1100 23rd Ave., E., Seattle, WA 98112.
20. McLennan, C.E. 1943. Antecubital and femoral venous pressure in normal and toxemic pregnancy. *American Journal of Obstetrics and Gynecology* 45:568-591.
21. Widlund, G. 1945. The cardiopulmonal function during pregnancy. *Acta Obstetricia et Gynecologica Scandinavica* 25 (Suppl 1), ch. VI:72-96.
22. Veal, J.R., and Hussey, H.H. 1947. The venous circulation in the lower extremities during pregnancy. *Surgery, Gynecology & Obstetrics* 72:841-847.
23. Wright, H.P., and Osborn, S.B. 1950. Changes in the rate of flow of venous blood in the leg during pregnancy, measured with radioactive sodium. *Surgery, Gynecology & Obstetrics* 90:481-485.
24. Lyons, H.A., and Antonio, R. 1959. The sensitivity of the respiratory center in pregnancy and after the administration of progesterone. *Transactions of the Association of American Physicians* 72:173-180.
25. Dahlstrom, H., and Ihrman, K. 1960. A clinical and physiological study of pregnancy in a material from northern Sweden, V. The results of work tests during and after pregnancy. *Acta Societatis Medicorum Upsaliensis* 65:305.
26. Ihrman, K. 1960. A clinical and physiological study of pregnancy in a material from northern Sweden, VIII. The effect of physical training during pregnancy on the circulatory adjustment. *Acta Societatis Medicorum Upsaliensis* 65:335-347.
27. Sovia, K., et al. 1964. Physical working capacity during pregnancy and effect of physical work tests on fetal heart rate. *Annales Chirurgiae et Gynaecologiae Fenniae* 53:187-196.
28. Ueland, K., Novy, J.M., and Metcalfe, J. 1969. Maternal cardiovascular dynamics, IV. The influence of gestational age on the maternal cardiovascular response to posture and exercise. *American Journal of Obstetrics and Gynecology* 104(6):856-864.
29. Hytten, F.E., and Leitch, I. 1971. *The physiology of human pregnancy.* Oxford: Blackwell Scientific.

30. Guzman, C.A., and Caplan R. 1970. Cardiorespiratory response to exercise during pregnancy. *American Journal of Obstetrics and Gynecology* 108(4):600-605.

31. Ueland, K., Novy, J.M., and Metcalfe, J. 1973. Cardiorespiratory responses to pregnancy and exercise in normal women and patients with heart disease. *American Journal of Obstetrics and Gynecology* 115(1):4-10.

32. Knuttgen, H.G., and Emerson, K. 1974. Physiological response to pregnancy at rest and during exercise. *Journal of Applied Physiology* 35(5):549-553.

33. Pomerance, J.J., Gluck, L., and Lynch, V.A. 1974. Physical fitness in pregnancy: Its effect on pregnancy outcome. *American Journal of Obstetrics and Gynecology* 119(7):867-875.

34. Sandstrom, B. 1974. Adjustments of the circulation to orthostatic reaction and physical exercise during the first trimester of primipregnancy. *Acta Obstetricia et Gynecologica Scandinavica* 53:105.

35. Erkkola, R. 1975. The physical fitness of the Finnish primigravidae. *Annales Chirurgiae et Gynaecologiae* 64:394-400.

36. Pernoll, M.L., Metcalfe, J., Schlenker, T.L., Welch, J.E., and Matsumoto, J.A. 1975. Oxygen consumption at rest and during exercise in pregnancy and postpartum. *Respiration Physiology* 25:285-293.

37. Pernoll, M.L., Metcalfe, J., Kovach, P.A., Wachtel, R., and Dunham, M.J. 1975. Ventilation during rest and exercise in pregnancy and postpartum. *Respiration Physiology* 25:295-310.

38. Seitchcck, K. 1976. Body composition and energy expenditure during rest and work in pregnancy. *American Journal of Obstetrics and Gynecology* 97(5):701-713.

39. Edwards, M.J., Metcalfe, J., Dunham, M.J., and Paul, M.S. 1981. Accelerated respiratory response to moderate exercise in late pregnancy. *Respiration Physiology* 45:229-241.

40. Artal, R., Platt, L.D., Sperling, M., Kammula R.K., Jilek, J., and Nakamura, R. 1981. Maternal cardiovascular and metabolic responses in normal pregnancy. *American Journal of Obstetrics and Gynecology* 140(2):123-127.

41. Clapp, J.F. 3rd, and Dickstein, S. 1984. Endurance exercise and pregnancy outcome. *Medicine and Science in Sports and Exercise* 16(6):556-562.

42. Morris, N., Osborn, S.B., Wright, H.P., and Hart, A. 1956. Effective uterine blood flow during exercise in normal and pre-ecplamptic pregnancies. *Lancet* ii:481-484.

43. Emmanouilides, G.C., Hobel, C.J., Yashiro, K., and Klyman, G. 1972. Fetal responses to maternal exercise in sheep. *American Journal of Obstetrics and Gynecology* 112(1):130-137.

44. Orr, J., Ungerer, T., Will, J., Wernicke, K., and Curet, L.B. 1972. Effect of exercise stress on carotid, uterine, and iliac blood flow in pregnant and nonpregnant ewes. *American Journal of Obstetrics and Gynecology* 114(2):213-217.

45. Curet, L.B., Orr, J.A., Rankin, H.G., and Ungerer, T. 1976. Effect of exercise on cardiac output and distribution of uterine blood flow in pregnant ewes. *Journal of Applied Physiology* 40(5):725-728.

46. Clapp, J.F. 3rd. 1978.1. Cardiac output and uterine blood flow in the pregnant ewe. *American Journal of Obstetrics and Gynecology* 130(4):419-423.

47. Clapp, J.F. 3rd. 1978.2. The relationship between blood flow and oxygen uptake in the uterine and umbilical circulations. *American Journal of Obstetrics and Gynecology* 132(4):410-413.

48. Clapp, J.F. 3rd. 1980. Acute exercise stress in the pregnant ewe. *American Journal of Obstetrics and Gynecology* 136(4):489-494.

49. Clapp, J.F. 3rd, Szeto, H.H., Larrow, R., Hewitt, J., and Mann, L.I. 1980. Umbilical blood flow response to embolization of the uterine circulation. *American Journal of Obstetrics and Gynecology* 138(1):60-67.

50. Chandler, K.D., and Bell, A.W. 1981. Effects of maternal exercise on fetal and maternal respiration and nutrient metabolism in the pregnant ewe. *Journal of Developmental Physiology* 3(3):161-176.

51. Clapp, J.F. 3rd, McLaughlin, M.K., Larrow, R., Farnham and Mann, L.I. 1982. The uterine hemodynamic response to repetitive unilateral vascular embolization in the pregnant ewe. *American Journal of Obstetrics and Gynecology* 144(3):309-318.

52. Naeye, R.L., and Peters, E.C. 1982. Working during pregnancy: Effects on the fetus. *Pediatrics* 69(6):724-727.

53. Lotgering, F.K., Gilbert, R.D., and Longo, L.D. 1983. Exercise responses in pregnant sheep: Oxygen consumption, uterine blood flow, and blood volume. *Journal of Applied Physiology: Respiration in Environmental Exercise Physiology* 55(3):834-841.

54. Smith, A.D., Gilbert, R.D., Lammers, R.J., and Longo, L.D. 1983. Placental exchange area in guinea pigs following long-term maternal exercise: A stereological analysis. *Journal of Developmental Physiology* 5(1):11-21.

55. Hohimer, A.R., Bissonnette, J.M., Metcalfe, J., and McKean, T.A. 1984. Effect of exercise on uterine blood flow in the pregnant Pygmy goat. *American Journal of Physiology* 246(2 pt 2):H207-H212.

56. Soiva, K., Salmi, A., Gronroos, M., and Peltonen, J. 1964. Physical working capacity during pregnancy and effect of physical work tests on foetal heart rate. *Annales Chirurgiae et Gynaecologiae* 53:187.

57. Pomerance, J.H., Gluck, L., and Lynch, V.A. 1974. Physical fitness in pregnancy: Its effect on pregnancy outcome. *American Journal of Obstetrics and Gynecology* 119:867-875.

58. Terada, M. 1974. Effect of physical activity before pregnancy on fetus of mice exercised forcibly during pregnancy. *Teratology* 10:141-144.

59. Erkkola, R., and Makela, M. 1976. Heart volumes and physical fitness of parturients. *Annals of Clinical Research* 8:15-21.

60. Dhindsa, D.S., Metcalfe, J., and Hummels, D.H. 1978. Responses to exercise in the pregnant pygmy goat. *Respiration Physiology* 32:299-311.

61. Longo, L., Hewitt, C.W., Lorijn, R.H.W., and Gilbert, R.D. 1978. To what extent does maternal exercise affect fetal oxygenation and uterine blood flow. *Science Abstracts, 25th Annual Meeting of the Society for Gynecologic Investigation*, Atlanta, GA, p. 7.

62. Clapp, J.F. 3rd, Szeto, H.H., Larrow, R., Hewitt, J., and Mann, L.I. 1981. Fetal metabolic response to experimental placental vascular damage. *American Journal of Obstetrics and Gynecology* 140(4):446-451.

63. Nelson, P.S., Gilbert, R.D., and Longo, L.D. 1983. Fetal growth and placental diffusing capacity in guinea pigs following long-term maternal exercise. *Journal of Developmental Physiology* 5(1):1-10.

64. Clapp, J.F. 3rd, and Dickstein, S. 1984. Endurance exercise and pregnancy outcome. *Medicine and Science in Sports and Exercise* 16(6):556-562.

65. Hon, E.W., and Hohlgemuth, R. 1961. The electronic evaluation of fetal heart rate: The effect of maternal exercise. *American Journal of Obstetrics and Gynecology* 81(2):361-371.

66. Soiva, K., Salmi, A., Gronroos, M., and Peltonen, J. 1964. Physical working capacity during pregnancy and effects of physical work tests on fetal heart rate. *Annales Chirurgiae et Gynaecologiae* 53:187-196.

67. Pokorney, J., and Rous, J. 1967. Effects of mother's work on foetal heart sounds. In J. Horskey (ed.), *Intrauterine dangers to the fetus*, NY: Excerpta Medica Foundation, p. 354.

68. Stembera, A.K., and Hodra, J. 1967. The "exercise test" as an early diagnostic aid for fetal distress. In J. Horsky (ed.), *Intrauterine dangers to the fetus*, NY: Excerpta Medica Foundation, p. 349.

69. Pomerance, J.J., Gluck, J., and Lynch, V.A. 1974. Physical fitness in pregnancy: Its effect on pregnancy outcome. *American Journal of Obstetrics and Gynecology* 119(7):867-875.

70. Dressendorfer, R.H., and Goodlin, R.C. 1980. Fetal heart rate response to maternal exercise testing. *The Physician and Sportsmedicine* 8:90.

71. Hauth, J.C., Gilstrap, L.C. 3rd., and Widmer, K. 1982. Fetal heart rate reactivity before and after maternal jogging during the third trimester. *American Journal of Obstetrics and Gynecology* 142(5):545-547.

72. Collins, C.A., Curet, L.B., and Mullin, J.P. 1983. Maternal and fetal responses to a maternal aerobic exercise program. *American Journal of Obstetrics and Gynecology* 145(6):702-707.

73. Artal, R., Romem, Y., Paul R.H., and Wiswell, R. 1984. Fetal brady-cardia induced by maternal exercise. *Lancet* 2(8397):258-260.

74. Matsumoto, J., Kaji, T., Takahashi, R., and Kikuchi, S. 1984. The effect of maternal exercise on the fetal heart rate. *Acta Obstetrica et Gynaecologia Japonica* 36(7):1057-1063.

75. American College of Obstetricians and Gynecologists. 1985. *ACOG home exercise programs: Exercise during pregnancy and the postnatal period.* Technical bulletin issued May 1985.

76. American College of Obstetricians and Gynecologists. 1994. *Exercise during pregnancy and the postnatal period.* Technical Bulletin no. 189, issue February 1994.

77. Melpomene Institute for Women's Health Research. 1987. *Selecting a prenatal exercise program.* Produced by K. Lohr of Melpomene Institute and T. Booth of Family Tree. Minneapolis, MN.

78. Reis, F.M., Fadalti, M., Florio, P., and Petraglia, F. 1999. Putative role of placental corticotropin-releasing factor in the mechanisms of human parturition [Review]. *Journal of the Society of Gynecologic Investigations* 6(3):109-119.

79. Hoffman, G.E., McDonald, T., Shedwick, R., and Nathanielsz, P.W. 1991. Activation of cFos in ovine fetal corticotropin-releasing hormone neurons at the time of parturition. *Endocrinology* 129(6):3227-3233.

80. Myers, D.A., Myers, T.R., Grober, M.S., and Nathanielsz, P.W. 1993. Levels of corticotropin-releasing hormone messenger ribonucleic acid (mRNA) in the hypothalamic paraventricular nucleus and proopiomelanocortin mRNA in the anterior pituitary during late gestation in fetal sheep. *Endocrinology* 132(5):2109-2116.

81. Swaab, D.F. 1995. Development of the human hypothalamus [Review]. *Neurochemical Research* 20(5):509-519.

82. Brewer, G.S., and Brewer, T.H. 1983. *The Brewer Medical Diet for normal and high-risk pregnancy.* NY: Simon and Schuster.

83. Crelin, E.S. 1969. The development of the bony pelvis and its changes during pregnancy and parturition. *Transactions of the New York Academy of Sciences* 31:1049.

84. Vullo, U.J., Richardson, J.K., and Hurvitz, E.A. 1996. Hip, knee and foot pain during pregnancy and the postpartum period. *Journal of Family Practice* 43(1):63-68.

85. Sweigard, L. 1974. *Human movement potential.* NY: Harper & Row.

CHAPTER 6

INTERACTIONS OF PREGNANCY AND EXERCISE

This chapter provides an in-depth examination of the research concerning the areas in which pregnancy and exercise act on each other. It is in the best interest of those designing and teaching health and fitness programs to have a clear and formidable understanding of maternal and fetal responses to exercise and the effects of pregnancy on the physiological measures used to assess exercise.

Reporting in the *Annals of Epidemiology* in 1996, Zhang and Savitz noted that of 9953 women who gave birth in 1988 and participated in a National Maternal and Infant Health (NMIH) Survey cross-sectional study, 42% reported exercising during pregnancy [1]. By extrapolation, this means that approximately 1.6 million women who delivered in 1988 exercised in some manner during their pregnancies (there were approximately 4 million live births each year in the United States in the late 1980s and early 1990s). In the NMIH Survey, walking was the most frequently reported activity (43% of those who exercised), with swimming (12%) and aerobics (12%) following in frequency. It was also reported by McGinnis in 1992 that approximately 38% of women of childbearing age regularly engaged in recreational physical activity [2]. Of women who exercise, Carpenter and Sady in 1988 and Clapp and Dickstein in 1984 reported that about half of those women who regularly engaged in moderate- to high-intensity, sustained cardiovascular activities planned to continue to do so through their pregnancies [3, 4].

There are significant numbers of pregnant women who are involved in physical activity, and we can expect to see these numbers grow. Statistics kept at the **www.cdc.gov/ nchs** Web site indicate the birthrate in the United States began to rise in 2000; health and fitness organizations are lobbying the public to increase activity. Health care providers are aware that exercise continued in pregnancy is safe for the fetus, is effective in alleviating maternal discomforts, and provides a good preparation for birth. As the next wave of research explores the impact of starting exercise within pregnancy, our ability to design activities will become increasingly refined. While there are still few studies that refer to this latter matter, in practice we know that with sensible precautions, women who begin exercise early enough in pregnancy and continue with regularity up to delivery also reap benefits.

Examining areas in which pregnancy and exercise interact makes it possible to gain the information necessary to make intelligent decisions on a case-by-case basis. The principal interactions of pregnancy and exercise occur in these areas: cardiovasculature and hemodynamics, thermoregulation, metabolism, respiration and acid-base balance, biomechanics, psychophysiological interactions, fetal responses, and pregnancy outcomes.

CARDIOVASCULATURE AND HEMODYNAMICS

The effect on cardiovasculature and hemodynamics of continuing aerobic exercise into and through a healthy pregnancy is enhancement of the oxygen and nutrient delivery system for both mother and fetus. Physically active women have significantly greater blood volumes than their inactive counterparts, with the normal accompaniment of increased vasculature, heart strength, cardiac output, and aerobic training effects. These factors, along with favorable changes in blood pressure, increased hemoglobin concentration, and increased placental function, augment the delivery system in a healthy, active woman. In addition, it appears that initiation of a moderate exercise regimen in early pregnancy also produces favorable adjustments.

Placenta

Two studies have demonstrated that placental volume and function are enhanced by aerobic exercise during the first and second trimesters. One study showed that regular recreational exercise performed by healthy women at or above baseline conditioning levels increases the rate of growth in placental volume in the second trimester of human pregnancy [5]. The other investigation demonstrated increases in the histomorphic parameters (including volume and proliferation of chorionic villi) associated with placental perfusion and transfer function, occurring mostly in early and mid pregnancy [6]. Speculation regarding underlying mechanisms centers on (1) stimulation due to the intermittent reduction in uterine blood flow during sustained activity at a training intensity and (2) increased blood volume and tissue vascularity associated with sustained exercise over a prolonged period of time.

In another study, Clapp et al. demonstrated that healthy, low-risk women without previous regular exercise histories who commenced moderate physical activity programs (three to five days per week) at eight weeks of pregnancy, and who continued exercising through the remainder of pregnancy, produced infants who were significantly longer and heavier and who had significant differences in body composition compared to infants of women who continued not to exercise [7]. The researchers note that the underlying mechanism is the significant increase in placental volume that is associated with exercise in pregnancy, most notably in the mid (second) trimester.

The uteroplacental unit is the cardiovascular organ that provides the interface between maternal and fetal circulations (see chapter 5). Placental development starts with the embryonic invasion of the maternal endometrium and the decidual reaction of the endometrium (uterine lining). Endometrial stromal cells enlarge with accumulated glycogen and lipids; the endometrial capillaries become dilated and congested and form sinusoids, which erode, allowing maternal blood to be accessed through membranes by the developing embryo's chorionic villi. This establishes a primitive circulation and creates a demand for increased blood volume. Around the eighth week, further circulatory developments occur, resulting in the fully developed placenta. Sustaining this unit requires a sufficient blood volume, approximately 40% above that in the nonpregnant state.

Should there be a uteroplacental insufficiency, a situation in which circulatory interface is not adequate to sustain appropriate fetal growth, exertion causes a strain on the delivery of oxygen and nutrients. No amount of cardiovascular conditioning on the mother's part will alleviate this situation. It can be caused by a number of conditions, such as undernutrition in the first trimester, smoking, drugs, genetic factors, or a variety of other factors including unidentifiable pathologies. In this case, usually a diagnosis of *intrauterine growth restriction* (IUGR) or *small for gestational age* (SGA) will be made by 20 weeks, and most exercise regimens will be declared inappropriate. There is no evidence in the literature that the fetuses of exercising women who receive such a diagnosis and cease exercise have worse outcomes than those of women who have not been active prior to receiving such a diagnosis. In practice it is advisable to inquire regularly of women participating in prenatal programs about the *fundal growth*—or external measurement of the uterus (from pubic bone to the *fundus,* or top of the uterus) taken by their care providers—to ensure that it is appropriate for them to continue an activity regimen that places demands on the cardiovascular system.

Shifts in Cardiovascular and Hemodynamic Measures

The increased blood volume associated with pregnancy is accompanied by increases in cardiac output and stroke volume, shown in the early studies cited in chapter 5. But the proportion of increase is not equal to the increase in blood volume, which results in an increase in resting pulse, a phenomenon that is well established in the literature in both cross-sectional and longitudinal studies [8-14]. It appears that maximal heart rates, when comparisons are made between pregnant women and nonpregnant controls, show no significant alterations due to pregnancy [15, 16]. When maximal heart rates are compared between pregnancy and the postpartum period, they are also not found to be influenced by pregnancy [11, 17, 18]. However, the effect of pregnancy on maternal heart rate is not established at submaximal effort levels. When heart rates of exercising pregnant women are compared to nonpregnant controls this yields an effect that is at odds with the results of comparing pregnant women to themselves postpartum [15].

Resting oxygen consumption in pregnancy is elevated, indicating the increased metabolic cost of pregnancy and the influence of progesterone [9, 10, 15, 18, 20]. Findings regarding oxygen consumption during submaximal exercise vary. Some studies have shown no difference when comparing pregnancy and postpartum values [21, 22]. Others studies show elevated levels during pregnancy compared with levels postpartum [18, 23, 24]. One study looked at oxygen consumption relative to body mass and found no difference between pregnant women and controls at rest; lower levels in pregnant women than in nonpregnant controls during exercise (probably due to the disproportional increases in tissue type in pregnancy, including fluid, placenta, and fetus); and no difference between pregnant and postpartum women, even with postpartum weight loss [15].

Elevations in cardiac output during rest are seen in pregnant women compared to both nonpregnant and postpartum controls [8, 13-15, 17, 22-26]. Significant and insignificant elevations of cardiac output during submaximal exercise are well supported in the literature [12, 14, 15, 17, 18, 21-24].

Findings on stroke volume in pregnant women are variable. Resting values were increased in one study when pregnant and nonpregnant subjects were compared [27] and in other studies when pregnant and postpartum women were compared [13-14, 18], but other researchers found no change in resting stroke volume in pregnancy versus the postpartum period [13, 24]. Findings are also mixed regarding whether or not exercise increases stroke volume in pregnancy, some studies finding no differences [21, 23] and others finding elevations in pregnancy [13, 14, 18]. Two studies have shown elevated stroke volume in postpartum subjects [12, 15].

Swimming and water aerobics are special cases. Immersion in water causes a redistribution of extravascular fluid into the vascular space [28-31]. Fluid enters the venous system, increasing the central blood volume [32], initiating an increase in cardiac output and stroke volume and consequently lowering the heart rate. With level of exertion controlled for, maternal heart rates have been shown to be significantly lower during running in water than during running on land [33], as would be predicted under these conditions. Maternal heart rates also tend to be lower following water exercise than following land exercise [34].

It is also the case that pregnancy enhances many of the delivery systems of cardiovascular conditioning, including its expansion of blood volume, the reduction of the risk of heart disease through estrogen's effect on lipids in the circulatory system, and the effect of progesterone and relaxin on the vasculature to lower blood pressure. In the nonpregnant population, the heart, arteries, and veins must be healthy—sturdy but flexible and open to permit the flow of blood—to deliver the needed additional supplies of nutrients during exercise. Among the well-known training effects of regular sustained aerobic exercise is the lowering of levels of low-density lipoproteins and very low-density lipoproteins (implicated in the development of arterial plaque), helping to maintain a clear pathway for blood. The vasculature becomes more elastic through exercise, also ensuring lowered resistance to the increased volume and rate of blood flow. The combined effect of these changes is to aid delivery of oxygen and nutrients to the major large muscle groups and to muscles of the extremities, which are called on to produce large bodily movements and manipulations of the environment. In response to the muscles' demand for nutrients, the cardiovasculature can respond rapidly in a fit individual.

In pregnancy, the hormone *relaxin* acts to relax vascular walls, which in a normal pregnancy results in a lowering of blood pressure. The advantages of this include lowered resistance for delivery of energy to competing systems (maternal and fetal), the affinity of maternal endometrial capillary arteries for small-scale hemorrhage to provide a platform for the *decidua basalis* or maternal placenta, and ease of vasodilation to improve cooling. These mechanisms are feto-protective. In exercising women, the combination of the effects of pregnancy and exercise may also lead to cautions concerning orthostatic hypotensive syndromes.

Hypotensive Syndromes

As a result of the relaxation of vasculature in pregnancy, detrimental orthostatic hypotensive syndromes can occur. During standing still in the third trimester, for example, maternal cardiac output is reduced by approximately 18% from that in a side-lying position [35]. Clearly, standing still for long periods of time is particularly dangerous.

While exercising in an upright weight-bearing alignment, the pregnant woman may find blood pooling in her fingers or lower legs after 15 to 20 minutes of sustained aerobic work, particularly in humid weather. It is very important to use a cool-down that includes repeated contractions of proximal muscles—that is, deep muscles close to the core of the body, such as those controlling movement and position in the iliofemoral joint, spine, abdomen, thorax, and shoulder girdle—in order to drive the blood back toward the heart and gut.

Similarly, but less dramatically, in the static supine position with legs extended (see figure 6.1 and sidebar, p. 102), cardiac output is reduced by approximately 9% in the second and third trimesters [35]. This latter effect has stirred the controversy about the advisability of strength exercises in the supine position (see the sidebar

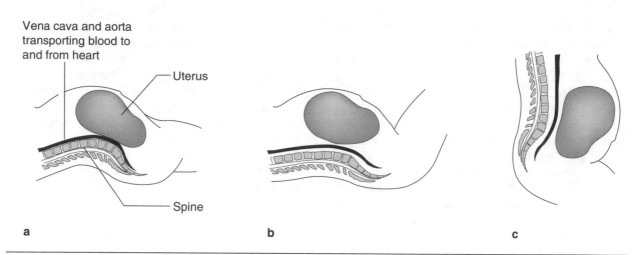

Figure 6.1 Supine position, right lateral views, (a) legs extended position, and (b) constructive rest position; (c) side-lying position, from above.

Supine Position During Pregnancy

Is it safe to do curl-ups in the supine position during the second and third trimesters?

In both 1985 and 1994, the American College of Obstetricians and Gynecologists (ACOG) in its bulletins regarding exercise and pregnancy issued warnings against lying in the supine position because of the risk of hypotensive syndrome (the weight of the uterus on the vena cava can cause blood pressure to drop). This idea has stirred controversy. Research has shown that a few minutes of supine exercise has no effect on fetal response, and there have been no reports linking supine exercise to adverse outcomes. The constructive rest position (supine, with knees bent and feet flat on the floor) has clear biomechanical advantages for learning correct abdominal patterning. In practice, women who are affected by hypotensive syndrome are often self-reporting—approximately one woman in 30 will be uncomfortable and unwilling to exercise on her back, even for a few minutes. In general, women can avoid the supine position by doing abdominal exercises on the hands and knees or on the side or by doing curl-downs. Occasionally, however, it is necessary to use the supine position for a minute or two to assess diastasis recti or to teach abdominal breathing.

Implications of Hypotensive Syndromes for Exercise Prescription

Hypotensive syndromes due to the relaxation of vasculature have a number of implications for exercise in pregnancy:

1. Women should limit supine exercise to 2 or 3 minutes and should perform supine exercise prior to aerobic exercise or cardiovascular conditioning activities. They should avoid the supine position in late pregnancy. There are many creative alternatives to exercises ordinarily done in the supine position, and these should be employed after the first trimester.

2. Less fit women should limit aerobic exercise duration on the feet at any one time to 20 to 30 minutes; more fit women should limit duration to 30 to 45 minutes.

3. Women exercising should avoid sudden changes of position or level.

4. They should include a thorough cool-down to prevent pooling of blood in the extremities.

5. During the second and third trimesters they should rest daily in the side-lying position to maximize blood flow.

above). Nesler's study demonstrated that 3 to 5 minutes of exercise in supine had no adverse effects [36]. It is important to note that no detriment to the fetus has been reported in the literature despite theoretical considerations. During supine exercise, the woman is moving and generally remains on her back (strictly speaking) for only

a few minutes at any one time. Pregnant women have sharp protective instincts concerning movements with which they are not comfortable or of which they are fearful. There is no record of women passing out; and in practice, approximately one woman in 30 declines to perform exercises in this position [37]. Placement of the uterus in relationship to the vena cava, the size and weight of the uterus, and the proportions of the woman also contribute to this situation.

In a study of handgrip and single- and double-leg extension strength exercises in both a supine (30° tilt) and a seated position, Avery et al. found that blood pressure responses of a small cohort of pregnant women in late gestation were similar to those of nonpregnant controls under all experimental conditions [38]. The researchers found moderate fetal bradycardia occasionally in the tilted position, suggesting that this position should be avoided in late pregnancy [38].

Hypertension, Pregnancy-Induced Hypertension, Preeclampsia, and Toxemia

Hypertensive disorders, the most common medical complication in pregnancy, have long been a contraindication for exercise. One prospective study recently looked at the effect of exercise on blood pressure in pregnant women with risk factors for hypertension in pregnancy, ranging from mild hypertension to gestational hypertensive disorders or a family history of hypertension. Women were recruited at 14 weeks gestation, observed for 4 weeks, and randomized into exercise and control groups. Following 10 weeks (18-28 weeks gestation) of exercise at a rate of perceived exertion level of 13 (mean MET [metabolic equivalent] level 4.7 with a standard deviation of 0.8) for 30 minutes three times per week, a strong trend toward lowered diastolic blood pressure was detected among the women at risk of hypertensive disorders who were in the exercise group [39].

Women with chronic hypertension prior to pregnancy, or blood pressure at least 140/90 before 20 weeks gestation, are at increased risk of *preeclampsia,* a serious hypertensive disorder of pregnancy. *Pregnancy-induced hypertension* (PIH) is defined as elevated blood pressure after 20 weeks of gestation in women who did not have elevated blood pressure prior to pregnancy. In some women this may be an early sign of preeclampsia, while others may need monitoring and attention to diet, exercise, and—most importantly—stress reduction.

The development of proteinuria (protein spilling into the urine), in addition to hypertension, is a sign of preeclampsia, and generally occurs after 20 weeks as well. However, changes in the vascular system may occur by week 14; among these are increased peripheral vascular resistance, reduced cardiac output, reduced plasma volume, and decreased glomerular filtration rate including retention of salt and water [40]. Risk factors associated with preeclampsia are listed below on the left.

These complications lead to reduced perfusion of the placenta and maternal kidneys, liver, and brain. The fetus can suffer IUGR and even hypoxia. Altered fatty acid composition, in addition to vasospasm and other vascular symptoms, probably explains the hyperlipidemia,

---

Risk Factors Associated With Preeclampsia

Chronic hypertensive disease

Chronic renal disease

Deficient prenatal care

Diabetes

Emotional stress

Family tendency

Lack of education

Lower socioeconomic status

Maternal age under 20 or over 35

Multiple pregnancy

Nulliparity

Poor nutrition

Previous history of preeclampsia

Trophoblastic disease

Kline, D.A. 1997. *Nutrition for women, Part I: Sexual and reproductive health.* Eureka, CA: Nutrition Dimension; Varney, H. 1996. *Varney's midwifery,* 3rd ed. Boston: Jones & Bartlett.

Complications of Preeclampsia

Fetal Complications

Growth restriction

Hypoxia

Prematurity

Death

Maternal Complications

Pulmonary edema

Placental abruption

Renal failure

Liver failure

Convulsions

Cerebral hemorrhage

Death

Kline, D.A. 1997. *Nutrition for women, Part I: Sexual and reproductive health.* Eureka, CA: Nutrition Dimension; Varney, H. 1996. *Varney's midwifery,* 3rd ed. Boston: Jones & Bartlett.

antioxidant deficiency, coagulation difficulties, and ischemia or infarctions of the uterus and placenta that occur in preeclampsia [41, 42]. At the end stage of this disorder, *eclampsia* or *toxemia,* the mother can suffer convulsions, organ failure, and death. This condition is the third leading cause of maternal mortality [40]. Complications of this disorder are shown in the sidebar on the bottom right of page 103.

The roles of calcium and magnesium in preeclampsia have been hotly debated. While a number of researchers believe that calcium is effective in preventing hypertension in pregnancy [43-47], others have shown that calcium supplementation does not change the incidence of preeclampsia [48, 49]. Calcium may be effective in reducing blood pressure; but it seems clear that, in and of itself, calcium will not prevent preeclampsia. Nonetheless, low levels of both calcium and magnesium are associated with preeclampsia.

The role of magnesium appears to be associated with its function as an activator of enzymes that are involved in membrane transport and integrity, as well as with its relationship to prostaglandins. Specifically, it is the ratio of prostacyclins (vasodilators) to thromboxanes (some of which are vasoconstrictors) that is dramatically altered in the case of low serum magnesium. Both prostacyclin and thromboxane substances are increased during a normal pregnancy. However, women who develop preeclampsia have much smaller increases in prostacyclin production than other women while thromboxane continues to rise at the same rate, thus increasing vasoconstriction and raising blood pressure.

The precursors of prostaglandins are fatty acids. Thromboxane 2 (a vasoconstricting prostaglandin) derives from omega-6 fatty acids, much more plentiful in many diets than omega-3 fatty acids, from which thromboxane 3 (a vasodilating prostaglandin) is derived. Altering the omega-3 fatty acid content of cells through dietary changes may reduce the risk of preeclampsia. Williams et al. found that women with the lowest levels of omega-3 fatty acids were 7.6 times more likely to have preeclampsia than those with the highest level [42].

Pregnancy-induced hypertension and preeclampsia remain somewhat elusive. Although factors other than nutrition underlie these phenomena, nutrition is a factor in the severity of such disorders. There are associations of malnutrition, lower socioeconomic status, and lack of education with increased risk of preeclampsia, as well as an association of stress and malnutrition with increased risk. Following a nutritional plan that includes adequate protein, particularly early in pregnancy, is one guideline usually given to women as a means of reducing the risk of developing severe hypertension. Especially women with a personal history or family history of hypertensive disorders need to take care to eat a healthy diet. The impact of moderate exercise on hypertensive disorders of pregnancy is an area of great interest, but one in which there is little research to date.

Uteroplacental Blood Flow

As noted in chapter 5, during the 1970s and early 1980s one of the major issues contributing to an extremely conservative attitude regarding exercise in pregnancy was the question of diversion of maternal blood flow away from the uterus to the skeletal muscles during moderate and vigorous activity. Animal research, conducted primarily on sheep, gave rise to the question of how much the blood flow could be diverted in humans before any detriment occurred, when in animals the answer seemed to be about 50% [50, 51]. Current speculation is that in moderate recreational exercise, the diversion is approximately 50% and that in competition it can be 70% to 80%.

Since the mid-1980s, researchers have continued to evaluate the effects of exercise on uterine blood flow in human subjects. Using Doppler echocardiogram technology, investigators have looked at both the systolic-to-diastolic (S/D) ratio and the pulsatility index (PI) of the uterine arteries during bicycle and aerobic dance exercise, with mixed results [52-56]. Three studies showed that the S/D ratio increased significantly with maternal exercise [53, 55, 56], while two studies did not [52, 54]. Those studies looking at PI also had varying results. Findings regarding umbilical arteries were in greater agreement, with no significant changes in the S/D ratio noted in all five studies, plus one by Veille et al. [57]. On the basis of current studies, Veille concludes that umbilical artery PI does not change because of maternal exercise in any time period studied, but does decrease with advancing gestational age [58]. There continues to be no documentation of detrimental fetal outcomes, on the basis of diversion of uterine blood flow, in healthy women who participate in regular moderate- to high-intensity exercise.

The probable primary reason for this lack of detrimental fetal outcome is the feto-protective, more-than-additive combination of increased blood plasma due to aerobic training effect and pregnancy [59-61]. This overexpansion reduces the fall in visceral blood flow and helps maintain fetal substrate delivery during exercise. The increased hematocrit associated with exercise, as well as compensatory mechanisms of the placenta in well-conditioned, highly fit women [5, 6], also helps account for the ability of the cardiovascular system to deliver needed nutrients. The authors of one study report fetal cerebral vasodilation induced by submaximal exercise [62], which they speculate could be a consequence of moderate fetal hemoglobin desaturation. This might indicate a physiologic mechanism that protects the fetal brain. They also report no significant alteration in uterine perfusion.

In a recent study, Clapp et al. tested the hypothesis that pregnancy increases portal vein blood flow and that regular exercise during pregnancy limits the shunting of blood flow away from the uterus in response to gravity (i.e., standing) or exercise-induced hemodynamic stress. The researchers concluded that portal vein flow increases significantly during pregnancy and that exercise training in mid and late pregnancy reduced the shunting of blood flow away from the uterus during exercise as well as improving recovery at 5 minutes postexercise [63].

Exercise Intensity

Determining aerobic exercise intensity in pregnancy is complicated by shifts in the customary measures used to figure both functional capacity and heart rate. Among a range of reports on maternal cardiovascular responses, those dealing with the capacity for maximal oxygen consumption and heart rate [64-69] provide no clear standards by which to establish general guidelines for recommended intensities on the basis of either a percentage of $\dot{V}O_2$max or a target heart rate range. Only one longitudinal research project has clearly delineated intensity levels for highly athletic pregnant women on the basis of pre-pregnancy capacities [61, 64]. In addition to the confounding factors that result from the pregnancy itself (changes in blood volume, resting heart rate, stroke volume, hemoconcentration, and plasma glucose patterns), pregnant women are subject to the same variants as the nonpregnant population, including genetic potential, age, previous and current conditioning, and lifestyle preferences.

In practice, the subjective measure of rate of perceived exertion has been useful in helping women establish an appropriate intensity level for themselves on any given day. Once a woman can establish a subjective moderate intensity (i.e., she feels she is working *somewhat hard* to *hard*), she may be able to establish a measurable heart rate range. However, she is still subject to day-to-day fluctuations in capacity dependent on her body's reaction to the pregnancy, as well as her age, training, and lifestyle.

A wide range of intensity levels may be appropriate for women during pregnancy, as figure 6.2 indicates. The left-hand column refers to low, moderate, and high intensities dependent on the measures given in the next three columns: RPE (rate of perceived exertion), % $\dot{V}O_2$max (functional capacity based on the percentage of the maximum oxygen consumption possible for a given individual), and heart rate. Lower intensities are appropriate for older women and those who are less active or

who have conditions that may require reduction of intensity levels (such as mitral valve prolapse or mild anemia)—or who are used to working harder but feel like taking it easy on a given day. Moderate intensity levels are appropriate for most women who are healthy and active.

Higher levels of intensity are appropriate only for competitive and professional athletes or dancers and for very active recreational exercisers. Women capable of working daily at a high intensity should be closely monitored by medical staff trained in exercise measurement and testing, as well as in fetal monitoring, for assessment of their own and their fetuses' responses to exertion.

Deconditioning

It is clear that individuals placed on bed rest rapidly become deconditioned, by as much as 25% in three weeks [70]. It is important to keep this in mind with women who must rest in bed or reduce the level of their activity during the first trimester, near the end of their pregnancy, or postpartum. Following bed rest, reconditioning is slow but steady, whether the individual is returning to exercise or simply to activities of daily living. Working at lower intensities and progressing gradually by increasing time, then intensity, are appropriate. Regaining a previous state of fitness takes longer than the deconditioning process [70] in the nonpregnant population. Although no information is available for the pregnant population, this is a commonly encountered situation, and a conservative approach is wise.

The traditional practice of prolonged hospital bed rest for conditions such as premature rupture of membranes, premature labor, and IUGR has been called into question [71]. While the major detriment has been assumed to be maternal muscle atrophy, lower birth weight among infants of mothers on prolonged bed rest compared to those of mothers who are returned to daily activities has been observed for these conditions [71]. In addition, women placed on bed rest for at least 20 hours per day for three weeks or more described a high level of physical, emotional, familial, and economic hardship resulting from the experience [72]. Clearly, high-intensity exercise is contraindicated in these situations, but a return to activities of daily living and perhaps low-intensity activities is worthy of further study.

Two studies conducted on rats indicate that when cardiovascular conditioning has occurred pre-pregnancy, cessation of exercise during early pregnancy negatively affects offspring viability [73, 74]. In one study, Vanheest and Rodgers sought to evaluate the effects of chronic endurance training on glucose and lipid homeostasis in diabetic rats and their offspring. Three groups were designated: the EE group exercised before and

Intensity	RPE[1]	Functional capacity ($\%\dot{V}O_2max$)	Heart rate[2] (beats/minute)
	very light		
		50%	100 to 120
			103 to 123
low			106 to 126
	fairly light		109 to 129
			112 to 132
		60%	115 to 135
			118 to 138
			121 to 141
	somewhat hard		124 to 144
			127 to 147
		70%	130 to 150
moderate			133 to 153
			136 to 156
	hard		139 to 159
			142 to 162
		80%	145 to 165
			148 to 168
			151 to 171
	very hard		154 to 174
			157 to 177
high		90%	160 to 180
			163 to 183
			167 to 187
	very, very hard	95%	170 to 190

[1]RPE refers to the Rate of Perceived Exertion, in this setting subjective description only has been used.

[2]Heart rates shown are for women in the age range 20 to 40. Those in the left column are likely values for women closer to 40 or less fit. Those in the right column are likely values for women closer to 20 or extremely fit. The correspondence of exercising heart rates and the percentage of functional capacity is a complex relationship dependent on genetic potential, training, and age, and further complicated by the responses of pregnancy.

Sources: Ann Cowlin, unpublished records of 241 prenatal exercise participants' heart rates and RPE, 1982-1997; American College of Sports Medicine. 1995. *Guidelines for exercise testing & prescription*, 6th ed., Philadelphia: Lea & Febiger; McArdle, W.D., Katch, F.I., and Katch, V.L. 1991. *Exercise physiology: Energy, nutrition and human performance*, 3rd ed., Philadelphia: Lea & Febiger. © 1996 Ann Cowlin. Used by permission.

Figure 6.2 Range of aerobic intensities for healthy pregnant women.

during pregnancy, the ES group exercised before pregnancy and ceased exercise at conception, and the SS group was sedentary before and during pregnancy. While responses to glucose and insulin tests were different between the EE and SS groups, and exercising before and during gestation did not reduce the viability of offspring, cessation of exercise in early pregnancy (ES group) negatively affected offspring viability. The number of offspring remaining viable in each group was EE = 17, ES = 0, SS = 14 [73].

In the second study, Houghton et al. investigated the effects of chronic running on fetal glycogen storage in rats trained during pre-pregnancy. They found that high-intensity exercise did not compromise fetal glycogen storage; however, chronic pre-pregnancy exercise and cessation of exercise at conception appeared to compromise fetal growth and development [74].

THERMOREGULATION

An early theoretical consideration in pregnancy research was the possibility of detrimental teratogenic effects (or heat-induced malformations) due to elevated core body temperatures associated with moderate- to high-intensity aerobic exercise. The risk of neural tube defects during the first trimester owing to this effect was considered grave. Exposure to elevated temperatures—such as a hot tub—in early pregnancy has been shown to have detrimental effects [75, 76]. However, no evidence of this phenomenon in association with exercise has been forthcoming [77, 78]. Research in the area [79, 80] has yielded the following findings:

1. Core temperature falls in the early stages of exercise during pregnancy, due in part to increased blood volume to carry heat away from the body core.
2. Pregnant women begin to perspire more rapidly under the same exercise conditions than nonpregnant women.
3. Greater skin area and increased vasculature allow added evaporation surface to promote cooling.
4. Pregnancy-induced increased ventilation promotes cooling.
5. Habitual exercisers' regulation of internal temperature is enhanced.

Because the fetus is incapable of its own heat dissipation, these adaptations are feto-protective.

Hydration During Exercise

A paramount concern during maternal exercise is hydration. The availability of water to contribute to the cooling process and to ensure adequate blood expansion is a fundamental principle that must be emphasized. Prior to participating in an exercise session, pregnant women should have 4 to 8 ounces of water and should have at least 2 to 4 ounces every 20 to 30 minutes once the session starts. The importance of consuming 2 quarts or more of water or other hydrating fluids per day cannot be overstated. Very active women should be encouraged to drink water until their urine is clear. During hot, humid weather, exercise should take place only in a cooled or air-conditioned environment.

Hydration in Labor

Research on gastric emptying shows that normal absorption of water or of sports drinks with less than 5% glucose or glucose-polymers is not affected by exercise as long as the intensity remains less than 70% $\dot{V}O_2$max. [81]. The intensity of labor rarely exceeds this limit. In practice, the consumption of 2 to 4 ounces of water or sports drink at 50° to 60° F, every 20 to 30 minutes, has a positive effect on muscle strength and endurance in ultradistance events (such as labor), despite the diversion of blood flow from the digestive organs. This information raises questions about the practice of withholding fluids and carbohydrates in labor.

METABOLISM

A number of metabolic processes are affected by pregnancy. The equation for energy balance that is maintained by the comparison between nutrient intake and exertion is complicated not only by the presence of the baby, but also by changes in the glycemic response. Availability of fuels has a profound impact on biochemistry, affecting reproductive function, stress responses, an adequate blood supply, and the immune system.

Hyperinsulinemia and Diabetes

The tendency toward *hyperinsulinemia* (increased frequency of insulin production) that has been noted in association with pregnancy [82] has two important implications for women who choose to exercise. First, because of changes in liver function that shift the balance between plasma glucose and insulin production in the pancreas, less plasma glucose is available to exercising muscles during pregnancy than at other times. As a result, fatigue may be more common and should be taken by the exercising pregnant woman as a sign that it is time to slow down, stop exercising, and eat. Because hyperinsulinemia is often a precursor to adult-onset *diabetes* (the condition in which carbohydrate metabolism is impaired and insulin production reduced or eliminated), and also because women with gestational diabetes are at high risk of diabetes mellitus in later life [83], newly pregnant women must understand the need to eat small amounts often, the need to eat enough protein to maintain steady blood sugar levels, and the importance of monitoring for gestational diabetes.

The second implication is that there is a tendency to add subcutaneous fat that is pronounced in sedentary or overfed individuals. Results of research on obesity indicate that defects in lipid oxidation and thermoregulation are tied to the balance of insulin and glucose production [84]. Because a major physiological priority in pregnancy is the nourishment and protection of the fetus, it is easy to see how human development has included a complex glycemic response that encourages storage of nutrients as fat and diversion of energy supplies from the mother to the fetus. The maternal endocrine system is in a state of chronic metabolic stress resulting from an increase in fuel delivery to the mother's circulation combined with hormonal actions that rapidly deplete available fuel; in this situation there are large fluctuations between postprandial and fasting blood glucose levels [85]. These changes result in insulin resistance and the development of gestational diabetes in a percentage of the population. Technically, *gestational diabetes* is an abnormal carbohydrate metabolism diagnosed in pregnancy, and a diagnosis of *diabetes mellitus* can be made only with a postpartum glucose test to confirm persistent glucose abnormality [86].

In the general population, exercise is associated with improved functions of carbohydrate and lipid metabolism. Consequently, exercise is being used as an adjunct treatment for both diabetes and obesity. This protection extends to pregnancy as well [87, 88], and both the Second and Third International Workshop-Conference on Gestational Diabetes Mellitus endorsed the concept of pregnant diabetic women pursuing an active lifestyle under medical supervision [89, 90]. The management of gestational diabetes through nutrition and exercise is well accepted [91, 92].

On a physiological basis, there is good reason to view exercise as a method of treating or managing gestational diabetes. A partial effect of pregnancy is the increased presence of hormones that have a diabetogenic effect—estrogen, progesterone, cortisol, prolactin, and human chorionic somatomammotropin [93]. While muscles participate in contraction-stimulated glucose transport, other factors such as catecholamines, corticosteroids, and thyroid and growth hormones affect this transport [93]. Following exercise, glucose tolerance is increased for some time, depending on insulin and contractile activity [94]. Benefits to a woman with gestational diabetes most likely are derived from insulin receptor regulation and improved insulin sensitivity [95-97], as well as a decrease in glucose-stimulated levels of serum insulin [98], as they are in the nonpregnant population.

Reports of the incidence of pregnant women with gestational diabetes mellitus vary with the criteria used to screen for this disorder; the figure ranges from 1.4% to 12.3% [99]. A distinction must be made between insulin-dependent and non-insulin-dependent diabetes. In either case, women must be carefully monitored; and fitness level, degree of carbohydrate disturbance, and other medical conditions must be taken into account. Insulin dependency requires close medical supervision. Individualized programs need to be created. Artal et al. have suggested that because of the higher level of carbohydrate utilization in non-weight-bearing compared to weight-bearing exercise, non-weight-bearing activities may be preferable for gestational diabetes clients [100]. In practice, we have found it helpful for these clients to augment land-based exercise classes with at least two cardiovascular sessions per week involving lap swimming, stationary cycling, or both.

Weight Gain, Obesity, and Diabetes

Clapp and Little's findings concerning maternal weight gain and fat deposition at low and high levels of maternal recreational activity help delineate the dose effect of physical fitness conditioning on the pattern of maternal weight gain, fat distribution, and birth weight. The researchers found that healthy, fit women who continued regular sustained recreational exercise throughout pregnancy at any level above a baseline for cardiovascular conditioning gained less weight and deposited less subcutaneous fat than women who stopped exercising, but this effect was limited to the latter portion of pregnancy [101]. Women who were fit prior to pregnancy and ceased exercise, or who dropped their levels of exercise during pregnancy below conditioning levels, showed increased weight gain and subcutaneous fat deposition. This may have reflected their failure to reduce excessive calorie intake as their exercise level dropped [101-104]. The exercising women also had lower-birth-weight infants, but this effect is primarily related to a having a leaner body mass. The increased birth weight of infants born to women who stopped exercising or who dropped their levels indicates the enhanced capacity of the placenta of a woman who exercises in the first half of pregnancy (discussed earlier) to deliver nutrients. If women stop exercising or decrease their level of activity, clearly they should reduce their caloric intake.

In recent research, Clapp and Kiess looked at the effect of exercise on pregnancy-associated increases in metabolic markers (tumor necrosis factor alpha and leptin) that reflect increases in fat mass and insulin resistance. They concluded that regular weight-bearing exercise during pregnancy suppresses the pregnancy-associated increases of both of these markers [105]. Monitoring these markers may some day help us prescribe exercise with more precision in women at risk of pregnancy-associated weight gain. As our ability to uncover metabolic markers and genetic predispositions improves, we are better able to specify which clients are at risk for weight gain. For example, recently Gutersohn et al. remarked in a letter to *Lancet* that first-time mothers of a particular genotype (the G protein beta3 subunit

825 TT genotype) are at high risk of obesity and postpregnancy weight retention if they do not exercise regularly [106].

Dye et al. have looked at the relationship among physical activity, obesity, and gestational diabetes, with interesting findings. Examining birth registry information for central New York State, they found that exercise was associated with reduced rates of gestational diabetes only among women with a pre-pregnancy body mass index greater than 33 [107]. Also, women of higher socioeconomic status who were obese and did not exercise were at significantly elevated risk of gestational diabetes compared with their counterparts of lower socioeconomic status [107].

Socioeconomic Status, Nutrition Status, and Type of Work

That women of lower socioeconomic status in a postindustrialized nation incur less gestational diabetes may reflect a symmetrical situation in developing countries, that is, women in less developed nations with fewer resources have more physically demanding lives than their more well-to-do counterparts. In a less developed nation, where food is not abundant or cultural norms restrict energy consumption, this lack of resources translates into more hours spent in standing work in the later stages of pregnancy accompanied by less nutrition. The results are less maternal weight gain, lower birth weights, and poorer neonatal outcomes [108]. In a developed nation, where food is abundant, women may need to engage in recreational activity as a means of establishing a healthy energy balance and reducing weight gain. The resultant energy expenditure may also be helpful in reducing the propensity for gestational diabetes.

The effect of standing physical work toward the end of pregnancy has been noted as a reason for poor outcomes since the end of the 19th century; and since that time, rest in the last few weeks of pregnancy has been suggested for women whose life or work situation requires them to engage in long periods of standing [109-111]. But the advent of recreational physical activity has produced an irony. Physically fit women—including those who do large amounts of weight-bearing activity—appear to be in a better situation to sustain fetal growth at the end of pregnancy than those who do standing physical work in an industrial or service job, or at home. Early findings regarding maternal fitness and birth weight, demonstrating no effect on birth weight due to physical activity, reinforced this thesis. Additionally, one of Erkkola's early studies, while not demonstrating a significant difference, did note a tendency to increased birth weight among fit mothers [112].

Additional findings have surfaced indicating that heavy physical working conditions have a negative effect on maternal weight gain and birth weight [113-115]. Other findings from the late 1980s and early 1990s suggested the possibility that exercise increases birth weight [116, 117]. As a result, there has been confusion about the implications for exercise prescription. The following papers provide insight into the situation and offer guidance to those designing programs and those seeking fruitful lines for future research.

Briend's thesis [108] correctly asserts that the impact of the two-legged upright posture in humans contributes to hypotensive syndromes and consequently to weight gain problems for the mother and fetus. Blood pooling in the legs and lack of a vigorous pumping action during standing for long periods of time inhibit the venous return of the blood supply. The advantage of vigorous weight-bearing exercise is the pumping action of the large muscles in the hip, buttocks, and trunk that help to drive the blood back into the core of the body. The type of activity associated with industrialization and service jobs such as waitressing or nursing, as well as that associated with housework, while often strenuous, does not produce the variation in limb (and thus blood vessel) arrangement or the large muscle actions necessary to move the blood. In addition, these physical jobs can be strenuous. Briend's thesis that this result is somewhat independent of nutrition also begs for attention, as we see prematurity and low birth weight in these situations in postindustrial nations as well as in developing countries. As a consequence of this knowledge, well-designed exercise programs include a variety of movement activities and a side-lying resting period.

Tafari et al. provide insight into the fetal-protective mechanisms at work in a situation of strenuous physical work and undernutrition. In a study conducted in Addis Ababa, Ethiopia, the researchers found that women who had lower-than-recommended calorie intakes and who participated in hard physical labor had significantly lower early-pregnancy body weights, lower gestational weight gains, and lighter newborn infants than less active mothers on similar low-calorie intakes [118]. The nonfetal portion of the maternal pregnancy weight gains, however, was more affected than birth weight by the level of the mother's physical activity [118], indicating that the utilization of nutrients favors the fetus in the case of maternal undernourishment and heavy physical work. The researchers surmise that there must be some metabolic adjustments that partially protect the fetus in this situation; the placenta appears to respond to the reduced maternal hepatic gluconeogenesis that accompanies fasting [119, 120] by an increased secretion of chorionic gonadotropin hormone, which enhances hypoaminoacidemia and hyperketonemia through its anabolic and lipolytic actions [121, 122]. Ketone bodies, free fatty acids, and perhaps lactate and pyruvate provide increased portions of the fetal fuel. The fetus utilizes ketones to form lipids and provide cellular energy [123, 124], and the fetal heart uses free fatty acids for energy [123]. While these actions do not totally compensate for maternal undernourishment, they do provide insight into compensatory metabolic mechanisms that favor the fetus. The extent to which the mother suffers loss of vital nutrient stores can be severe, forming a powerful incentive for ensuring that maternal nourishment is adequate.

Stress

Stress, anxiety, and tension are hallmarks of life at the start of the 21st century. The body's response to stress affects metabolism through endocrine function, resulting in physical changes such as infertility and psychophysiologic responses such as obsessive behavior. Associated with both daily difficulties and major life events, anxiety is a generalized apprehension that affects sense of self [125], behavior [126], and emotional tone and autonomic functions [127]. *State anxiety* (A-State) is the transitory, event-associated affect such as that experienced before a test. *Trait anxiety* (A-Trait) has to do with idiosyncratic anxiety proneness, such that an individual who is said to be high in A-Trait responds to stressful situations with a high level of state anxiety [128].

Stress and Exercise

During the 1970s and 1980s, the work of Morgan and others established the association of acute vigorous exercise with the reduction of state anxiety and blood pressure [129-134]. Among the overall findings are that while there is an association, cause and effect remain to be shown, and results are inconsistent. Specifically, a "timeout," rest, or distraction may be associated with just as great a quantity of reduction, but not as long a duration as is associated with exercise; non-cultic meditation is also effective; and cluster intervention methods (coupling exercise with other modalities) may be most effective. The majority of this research has been conducted on men, and appropriate research on women in this area is greatly needed. Results of studies to determine whether women and men experience the same anxiety reduction in association with exercise are mixed [135, 136].

Research does seem to indicate that long-term fitness training may be helpful in reducing trait anxiety [135-137]. It seems to be important to employ exercise of moderate or high cardiovascular intensity on a regular, sustained basis in order to achieve this effect. In other words, the type and amount of activity required to produce aerobic conditioning may be associated with reducing trait anxiety as well.

Stress and Childbearing

Pregnant and postpartum women, particularly first-time mothers, are involved in a major life event, and the potential for anxiety is great. Specific questions, such as how a cup of coffee or an angry reaction to an event might be affecting the fetus, as well as general questions, such as whether the baby will be healthy or the pregnant woman will be a "good" mother, can assail the mind of the mother-to-be, making pregnancy a potential time of both high state anxiety and high trait anxiety. In addition, life stressors—financial, interpersonal, or medical problems—can add to distress and anxiety, which in turn can adversely affect outcome.

When researchers took monthly measures of daily stress *(hassles),* state anxiety, and pregnancy-specific stress and assessed lifestyle behaviors by trimesters, they found correlations between these factors and complications over the course of the pregnancy and the birth process, with primiparas (first-time mothers) more likely to experience complications than multiparas [138]. In another study, in an ethnically diverse sample of low-income women, the effects of stress, social support, and labor and delivery experiences on postpartum depression were assessed and found to account for 45% of the variance in postpartum depressed mood [139].

The negative effects of stress include increased probability of PIH [140], decreased maternal well-being, and increased somatic complaints [141]. Stress is also a significant predictor for spontaneous preterm delivery and low birth weight [142]. One study showed that while psychosocial factors (depression, trait anxiety, stress, mastery, self-esteem, and social support) played a role in the etiology of low prenatal weight gain among white women, there was no such effect among black women [143]. Another study, examining 1150 women from six ethnic groups, indicated that living in public housing and believing that chance plays a major role in health status were negatively associated with birth weight; having a stable residence was positively associated with birth weight [144]. Although the specific causes for negative birth outcomes may vary from group to group, there is evidence that stress, anxiety, and life tensions play a major role.

In practice, one of the questions prenatal exercise instructors encounter is whether or not the benefits of exercise that accrue for nonpregnant persons will also accrue in pregnancy. The extent to which exercise has a salubrious effect on stress or anxiety during pregnancy is a good question. There is a relationship between the mediation of stress by corticotropin-releasing hormone (CRH) and opioid peptides (beta-endorphins), and the effect of stress on disturbed reproductive function (disrupted menstruation, parturition [birth], and lactation)

[145, 146]. During labor, corticotropin and beta-endorphin are found at the levels seen in athletes during maximal exercise; in addition, the placenta produces increasing amounts of CRH toward the end of pregnancy, signaling that the placenta may be involved in adaptive stress mechanisms to help mother and fetus withstand the stress of labor [145]. How exercise influences this equation is unknown, although it would seem theoretically possible that exercise could act to help mediate the stress of labor.

In a small sample, Rauramo et al. found that the responses of stress hormones and placental steroids in late-pregnancy exercisers were similar to those in nonpregnant exercisers [147]. Although the researchers found some incidence of uterine contractions brought on by increased levels of norepinephrine, the increase in epinephrine mitigates this effect, and regular contractions did not start in any subjects [147]. Berkowitz et al. found that women who participated in recreational activities had a decreased risk of spontaneous preterm birth [148].

Another exercise factor that might mitigate stress is a group exercise setting. Clearly, social support is a valuable tool in the effort to avoid low maternal weight gain, premature birth, and low birth weight that may result from, or be exacerbated by, anxiety, stress, or life tensions [138-144, 149, 150]. Women who participate in well-run group prenatal exercise programs report that the group support is at least as important to their well-being as the actual exercise component [151].

In an uncontrolled study, Berger and Owen compared exercise modalities and obtained different results depending on the conditions under which the exercise took place [152]. The findings led the researchers to suggest that for exercise to reduce stress it must be enjoyable, aerobic, devoid of competition, predictable, and repetitive [152]. The release of stress hormones during exercise is related to both intensity and psychotropic effects. During the ergotropic response (fight or flight), increased levels of norepinephrine contribute to uterine irritability. This response is often present in competitive exercise situations. In practice, we have found that during periods of rapid uterine growth (often in weeks 24-34), it is helpful to avoid work or exercise environments in which the ergotropic response is activated.

Relaxation

By contrast, the trophotropic response—or relaxation response—is marked by an organizing alpha brain wave, leading to a sense of calm alertness and a reduction in stress response [153]. Athletes who develop the capacity to remain relaxed during strenuous work by using an associative mental focus are at less risk for injury [154]. This has profound implications for the design of prenatal exercise activities.

Relaxation has long been a tenet of childbirth education. Because labor is generally a long process, the body's natural ability to operate in a low-energy state is very useful leading up to the actual birth. In early labor, adrenaline inhibits the release of *oxytocin,* the hormone responsible for uterine contraction, so that being relaxed promotes the labor process. Later, as birth approaches, an interesting reversal takes place and adrenaline stimulates oxytocin to produce the *ejection reflex,* which enables the uterus to expel the baby [155]. Contemporary life rarely poses opportunities for relaxation, and childbirth preparation classes usually occur only toward the end of a pregnancy. So it falls to exercise instructors and personal trainers to incorporate regular practice of relaxation techniques into their pregnant clients' regimens.

Energy Needs and Nutrition

Two factors related to maternal nutrition have been shown to affect birth weight. These are pre-pregnancy weight and weight gain during pregnancy [156, p. 317]. Women who are severely underweight at the start of pregnancy and those who gain insufficient weight during pregnancy are at risk for delivering a small-for-gestational-age infant. Smoking, drugs, maternal disease, and the length of gestation also affect birth weight. Babies who are small for gestational age are at increased risk for perinatal mortality, small head circumference, mental retardation, cerebral palsy, learning disabilities, visual and hearing defects, neurological defects, and poor infant growth and development [156, p. 317]. It is obviously in the best interest of the child for the mother to be well nourished.

Pregnancy and exercise each require energy beyond regular survival levels. Both the National Research Council, Food and Nutrition Board's recommended daily allowance (RDA) and the ACOG recommendation are for an additional 300 kilocalories per day above other energy requirements [157, 158]. This is a generally accepted amount. Early in pregnancy, the body uses energy for expanding blood volume and vasculature, increasing hormone production, and stepping up organ function to handle the added demands of pregnancy. Later, the fetus requires energy for its metabolic processes. Caloric requirements for exercise are in addition to those required for pregnancy. Women who are underweight, or whose nutrition is insufficient, or who are under nutritional stress (adolescents, those with certain disorders, or those with substance abuse problems) require even more added calories. Sufficient maternal calories is a paramount issue.

The foundation of cell growth is protein. Many experts believe that protein is the key macronutrient to track in pregnant women but disagree about how much protein is required. Both the RDA and the

ACOG recommendation are for an added 10 grams of protein per day per infant, for a total of approximately 60 grams for a healthy, midsize mother-to-be carrying one baby. However, there are other points of view on this issue. In the 1940s, Harvard researcher Bertha Burke found that a diet that included a base of 75 grams of protein per day (along with other adequate nutrition) was protective against underweight and other infant disorders [159]. The Brewer Medical Diet for Normal and High-Risk Pregnancy calls for 100 to 120 grams total because protein is stored in pregnancy and therefore the amount eaten is not the same as the amount available [160]. The Brewers were also the first to suggest that lack of adequate protein is a contributing factor to the development of preeclampsia or PIH. In practice, when women feel tired and have daily nausea in early pregnancy, increasing protein intake and eating small amounts often throughout the day are helpful methods, both for relieving symptoms and for reducing the risk of hypertension later.

Nutrition for Women Who Exercise While Pregnant

The following simple, practical guidelines are helpful to women who exercise during their pregnancies:

1. A regular supply of simple and complex carbohydrates (fruits, vegetables, grains) with a protein complement (milk, meat, poultry, fish, legumes in combination) is essential. The woman should take in 200 to 300 kilocalories every 2 to 3 hours, depending on gestational stage, her size, and level of activity. She should eat a wide variety of foods. Approximately 70 to 90 grams of protein per day for a woman carrying a single baby, spread among the various meals, is essential, along with a minimum of 2 quarts of water to maintain an adequate blood supply. She should eat high-quality fats, such as olive or canola oil, avocados, nuts, and seeds.

2. It is critical to pay careful attention to fatigue when exercising. Women should stop exercising at the point of muscle fatigue, and should not begin exercise when even mildly fatigued. Watered juice or sports drinks are encouraged during the workout.

3. Alternating cycles of activity, nutrition, and rest/relaxation are beneficial, as this allows the body systems time to complete metabolic processes and maximize circulation.

Not only is protein needed to help create the baby and meet the mother's needs; the expansion of blood volume must also be maintained. If about 300 kilocalories is to be added to the daily intake but only 10 grams (40 calories, or 12.5%) is protein, this hardly seems sufficient to achieve all the purposes for which protein is needed, especially in an exercising mother-to-be. On the other hand, eating more than 100 grams of protein per day is probably necessary only for a pregnant athlete with a heavy workout schedule. Keeping all this information in mind, in practice we have found that recommending an added 30 grams of protein per day per baby, for a total of approximately 70 to 90 grams per day with a single fetus or 100 to 120 grams with twins, produces good results.

Immune System Responses

It has been established that there are sex differences in immune function [161-167]. While women's response to viruses and parasitic infections is more active than men's [167], their cell-mediated immune responses are less vigorous [166]. Women, by far, are more susceptible to all of the diseases of the immune system, and the impact of gonadal hormones on immunologic function appears to be mediated through special receptors [168]. Findings show that estrogen stimulates transcriptional regulation of the CRH gene, which is the likely source of the sex differences in the immune/inflammatory reaction and the prevalence of autoimmune disorders in women [169]. Corticotropin-releasing hormone coordinates the stress response and immune/inflammatory reaction [170].

In pregnancy, the intensity of immune responses is blunted [171-173]. It has been known for some time that during pregnancy, although lupus erythematosus increases in the first trimester, it normalizes later [174], and that the symptoms of rheumatoid arthritis abate in pregnancy [175]. During the secretory phase of the menstrual cycle, progesterone fosters the production of immunological suppressor substances by the proliferative endometrium without affecting the secretory endometrium during the time when implantation might occur [176]. Natural killer cell activity is depressed just prior to ovulation [177]. These and other mechanisms are responsible for a complex relationship between sex hormones and immune function. Theoretically, it makes sense that the female body would have the ability to depress immune function in order to tolerate the presence of foreign DNA belonging to the fetus. Unfortunately, the price appears to be an increased susceptibility to autoimmune disorders.

The relationship between exercise and immune function in the nonpregnant population is itself a new subject about which little is known. How exercise in pregnancy might affect women's immune system is an interesting question that we will need longitudinal data to answer. Hopefully, research in this area will be forthcoming.

RESPIRATION AND ACID-BASE BALANCE

As we saw in chapter 5, ventilation and ventilatory responses to exercise are affected by pregnancy. Although some of the mechanisms are understood and effects have been validated for some time, there continue to be questions regarding the various responses. One key issue is whether data for pregnant exercisers versus nonpregnant exercisers, or data for pregnant exercisers versus the same exercisers postpartum, produce a more accurate picture of the situation. Further, it is not completely clear when postpartum comparisons should be made in order to reflect true values.

In submaximal testing, Jaque-Fortunato et al. found significantly higher ventilation ($\dot{V}E$), ventilatory frequency (VF), ventilatory equivalent for oxygen ($\dot{V}E/\dot{V}O_2$), and ventilatory equivalence for carbon dioxide ($\dot{V}E/\dot{V}CO_2$) in pregnant exercisers versus nonpregnant controls [178]. In comparisons of pregnant exercisers versus themselves at a mean postpartum period of 12 1/2 weeks, however, the pregnant exercisers had higher tidal volumes rather than higher VF [178]. Plasma lactate levels were higher at rest in pregnant women compared with themselves postpartum, did not differ at rest between pregnant women and nonpregnant controls, and did not differ in either comparison during submaximal exercise, leading to the conclusion that CO_2 elevations during exercise in pregnancy do not appear to be caused by an elevated bicarbonate buffering response to elevated plasma lactate levels [178].

Another issue is the effect of conditioning on exercise test responses. Wolfe et al. have found that in fit women, including those who become fit in the course of the pregnancy, maximal aerobic power and the capacity for sustained submaximal exercise are greater than in nonexercising pregnant women [179]. Regular exercise also contributes to the preservation of anaerobic working capacity in late gestation [179], clearly an attribute for the second stage of labor commonly known as the pushing stage. When comparing physically active pregnant women (mean gestational age 33 weeks) with nonpregnant controls, Kemp et al. found that the pregnant group had reduced partial pressure of O_2 (PCO_2) and weak acid concentrations, which are important mechanisms to regulate hemoglobin concentration and maintain a less acidic plasma environment at rest and after exercise in late gestation [180]. In addition, Ohtake and Wolfe have found that cardiovascular conditioning reduces both ventilatory demand and respiratory perception of effort in late gestation [181].

The practical reality of pregnancy is that toward the end of the first trimester, many women experience an uncomfortable tendency to hyperventilate that results from the effects of increasing levels of progesterone as the placenta takes over from the corpus of pregnancy as the primary progesterone producer. The hyperventilation phenomenon appears to be mediated by estrogen-dependent progesterone receptors in the hypothalamus that affect the respiratory control center in the medulla oblongata [182]. This increase is tied to lowering levels of carbon dioxide and increasing oxygen levels that benefit the fetus. The increased metabolic activity in pregnancy causes an increase in carbon dioxide levels, and hyperventilating lowers the carbon dioxide level.

As pregnancy progresses, the upward growth of the uterus puts pressure on the diaphragm. There is some widening of the rib cage, and the total effect is a reduction in functional residual volume. This may cause a sense of difficulty with breathing or labored breathing. Some women tend to hyperventilate as a response. Difficulty breathing for this reason or as a consequence of the effect of progesterone falls under the heading of *dyspnea*. Even women who are very fit may experience these sensations. To alleviate the symptoms, women should breathe slowly and deeply, taking advantage of intercostal expansion, and slow down if they are moving about. Toward the end of pregnancy, sedentary women are disadvantaged by increasing plasma lactate levels, which do not occur in fit women.

BIOMECHANICS

The potential for damage to the woman's neuromusculoskeletal structure in pregnancy and the postpartum period is great. Shifts in the center of gravity forward and slightly up destabilize her posture and realign the carriage of weights and forces through her joints, predisposing nerves, muscles, bones, and connective tissues to damage. Increased levels of relaxin and elastin further aggravate this situation. Chapter 5 outlines major postural and biomechanical changes that result from these conditions.

These changes occur gradually and can be responsible for a great many discomforts over the course of the pregnancy. Although very little research in this area exists, we do have some good anecdotal information that helps set guidelines. Clapp notes that the women he tests in his lab who exercise at a moderate or vigorous level regularly throughout pregnancy report few discomforts [183].

The author and colleagues who work in the prenatal exercise field have similar empirical evidence. In addition, we find patterns in the problems that do occur and have catalogued methods for dealing with them.

General Guidelines for Countering the Effects of Gravity on Joint Mechanics

The brain receives a continuous supply of afferent information about the shifting postural dynamic and eventually accepts the altered arrangement and balance of body segments. Feedback from cutaneous, joint, and muscle receptors is involved in this process. By the end of pregnancy the brain has reconfigured its image of the body in balance.

The first step in helping with joint mechanics during pregnancy is to be sure to account for the physics of pregnancy in the design of individual exercises by countering the negative effects of gravity on the pregnant physiognomy. During prenatal exercise, the following guidelines aid in the design of exercises to relieve structural stresses:

1. The woman can strengthen muscles that are over-stretched (hamstrings, gluteals, abdominals, and upper back).
2. She can stretch muscles that are shortened (psoas, low back, and chest).
3. Centering activities (physical balance and mental calm) promote efficient alignment and motion.
4. Resting in the side-lying position when muscle fatigue occurs (after appropriate cool-down) eliminates most of the negative effects of gravity.

Common Nerve Compression Syndromes

Pregnant woman are particularly subject to nerve compression syndromes, including carpal tunnel syndrome and sciatica. Methods to alleviate these problems during pregnancy include the following:

1. Stabilize and elevate the affected part.
2. Avoid weight bearing on the affected part.
3. Avoid extreme range of motion.

A number of practical, noninvasive, nonmedical procedures can be effective within a class or workout session. For arm, wrist, or hand problems, it is advisable to include movements that gently open the front of the chest and shoulder by bringing the arm upward and slightly back; rotator cuff exercises to balance the shoulder joint and upper spine; and gentle wrist rotation to reduce compression on the radial and ulnar nerves. If edema in the wrist is a factor, the woman should bring the thumb and little finger together. This creates a pocket of space at the inside of the wrist to relieve compression on nerves and blood vessels. For sacroiliac (SI) joint slippage or severe sciatica (nerve impinged and swollen), women need to see a physical therapist or other qualified bodywork professional. For less severe symptoms, exercises are outlined in chapter 8 (see "Special Exercises for Pregnancy"). During relaxation it is also useful to focus on releasing the muscles surrounding the joints in the region of the insertion of affected nerves into the spine: that is, cervical spine, upper back, chest, and shoulder for carpal tunnel syndrome, or lumbar spine and sacroiliac and iliofemoral joints for sciatica.

Low Back and Pelvic Discomfort

Low back and pelvic discomforts are common in pregnant women. Ostgaard et al., examining reduction of back and posterior pelvic pain, found that in their cohort of 407 pregnant women enrolled consecutively in their study, 47% had serious back or posterior pelvic pain at some point in pregnancy [184]. The researchers concluded that individually designed programs were more effective than group work and that differentiation between low back and posterior pelvic pain was essential [184]. A large percentage (82%) of the women with this problem also experienced reduction of posterior pelvic pain with the use of a nonelastic pelvic support [184]. In practice, we have found such supports helpful during aerobic dancing, especially for women in the second, third, or fourth pregnancy and women who have particularly relaxed connective tissue. In addition, even in a group class setting, it is important to take time with individuals to uncover precisely where their discomfort lies, so that whoever will be doing the therapy has a clear and accurate picture of the biomechanical situation.

In a study to assess causes and effective treatment of low back pain in pregnancy, McIntyre and Broadhurst tested all women attending a rural general practice for prenatal care and identified 20 patients as having low back pain. Three were diagnosed with the iliolumbar ligament as the source, and in the others the source was the SI joint. After three visits involving mobilization of the SI joint and home exercise, 15 reported no pain and the remainder a reduction of 50% [185]. Andrews and O'Neil found the pelvic tilt exercise helpful in relieving pelvic ligament pain [186]. The pelvic tilt mobilizes the SI joint, iliofemoral joint, and lumbar spine and also functions as an abdominal strengthener.

These findings resonate with practical experience. When queried as to the exact location and nature of their sensations, three-fourths of exercise clients in the author's practice reporting low back or posterior pelvic pain describe a feeling of a "hitch," "slippage," or "catching" in the SI joint region. Such movements as pelvic tilts, rocks, and rotations in a variety of starting postures, in addition to deep abdominal strengthening, have all been useful in relieving this joint dysfunction. Because of the forward momentum of the sacral region of the spine as the uterus increases in size and weight, it is logical that a dysfunction could easily occur in this region. Restoration of normal alignment of the facets of the SI joint through mobilization alleviates much discomfort, and exercises to help maintain mobility provide long-term assistance.

The alleviation of joint discomfort through strength and flexibility exercises is a common practice. In addition, balancing strength and elasticity among the muscles that control a given joint tends to balance and protect the joint. Physical balance is one of the components of centering. When the joints are balanced, the neuromusculature is less busy with remaining upright than when misalignment or unbalanced muscle development places demands on the superficial skeletal muscles—which fatigue over time—to help maintain upright as well as to cause movement in space. Instead, when joints are balanced, incipient contractions of deep muscle fibers nearest the joint centers are the primary righting mechanism. When balanced and relaxed, the individual is centered. Movement or behavior goals are easily and efficiently achieved as there is less physiological stress within the system to claim the brain's attention [187-189].

The possibility that hormones play a role in low back discomfort also exists. In a study of postmenopausal women, researchers found a small but significant effect on the prevalence of low back pain among women taking hormone replacement therapy [190]. While the authors speculate that their finding may be of minor clinical importance in menopause, it is possible that the effect of hormones on joints and ligaments plays a role in low back pain in a sufficient number of women at varying times in their lives, including pregnancy, that it should be taken into consideration in evaluations of low back discomfort. Inquiring about the discomfort during menses often provides insight into this matter.

Upper Back Fatigue

Another form of discomfort that is seen is upper back fatigue, due to increasing kyphosis and the weight of enlarging breasts. It is critical to assess this situation to make sure there is no underlying medical or neurological problem and, if there is not, to develop a strengthening program for the upper back. This situation can become aggravated following birth if the strength to maintain healthy spine alignment is not developed, because nursing reinforces the kyphotic posture.

Knee Pain

Two other difficulties are important to consider in the prenatal period, although the greatest problems are often experienced postpartum. One is the effect of changing alignment on the knees, and the second is the integrity of the pelvic floor and the incidence of related pelvic pain and incontinence. As mentioned in chapter 5, Vullo et al. have noted the tendency for lower leg pain to occur in the later stages of pregnancy and postpartum, and the researchers believe it is attributable to biomechanics as opposed to hormonal influences [191]. In practice, the author finds postpartum knee pain among women who have difficulty complying with the requirement to increase hamstring strength. Dumas and Reid found that although increases in hormone-related laxity of the knee cruciate ligaments during pregnancy do occur, minimal to moderate weight-bearing exercise did not result in any further measurable increase in laxity, and that the pregnancy-related increase had significantly lessened at four months postpartum [192]. Longitudinal studies of the relationship between exercise in pregnancy and long-term biomechanical consequences are needed.

Pelvic Floor Integrity

Pelvic floor integrity is critical to women. While the muscle group and bone structure of the pelvic area has not been commonly taught in regard to exercise, this is a significant area of knowledge for those who seek to work with women. Descriptions of the structures and muscles involved appear in chapter 5. Two issues emerge in relation to pelvic floor function associated with exercise. One is the occurrence of incontinence in competitive female athletes. The other is pelvic floor muscle exercises to prevent, rehabilitate, or ameliorate trauma to the pelvic floor—particularly in relation to birth—and its consequences for related organs: the uterus, rectum, and bladder.

One of the unfortunate aspects of upright posture is stress to the pelvic floor. A ramification of this for athletes is that in some sports, particularly in high-impact sports, lack of development of the pelvic floor muscles is disadvantageous. The rate of occurrence of incontinence among women athletes is not known; however, discussion of the situation has begun in the literature [193-195].

The issues surrounding trauma to the pelvic floor region are too many to enumerate here. Major questions concerning pelvic floor exercise in relation to pregnancy and birth include the following:

1. What can pregnant women do to prevent or minimize traumatic effects to their pelvic floor during birth?
2. When is exercise indicated as a prescription for repair or rehabilitation?
3. What key factors does the exercise instructor or personal trainer need to know about to assist women with pelvic floor exercise?

In relation to the first question, a woman must recognize that, even though she may do everything possible to prevent pelvic trauma, circumstances such as a congenital anomaly, surgical intervention in labor, medical emergency, or poorly handled delivery could affect her pelvic floor integrity.

Preparing the muscles for delivery requires both contraction and relaxation of the superficial connections of the pubis, ischial tuberosities, and coccyx, as well as the deeper levator and sphincter muscles. In addition, strengthening the transverse abdominal muscle facilitates the pushing or bearing-down action directed at the pelvic outlet [196]. The trajectory of effort from the diaphragm must "bounce" off the rigid, isometrically contracted transverse muscle at the appropriate angle and toward the specific outlet in question—rectum, vagina, or urethra.

Regarding the second question—indications for pelvic floor exercises—urinary incontinence is often the first indicator. But, urinary incontinence may be affected by congenital defects in the bladder or by smooth muscle (detrusor) malfunction as well as weak musculature. The detrusor contracts as the pelvic floor muscles relax, maintaining the ureter in alignment as it drops to allow the release of urine. Women who have good muscle isolation and strong pelvic contractions but experience incontinence may need attention to the detrusor [197]. The author finds that using the image shown in figure 6.3 is effective in helping women grasp the functioning of the detrusor.

Incontinence often results from specific damage to muscles, fascia, and nerves of the pelvic floor during childbirth [198-202]. Controversy surrounds the issue of whether *epidural anesthesia* (combinations of narcotics and muscle relaxants introduced into the epidural compartment of the ascending spinal cord via needle) [203, 204] or *episiotomy* (the practice of surgically cutting the perineum to speed delivery) [205] contributes to complications resulting in incontinence. In addition, the role of the care provider and her or his technique of delivery is controversial, with both medical training and medical management of labor coming under fire [206-209].

One of the key factors for fitness professionals to know about in regard to pelvic floor exercises—the third question—is that they are most effective in cases of urinary stress incontinence. For treatment of genuine urinary stress incontinence caused by weak pelvic floor muscles, *Kegels*—or pelvic floor muscle exercises first described in 1948 by Dr. Kegel [210]—have been used successfully since their introduction, with a significant improvement and/or cure rate of about 50% and poor motivation on the client's part as a common reason for failure [211]. Since their introduction, these exercises have become a staple of childbirth education; but as with any physical exercise, they need to be practiced regularly and over a longer period of time than childbirth education courses usually allow. Kegels have been shown to be effective for preventing complications of labor and maintaining pelvic floor integrity (assuming a well-managed labor) [206] and for development of appropriate muscle strength postpartum [212, 213]. Besides Kegel exercises, vaginal weight cones have also been shown to be effective in treating genuine stress incontinence, although client compliance with cones is lower than with exercise [214].

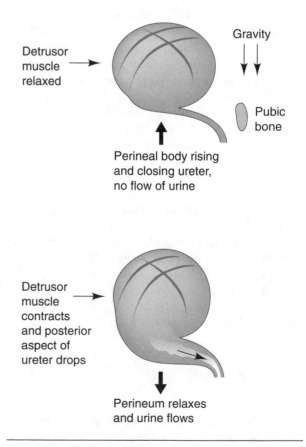

Figure 6.3   Visual aid for detrusor functioning.

Treatment of urinary incontinence, anal incontinence, or organ prolapse must be medically supervised.

PSYCHOPHYSIOLOGICAL INTERACTIONS

That exercise (including aerobic activities; strength or resistance work; flexibility, coordination, and balance exercises; centering, relaxation, and imagery) is valuable for health is well accepted [187, 215, 216]. That exercise of various types plays a role in mental and emotional well-being is becoming accepted. The cause and effect of this latter association, however, are difficult to establish. Some aspects, such as the role of exercise in the balance of compounds (norepinephrine, dopamine, and serotonin) that contribute to relief of depression [217], the role of activities that encourage concentration as a distraction and relief from stress [218], and the association of exercise with stress reduction described earlier, have been examined.

The concept of physical activity as an element that contributes to the *wholistic*—or *holistic* or *organismic*—well-being of the human organism gained credence near the end of the 20th century. Mechanisms that contribute to the phenomenon include these:

1. Relaxation through reduction of muscle tension
2. Reduction of elevated blood pressure and provision of other cardiopulmonary benefits through the cardiovascular and metabolic enhancement of the oxygen delivery system
3. Advantageous changes in brain chemistry and activity
4. Weight control, particularly changes toward a leaner body mass that contribute to healthy cell metabolism and good organ function

In addition, movement—or physical behavior—is the medium of sensorimotor enhancement. Through movement the individual experiences herself repeatedly over time and develops a sense of validation. The homunculus—or "little person"—that is created in the sensory cortex of the brain is the physical self as experienced and therefore the foundation of self-image. During pregnancy and the postpartum period, when identity is changing dramatically in both physical reality and the psyche, participation in self-creation through movement helps women maintain the connection between their inner and outer selves.

Women who participate in group exercise designed especially for pregnant or postpartum women and their infants also benefit from the support of other women, as described earlier. In addition, the significance of female support in labor is well documented [219, 220]. Whether the benefit derives from the mere reassurance provided by an experienced woman, from a culturally learned ability to be supportive, or from some as yet unquantified attribute of women, the support of women is a clear advantage when one is facing difficult challenges such as becoming a mother.

Increasingly, activity/support groups are being used with pregnant adolescents, adolescent mothers, and disadvantaged women. Much of the work centers on the ability of activity to bind women into a community, enhance their parenting skills, and improve their self-efficacy, as well as to develop physical strength and presence. Outcomes of adolescent mothers involved in parenting programs of this type through their school are excellent, with few low-birth-weight infants, longer spaces between the first and second child than the average for this group, and a tendency to complete at least their high school education [221].

FETAL RESPONSES

As technology improves, we are seeing ever more clearly into the environment in which fetal growth takes place. Is it a safe place? And how does the fetus respond when the mother exerts herself? More answers will be forthcoming, but already some information has been obtained.

Fetal Cardiovascular and Hemodynamic Response

The fetal heart rate normally accelerates but maintains variability during and after exercise [3, 222-228]. A number of factors influence the extent of change in fetal heart rate during and following exercise, among them gestational age and exercise type, intensity, and duration. Accelerations of a few to 20 beats per minute for periods up to 30 to 90 minutes following the exercise session are not uncommon. Reports of greater increases in fetal heart rate (and maternal temperature) after higher-intensity or longer-duration exercise have been noted, but no adverse fetal heart changes [78] in healthy pregnancies. One study notes "signs of transient fetal impairment" including adverse fetal heart and movement changes after very heavy exercise [229]; however, this study employed a different interpretation of exercise levels than other studies.

Improvements in ultrasound technology since the late 1980s have led to an increasingly clearer picture of fetal heart response to exercise. Two studies published in this period shed doubt on prior findings indicating that fetal bradycardia might be a fairly common response to maternal exercise. These studies pointed out that previous research involved the use of Doppler ultrasound to monitor the fetal heart rate, which resulted in recording the maternal cadence on the treadmill or stationary cycle ergometer [3, 230]. As this cadence is often 60 to 80 revolutions per minute, it was commonly mistaken for significant deceleration of the fetal heart or bradycardia. State-of-the-art monitoring now involves the use of ultrasound imaging. Transient fetal bradycardia may occur in a small percentage of cases of maximal exertion, but no ill effects have been observed to date as a result [231]. Two studies documenting fetal bradycardia both involved untrained women in rapidly progressing cycle ergometry near maximal capacity, suggesting that it is possible to induce a reduction in availability of fetal oxygen in the unconditioned population during acute strenuous exertion [3, 232].

Two studies present interesting but difficult-to-interpret findings regarding fetal hemodynamics. Bonnin et al. found slight fetal cerebral vasodilation, which could be due to fetal hemoglobin desaturation, in submaximal maternal exercise, although there was no significant alteration in uterine perfusion [62]. Sjostrom et al. obtained similar findings, with significantly higher PI values in the umbilical artery, significantly lower PI values in the fetal middle cerebral artery, and significantly lower cerebro-umbilical PI ratios, suggesting a shift in blood distribution in favor of the fetal brain in mothers with high trait anxiety scores [233].

Placental Function and Birth Weight

Assuming that uteroplacental function is sufficient, the pattern of maternal activity in the last trimester and the maternal nutritional status probably account for varying reports of birth weight among infants of women who habitually exercise during pregnancy. How much activity a woman undertakes and at what level during the final months of gestation may have a profound effect on birth weight; continuing high-intensity exercisers produce infants with low body fat levels that account for the reduced birth weight (as opposed to small-for-gestational age structure and weight). Women who reduce or cease exercise during the final months—a common tendency—may produce high-weight infants because placental function has been well established and the fetus has little competition for nutrients during the restriction in exercise level. Unpublished data by Clapp substantiate this view: women who exercised at high intensities during the later months of pregnancy gave birth to low body fat infants regardless of whether they had exercised at high or low intensities during the earlier months, while women who exercised at low intensities in the later months gave birth to higher body fat infants regardless of the intensity at which they had exercised earlier [183]. All women in this study who exercised throughout pregnancy had large placentas.

Fetal Movement

Findings concerning fetal body or breathing movements have been small and inconsistent [223, 227, 228]. In group classes, we have found that mothers are most aware of fetal movement during relaxation, at which time they frequently report high levels of fetal activity, or during strength and flexibility activities. There are no reports in the literature of detrimental fetal outcomes in this regard. Interestingly, there is a report that fetuses of mothers with relatively high trait anxiety spent significantly more time in quiet sleep and exhibited less gross body movement when in active sleep in the final weeks of gestation compared to fetuses of mothers with low trait anxiety [234].

Feto-Protections

Clearly, many mechanisms that protect the fetus are at work in pregnancy. In addition, although this might seem counterintuitive, many of the mechanisms of vigorous exercise also appear to protect the fetus. Cardiovascular, thermoregulatory, metabolic, and respiratory responses seem to enhance the environment in which the fetus grows.

PREGNANCY OUTCOMES

Many magnificent physiological adaptations occur in pregnancy, which the body perceives as work. In response to the demands of the developing fetus in a normal pregnancy, the body increases blood volume; raises resting heart rate; increases stroke volume; strengthens the heart muscle; reduces vascular tension; increases vasculature, ventilation, and respiration; and changes the glycemic response to favor energy conservation. These adaptations are protective mechanisms to ensure that the fetus is supplied with necessary nutrients. Some of these adaptations are also present in the body's response to sustained exercise, athletics, or dance, which are also perceived by the body as work. An exception is the resting heart rate, which normally decreases during the conditioning process in the nonpregnant population.

The prevailing view in medicine and exercise physiology, based on current and historically relevant research, is that maternal adaptations of pregnancy, including changes in cardiovasculature, hemodynamics, metabolism, acid-base balance, thermoregulation, respiration, and biomechanics, can be augmented by regular moderate exercise without fetal detriment [235-240]. The physical gains in strength, endurance, flexibility, and motor control that accrue through exercise, coupled with associated gains in self-awareness, confidence, mental discipline, and attention to healthy behavior (good hydration and nutrition, avoidance of smoking or drugs), predictably result in physically and mentally enabled individuals. The physiological processes that elicit these attributes account for the benefits of exercise in the childbearing period.

During a well-designed moderate- to high-intensity exercise program, the ability of the body to deliver and use oxygen and nutrients, and to move with strength, elasticity, balance, coordination, and efficiency, improves a great deal. As a result of this training effect, the body is not stressed very much when working at a lower intensity. This is a considerable benefit in sustaining low- to moderate-intensity ultradistance endurance activities such as pregnancy, labor, birth, and nursing.

Early-Pregnancy Outcomes

Regular exercise can also enhance feto-protective mechanisms, providing there is no uteroplacental insufficiency or life-threatening disorder. There is no evidence that exercise contributes to congenital anomalies, spontaneous abortion, placental abruption, IUGR, PIH, or fetal demise [236, 241]. Rather, there may be a slight protective factor for some of these conditions [242].

Birth Outcomes

Women who participate in regular exercise throughout their pregnancies report lower levels of perceived exertion during pregnancy and labor, experience less discomfort, and recover more quickly than those who do not exercise or who stop exercising during pregnancy [243]. Findings concerning length of labor, cesarean rates, birth weight, and Apgar scores are mixed, as shown in table 6.1 [244-249]. While discrepancies undoubtedly result in part from differences in methodology among studies, it is the case that birthing practices vary from place to place and that these variations explain some of the differences found from study to study. At one Illinois hospital, for example, it was shown that given certain labor situations, cesarean rates varied among physicians from 19% to 42% [250]. Thus it can be difficult to measure the effect of an activity regimen on the cesarean rate. However, two of the studies in table 6.1 do demonstrate highly significant differences in cesarean rates between nonexercise controls and high-intensity recreational exercisers [246, 247] that are difficult to ignore. Also, a recent study on aerobic exercise participation during the first two trimesters and type of delivery in first-time mothers demonstrated that sedentary women were 4.5 times as likely as the exercising mothers to deliver by cesarean [251].

In practice, the author and her colleagues have noted a cesarean rate among our local group prenatal exercise participants significantly below local hospital rates over a 15-year period of tracking these rates. While these are not publishable data, they are significant and consistent enough to reassure those who inquire into the safety of our local programs. Collection of this information on a nationwide basis is under way for all programs developed under our auspices, as is collection of other birth-related information such as episiotomy and epidural rates, use of forceps, augmented induction of labor, and length of hospital stay. Any scientific inquiry into these rates is complicated and difficult, and perhaps not truly feasible given the effect of local birthing practices.

Neonatal and Infant Outcomes

Preliminary evidence also suggests that fetal heart rate abnormalities, cord entanglement, and the presence of meconium and erythropoietin levels are significantly reduced for babies of exercising women [236, 242, 252, 253]. Because these conditions are classic signs of hypoxia, or fetal distress, in labor, it would appear that regular prenatal exercise could potentially be used to lower the incidence of fetal distress. In addition, although there is no increase in gestations of less than 260 days, there may be less postdate gestations [242, 254]. The incidence of low Apgar scores is reduced among infants of exercising mothers, and there is no indication of neurological or physical deficit [242, 255, 256]. The Apgar score is a rating given to a newborn at 1 and 5 minutes after birth with respect to color, cry, muscle tone, respirations, and reflexes (0 to 2 points for each of the five items). The higher the score, the better the condition of the newborn. Clapp has shown that although women who engage in high levels of endurance exercise during pregnancy may have infants whose birth weight is reduced compared to controls, most of that reduction is due to low body fat, not stature [257]. The head circumferences and lengths of these infants are normal. Further, Clapp has published data demonstrating that in the group he followed through the first year of infancy, all morphometric parameters were similar and there were no significant differences in psychomotor or mental scales between the two groups (exercising mothers and controls) of 1-year-olds [258].

Clapp has also published research concerning morphometrics and psychomotor and mental function of 5-year-olds whose mothers had or had not exercised during pregnancy. The data showed that motor, integrative,

Table 6.1   Research Findings Regarding Exercise and Labor Outcomes

Author(s)	Focus	Length of labor/stage	Cesarean rate(s)	Birth weight*	Apgar
Pfeifer 1951 [244]	Effect of athletics on outcomes	Fit women have shorter labors.	N/A	N/A	N/A
Pomerance, et al. 1974 [245]	Effect of fitness on outcome	Fit women have shorter labors.	N/A	N/A	N/A
Hall and Kaufmann 1987 [246]	Effect of level of fitness on outcome	No significant difference between exercisers and controls.	Control: 28.1% Low exercise level: 23.1% Medium exercise level: 19.0% High exercise level: 6.7%	3,359 3,471 3,445 3,510	1 min: 8.6 5 min: 9.3 1 min: 8.8 5 min: 9.1 1 min: 8.7 5 min: 9.5 1 min: 8.9 5 min: 9.6
Clapp 1990 [247]	Effect of running/ aerobics on outcome	*Mean active (> 4 cm) labor:* Control: 382 min Exercisers: 264 min *Mean active first stage:* Control: 302 min Exercisers: 223 min	Control: 30% Exercisers: 6%	3,776 3,369	1 min: <7/25% 1 min: <7/14%
Botkin and Driscoll 1991 [248]	Effect of aerobic exercise on outcome	No difference in first or third stages. *Second stage:* Control: 59 min Exercisers: 27 min	N/A	†	†
Kardell and Kase 1998 [249]	Compare high-intensity vs. medium-intensity training	High-intensity exercise results in longer labors.	N/A	†	†
Bungum, et al. 2000 [251]	Effect of aerobic exercise on type of delivery in first-time mothers	N/A	Odds of cesarean for sedentary women are 4.5 times greater than for those who exercised in first 2 trimesters.	N/A	N/A

* Mean weight in grams.
† No significant difference.

and academic readiness skills of the children of exercising mothers were similar to those of controls, but that the offspring of exercising mothers performed significantly better on the Wechsler Preschool and Primary Scale of Intelligence-Revised test and tests of oral language skills [259]. The interpretation of this information is tricky, however. Results could be strongly influenced by the lifestyle of mothers who choose to exercise regularly and vigorously, including the mother's nurturing style, the child's interaction with other significant adults such as care providers or grandparents, or attention to diet.

Other factors might include genetics, as well as the influence of motion and sound on the fetus in utero while the mother is exercising.

Maternal Benefits

Information concerning maternal adaptations and benefits was presented earlier in the chapter. There are, however, a couple of other pieces of information to consider. One is that weight-bearing exercise during adolescence and the childbearing years is highly protective of bone density in the postmenopausal years and thus preventative for osteoporosis. Although direct information is lacking, there is no reason to suspect that exercising pregnant or postpartum women fall outside this parameter, provided they have adequate calcium and vitamin D in their diets. Another, similar issue is cancer prevention. Clearly the childbearing years play a significant role in the additive effect of healthy behaviors that are instrumental in preventing cancer.

Physical Conditioning for Labor

If it can be conclusively shown that compared to a non-fitness approach, physical fitness enhances a woman's potential for a labor that is less noxious, requires fewer interventions of medical technology, and provides her with more coping skills that empower her in her birth, this information will be of great interest to the public health sector and health insurance industry. The network of professionals who work in this area continue to pursue improving prenatal exercise programs in part because they see the effects of their work with participants, who are almost universally grateful for a physical fitness preparation for labor, birth, and recovery.

Most of the information available on the advantages of prenatal exercise comes from research on women who are fit and healthy prior to conception and who maintain fitness and a healthy lifestyle throughout their pregnancies. The extent to which women who are sedentary prior to their pregnancies can benefit from a supervised exercise regimen, and at what level of activity, is under investigation [242, 260]; but clearly, physical conditioning is possible. One study demonstrates that previously sedentary women benefit from aerobic conditioning, showing increases in maximal aerobic power and submaximal duration, as well as preservation of anaerobic working capacity in late gestation [260]. All these effects are valuable assets during the prolonged, low-intensity endurance test of the first stage of labor followed by the strength test of the second (pushing or expulsion) stage.

Pain Management

Persons who participate in regular exercise, athletics, or dance demonstrate psychophysiological adaptations, including a sense of well-being, as discussed previously. Another adaptation can be relief from discomfort [261, 262]. Two factors appear to play significant roles in this phenomenon. First, brain chemistry has a role in the mitigation of what is commonly referred to as *pain*. Secondly, the self-efficacy of persons with extensive experience of their bodily sensations in physical activity affects how they use this information to improve their performance or achieve their goals.

Pain is an interesting phenomenon. Jessell and Kelly remark on the confusion between the terms *nociception* and *pain*. Nociception is the reception of signals in the central nervous system activated by neural receptors that provide information about tissue damage; *pain* is a more pervasive somatosensory experience that signals danger and contains a high emotional content based on experience and environment [263]. Nociception is also modulated by descending pathway activity, so that the perception of what we call pain is a complex series of neurological and cognitive responses. Jessell and Kelly detail three avenues of effective pain treatment that follow from current understanding of the phenomenon of pain. First, recognition that the balance of activity in large and small fibers is a contributory factor in transmission of pain signals has led to the use of dorsal column (certain ascending pathways) and transcutaneous electrical nerve stimulation for some peripheral pain. Second, the finding that stimulation of specific brain sites produces an analgesic effect is leading to better methods of controlling pain through activation of endogenous chemical systems. And third, the discovery that opiates applied directly to the spine have a powerful analgesic effect has led to the use of intrathecal and epidural applications of opiates.

The role of physical activity in this area relates largely to the second finding, that concerning stimulation of endogenous relief. The presence of naturally occurring beta-endorphins as a response to certain types of exertion is an example. At present, it appears that the level of beta-endorphins, while somewhat stimulated by the aerobic component of exercise, is primarily stimulated by fatigue, discomfort, and/or anaerobic activity [264]. Clearly, genetics and components of exercise other than aerobic fitness play fundamental roles in the capacity of the exerciser to deal mentally with noxious sensation.

A survey published in 1978 sheds light on how the ability to deal constructively with pain may work. In comparing average marathon runners with exceptional marathon runners, W.P. Morgan discovered that the average runners tended to dissociate from their bodies, while the exceptional runners tended to associate with their body sensations [265]. The average marathoners created elaborate schemes (e.g., designing and constructing buildings) to distract themselves from discomfort, often fearing *the wall*—the 20-mile mark in the 26-mile race where many runners experience severe distress. The exceptional runners, on the other hand, claimed that *the wall* was a myth and that you ran into it only if you weren't paying attention to your body, monitoring its discomforts, staying relaxed, and making necessary adjustments in your form.

A culture that does little to differentiate sensation beyond the distinction between pain and pleasure puts its members at a disadvantage. From such a standpoint, if a sensation is not immediately pleasurable, the only other choice is pain. In fact, though, a great many other bits of information may be involved (such as pressure, falling, lengthening, speed, or balance) that—if the mental environment were willing—could be interpreted without the emotional tag of pain. What one person might call a *pain,* a highly skilled athlete or dancer might call a *tight spot* or *tense area*—and then the highly skilled person might make some adjustment in form to relieve the discomfort. This capacity to sense, compute, and modify movement is an aspect of the phenomenon of *attention* [266]. By directing attention to goals of being relaxed, fluid, and balanced and achieving the desired movement (such as releasing a baby from one's body), it is possible to acquire the mental state that promotes ease of movement even under difficult circumstances [187, 267-269].

Recreational physical activity, like childbirth, involves sensations that are brought on in a voluntary way. Research on women's views of fulfillment in the birth process supports the theory that sensation associated with difficult but purposive physical events may bear the title *pain,* but has a different emotional content than pain associated with nonvoluntary body trauma [270]. All of this information, taken together, points to mindful movement as an important exercise element of the physical preparation for birth.

REFERENCES

1. Zhang, J., and Savitz, D.A. 1996. Exercise during pregnancy among US women. *Annals of Epidemiology* 6(1):53-59.
2. McGinnis, J.M. 1992. The public health burden of a sedentary lifestyle. *Medicine and Science in Sports and Exercise* 4:S196-S200.
3. Carpenter, M.W., Sady, S.P., Hoegsberg, B., Sady, M.A., Haydon, B., Cullinane, E.M., Coustan, D.R., and Thompson, P.D. 1988. Fetal heart rate response to maternal exertion. *Journal of the American Medical Association* 259:3006-3009.
4. Clapp, J.F. 3rd, and Dickstein, S. 1984. Endurance exercise and pregnancy outcome. *Medicine and Science in Sports and Exercise* 16(6):556-562.
5. Clapp, J.F. 3rd, and Rizk, K. 1992. Effect of recreational exercise on midtrimester placental growth. *American Journal of Obstetrics and Gynecology* 167(6):1518-1521.
6. Jackson, M.R., Gott, P., Lyle, S.F., Ritchie, J.W., and Clapp, J.F. 3rd. 1995. The effects of maternal aerobic exercise on human placental development: Placental volumetric composition and surface areas. *Placenta* 16(2):179-191.
7. Clapp, J.F., et al. 2000. Beginning regular exercise in early pregnancy: Effect on fetoplacental growth. *American Journal of Obstetrics and Gynecology* 183:1484-1488.
8. Robson, S.C., Hunter, S., Boys R., and Dunlop, W. 1989. Serial study of factors influencing changes in cardiac output during human pregnancy. *American Journal of Physiology* 256:H1060-H1065.
9. Artal, R., Wiswell, R., Romem, Y., and Dorey, F. 1986. Pulmonary responses to exercise in pregnancy. *American Journal of Obstetrics and Gynecology* 154:378-383.
10. Lotgering, F.K., Van Doorne, M.B., Struijk, P.C., Pool, J., and Wallenburg, H.C. 1991. Maximal aerobic exercise in pregnant women: Heart rate, O2 consumption, CO2 production, and ventilation. *Journal of Applied Physiology* 70:1016-1023.
11. McMurray, R.G., Hackney, A.C., Katz, V.L., Gall, M., and Watson, W.J. 1991. Pregnancy-induced changes in the maximal physiological responses during swimming. *Journal of Applied Physiology* 71:1454-1459.
12. Morton, M., Paul, M., Campos, G., Hart, M.V., and Metcalfe, J. 1985. Exercise dynamics in late gestation: Effects of physical training. *American Journal of Obstetrics and Gynecology* 152:91-97.
13. Pivarnik, J.M., Lee, W., Clark, S.L., Cotton, D.B., Spillman, H.T., and Miller, J.F. 1990. Cardiac output responses of primigravid women during exercise determined by the direct Fick technique. *Obstetrics and Gynecology* 75:954-959.
14. Ueland, K., Novy, M.J., Peterson, E.N., and Metcalfe, J. 1969. Maternal cardiovascular dynamics IV. The influence of gestational age on the maternal cardiovascular response to posture and exercise. *American Journal of Obstetrics and Gynecology* 104:856-864.
15. Khodiguian, N., Jaque-Fortunato, S.V., Wiswell, R., and Artal, R. 1996. A comparison of cross-sectional and longitudinal methods of assessing the influence of pregnancy on cardiac function during exercise. *Seminars in Perinatology* 20(4):232-241.
16. Sady, S.P., Carpenter, M.W., Sady, M.A., Haydon, B., Hoegsberg, B., Cullinane, E.M., Thompson, P.D., and Coustan, D.R. 1988. Prediction of VO$_2$max during cycle exercise in pregnant women. *Journal of Applied Physiology* 65:657-661.
17. Sady, S.P., Carpenter, M.W., Thompson, P.D., Sady, M.A., Haydon, B., and Coustan, D.R. 1989. Cardiovascular response to cycle exercise during and after pregnancy. *Journal of Applied Physiology* 66:336-341.
18. Sady, M.A., Hadon, B.B., Sady, S.P., Carpenter, M.W., Thompson, P.D., and Coustan, D.R. 1990. Cardiovascular response to maximal cycle exercise during pregnancy at two and seven months post partum. *American Journal of Obstetrics and Gynecology* 162:1181-1185.
19. Clapp, J.F. 3rd, Seaward, B.L., Sleamaker, R.H., and Hiser, J. 1988. Maternal physiologic adaptations to early human pregnancy. *American Journal of Obstetrics and Gynecology* 159:1456-1460.
20. Rees, G.B., Pipkin, F.B., Symonds, E.M., Patrick, J.M. 1990. A longitudinal study of respiratory changes in normal human pregnancy with cross-sectional data on subjects with pregnancy-induced hypertension. *American Journal of Obstetrics and Gynecology* 115:4-10.
21. Knuttgen, H.G., and Emerson, K. 1974. Physiological responses to pregnancy at rest and during exercise. *Journal of Applied Physiology* 36:549-553.
22. Guzman, C.A., and Caplan, R. 1970. Cardiorespiratory response to exercise during pregnancy. *American Journal of Obstetrics and Gynecology* 108:600-605.
23. Carpenter, M.W., Sady, S.P., Sady, M.A., Haydon, B., Coustan, D.R., and Thompson, P.D. 1990. Effect of maternal weight gain during pregnancy on exercise performance. *Journal of Applied Physiology* 68:1173-1176.
24. Ueland, K., Novy, M.J., and Metcalfe, J. 1973. Cardiorespiratory responses to pregnancy and exercise in normal women and patients with heart disease. *American Journal of Obstetrics and Gynecology* 115:4-10.
25. Bader, R.A., Bader, M.E., Rose, D.J., and Braunwald, E. 1955. Hemodynamics at rest and during exercise in normal pregnancy as studied by cardiac catheterization. *Journal of Clinical Investigation* 34:1524-1536.
26. Spatling, L., Fallenstein, F., Huch, A., Huch, R., and Rooth, G. 1992. The variability of cardiopulmonary adaptation to pregnancy at rest and during exercise. *British Journal of Obstetrics and Gynecology* 99 (Suppl 8):1-40.

27. Capeless, E.L., and Clapp, J.F. 3rd. 1989. Cardiovascular changes in early phase of pregnancy. *American Journal of Obstetrics and Gynecology* 161:1449 1453.

28. Epstein, M., Norsk, P. Loutzenhier, R., and Aonke, P. 1987. Detailed characterization of a tank used for head-out water immersion in humans. *Journal of Applied Physiology* 63:869-871.

29. Epstein, M. 1984. Renal, endocrine and hemodynamic effects of water immersion in man. *Contributions to Nephrology* 41:174-188.

30. Epstein, M., Miller, M., and Schneider, N. 1974. Depth of immersion as a determinant of the natriuresis of water immersion. *Proceedings of the Society for Experimental Biology and Medicine* 146:562-566.

31. Epstein, M., Duncan, D.C., and Fishman, L.M. 1972. Characterization of the natriuresis caused in normal man by immersion in water. *Clinical Science* 43:275-287.

32. Miki, K., Pazik, M.M., Krasney, E., Hong, S.K., and Krasney, J.A. 1987. Thoracic duct lymph flow during head-out water immersion in conscious dogs. *American Journal of Physiology* 252:782-785.

33. Svedenhag, J., and Seger, J. 1992. Running on land and in water: Comparative exercise physiology. *Medicine and Science in Sports and Exercise* 10:1155-1160.

34. Katz, W.J., McMurray, R., Goodwin, W.E., and Cefalo, R.C. 1990. Nonweightbearing exercise during pregnancy on land and during immersion: A comparative study. *American Journal of Perinatology* 7:281-284.

35. Clark. S.L., Cotton, D.B., Pivarnik, J.M., Lee, W., Hankins, G.D., Benedetti, T.J., and Phelan, J.P. 1991. Position change and central hemodynamic profile during normal third-trimester pregnancy and postpartum. *American Journal of Obstetrics and Gynecology* 164(3):883-887.

36. Nesler, C.L., Hassett, S.L., Cary, S., and Brooke, J. 1988. Effects of supine exercise on fetal heart rate in the second and third trimester. *American Journal of Perinatology* 5(2):159-163.

37. Cowlin, A.F. (ed). 1996. *Dancing Thru Pregnancy and AfterDance Perinatal Health and Fitness Instructors' Manuals*. Stony Creek, CT: DTP.

38. Avery, N.D., Stocking, K.D., Tranmer, J.E., Davies, G.A., and Wolfe, L.A. 1999. Fetal responses to maternal strength conditioning exercises in late gestation. *Canadian Journal of Applied Physiology* 24(4):362-376.

39. Yeo, S., Steele, N.M., Chang, M.C., Leclaire, S.M., Ronis, D.L., and Hayashi, R. 2000. The effect of exercise on blood pressure in pregnant women with a high risk of gestational hypertensive disorders. *Journal of Reproductive Medicine* 45(4):293-298.

40. Newman, V., and Fullerton, J.T. 1990. The role of nutrition in the prevention of preeclampsia. Review of the literature. *Journal of Nurse Midwifery* 35(5):282-291.

41. Sibai, B.M., Gordon, T., Thom, E., Caritis, S.N., Klebanoff, M., McNellis, D., and Paul, R.H. 1995. Risk factors for preeclampsia in healthy nulliparous women: A prospective study. *American Journal of Obstetrics and Gynecology* 172:642-648.

42. Williams, M.A., Zingheim, R.W., and King, I.B. 1995. Omega-3 fatty acids in maternal erythrocytes and risk of preeclampsia. *Epidemiology* 6(3):232-237.

43. Bucher, H.C., Guyatt, G.H., Cook, R.J., Hatala, R., Cook, D.J., Lang, J.D., and Hunt, D. 1996. Effect of calcium supplementation on pregnancy-induced hypertension and preeclampsia: A meta-analysis of randomized controlled trials. *Journal of the American Medical Association* 275:1114-1117.

44. Purwar, M., Kilkarni, H., Motghare, V., and Dhole, S. 1996. Calcium supplementation and prevention of pregnancy induced hypertension. *Journal of Obstetrics and Gynecology Research* 22:425-430.

45. Carroli, G., Duley, L., Belizan, J.M., and Villar, J. 1994. Calcium supplementation during pregnancy: A systematic review of randomized controlled trials. *British Journal of Obstetrics and Gynecology* 101:753-758.

46. Ito, M., Koyama, H., Ohshige, A., Maede, T., Yoshimura, T., and Okamura, H. 1994. Prevention of preeclampsia with calcium supplementation and vitamin D3 in an antenatal protocol. *International Journal of Gynaecology and Obstetrics* 47:115-120.

47. Belizan, J., and Villar, J. 1980. The relationship between calcium intake and edema, proteinuria and hypertension-gestosis: An hypothesis. *The American Journal of Clinical Nutrition* 33:2202.

48. Levine, R.J., Hauth, J.C., Curet, L.B., Sibai, B.M., Catalano, P.M., Morris, C.D., DerSimonian, R., Esterlitz, J.R., Raymond, E.G., Bild, D.E., Clemens, J.D., and Cutler, J.A. 1997. Trial of calcium to prevent preeclampsia. *New England Journal of Medicine* 337(2):69-76.

49. Sanchez-Ramoz, L., Adair, C.D., Kaunitz, A.M., Brianes, D.K., DelValle, G.D. and Delke, I. 1995. Calcium supplementation in mild preeclampsia remote from term: A randomized double-blind clinical trial. *Obstetrics and Gynecology* 85:915-918.

50. Longo, L.D., et al. 1978. To what extent does maternal exercise affect fetal oxygenation and uterine blood flow? *Science Abstracts, 25th Annual Meeting of the Society for Gynecologic Investigation*, p. 7 (or Federation Proceedings 37:905.).

51. Lotgering, F.K., Gilbert, R.D., and Longo, L.D. 1983. Exercise responses in pregnant sheep: Oxygen consumption, uterine blood flow and blood volume. *Journal of Applied Physiology* 55:834-841.

52. Baumann, H., Huch, A., and Huch, R. 1989. Doppler sonographic evaluation of exercise-induced blood flow velocity and waveform changes in fetal, uteroplacental and large maternal vessels in pregnant women. *Journal of Perinatal Medicine* 17:279-287.

53. Morrow, R.J., Ritchie, J.W.K., Bull, S.B. 1989. Fetal and maternal hemodynamics response to exercise in pregnancy assessed by Doppler ultrasound. *American Journal of Obstetrics and Gynecology* 160:138 140.

54. Erkkola, R.U., Pirhonen, J.P., and Kivijarvi, A.K. 1992. Flow velocity waveforms in uterine and umbilical arteries during submaximal bicycle exercise in normal pregnancy. *Obstetrics and Gynecology* 79:611-615.

55. Hackett, G.A., Cohen-Overbeek, T., and Campbell, S. 1992. The effect of exercise on uteroplacental Doppler waveforms in normal and complicated pregnancies. *Obstetrics and Gynecology* 79:919-923.

56. Asakura, H., Nakai, A., Yamaguchi, M., Koshino, T., and Araki, T. 1994. Ultrasonographic blood flow velocimetry in maternal and umbilical arteries during maternal exercise. *Acta Obstetrica et Gynaecologia Japonica* 46:308-314.

57. Veille, J.C., Bacevice, A.E., Wilson, B., et al. 1989. Umbilical artery waveforms during bicycle exercise in normal pregnancy. *Obstetrics and Gynecology* 73:957-996.

58. Veille, J.C. 1996. Maternal and fetal cardiovascular response to exercise during pregnancy. *Seminars in Perinatology* 20(4):250-262.

59. Pivarnik, J.M., Mauer, M.B., Ayres, N.A., Kirshon, B., Dildy, G.A., and Cotton, D.B. 1994. Effects of chronic exercise on blood volume expansion and hematologic indices during pregnancy. *Obstetrics and Gynecology* 83(2):265-269.

60. Clapp, J.F. 3rd. 1994. The athletic woman: A clinical approach to exercise during pregnancy. *Clinics in Sports Medicine* 13(2):443-458.

61. Clapp, J.F. 3rd. 1994. Exercise in pregnancy and the postpartum period: Review of research findings on maternal and fetal outcome, *Perinatal Health and Fitness Network Lecture Series*, New Haven, CT, Yale-New Haven Hospital, June 25, 1994.

62. Bonnin, P., Bazzi-Grossin, C., Ciraru-Vigneron, N., Bailliart, O., Kedra, A.W., Savin, E., Ravina, J.H., and Martineaud, J.P. 1997. Evidence of fetal cerebral vasodilation induced by submaximal maternal exercise in human pregnancy. *Journal of Perinatal Medicine* 25(1):63-70.

63. Clapp, J.F., Stepanchak, W., Tomaselli, J., Kortan, M., and Faneslow, S. 2000. Portal vein blood flow—effects of pregnancy, gravity and exercise. *American Journal of Obstetrics and Gynecology* 183(1):167-172.

64. Clapp, J.F. 1989. Oxygen consumption during treadmill exercise before, during, and after pregnancy. *American Journal of Obstetrics and Gynecology* 161(6):1458-1464.

65. Clark, S.L., Cotton, D.B., Lee, W., Bishop, C., Hill, T., Southwick, J., Pivarnik, J., Spillman, T., DeVore, G.R., and Phelan, J. 1989. Central hemodynamic assessment of normal term pregnancy. *American Journal of Obstetrics and Gynecology* 161(6):1439-1442.

66. Lotgering, F.K., Struijk, P.C., van Doorn, M.B., and Wallenburg, H.C. 1992. Errors in predicting maximal oxygen consumption in pregnant women. *Journal of Applied Physiology* 72(2):562-567.

67. McMurray, R.G., Hackney, A.C., Katz, V.L., Gall, M., and Watson, W.J. 1991. Pregnancy-induced changes in the maximal physiological responses during swimming. *Journal of Applied Physiology* 71(4):1454-1459.

68. Pivarnik, J.M., Lee, W., Clark, S.L., Cotton, D.B., Spillman, H.T., and Miller, J.F. 1990. Cardiac output responses of primigravid women during exercise determination by the direct Fick technique. *Obstetrics and Gynecology* 75:954-959.

69. van Doorn, M.B., Lotgering, F.K., Struijk, P.C., Pool, J., and Wallenburg, H.C. 1992. Maternal and fetal cardiovascular responses to strenuous bicycle exercise. *American Journal of Obstetrics and Gynecology* 166(3):854-859.

70. Saltin, B., Blomqvist, G., Mitchell, J.H., Johnson, R.L. Jr., Wildenthal, K., and Chapman, C.B. 1968. Response to exercise after bed rest and after training. *Circulation* 38 (Suppl II):1-78.

71. Maloni, J.A., et al. 1993. Physical and psychosocial side effects of antepartum hospital bed rest. *Nursing Research* 42(4):197.

72. Schroeder, C.A. 1996. Women's experience of bed rest in high-risk pregnancy. *Image* 28(3):253-258.

73. Vanheest, J.L., and Rodgers, C.D. 1997. Effects of exercise on diabetic rats before and during gestation on maternal and neonatal outcomes. *American Journal of Physiology* 273(4, Pt. 1):E727-E733.

74. Houghton, P.E., Mottola, M.F., Messapelli, J., Vandermolen, R., and Christopher, P.D. 1997. Glycogen storage in fetuses of trained pregnant rats. *Canadian Journal of Applied Physiology* 22(4):384-393.

75. Edwards, M.J. 1986. Hyperthermia as a teratogen: A review of experimental studies and their clinical significance. *Teratogenesis, Carcinogenesis, and Mutagenesis* 6(6):563-582.

76. Milunsky, A., Ulcickas, M., Rothman, K.J., Willett, W., Jick, S.S., and Jick, H. 1992. Maternal heat exposure and neural tube defects. *Journal of the American Medical Association* 268:882-885.

77. Artal-Mittlemark, R., Wiswell, R., Drinkwater, B. (eds.). 1990. *Exercise in pregnancy*, 2nd ed. Baltimore: Williams & Wilkins.

78. O'Neill, M.E. 1996. Maternal rectal temperature and fetal heart rate response to upright cycling in later pregnancy. *British Journal of Sports Medicine* 30(1):32-35.

79. Clapp, J.F., Wesley, M., and Sleamaker, R.H. 1987. Thermoregulatory and metabolic responses to jogging prior to and during pregnancy. *Medicine and Science in Sports and Exercise* 19:124-130.

80. McMurray, R.G., Katz, V.L., Meyer-Goodwin, W.E., and Cefalo, R.C. 1993. Thermoregulation of pregnant women during aerobic exercise on land and in the water. *American Journal of Perinatology* 10(2):178-182.

81. Mitchell, J.B., Costill, D.L., Houmard, J.A., Flynn, M.G., Fink, W.J., and Beltz, J.D. 1984. Effects of carbohydrate ingestion on gastric emptying and exercise performance. *Medicine and Science in Sports and Exercise* 20(2):110-115.

82. Clapp, J.F., and Capeless, E.L. 1991. The changing glycemic response to exercise during pregnancy. *American Journal of Obstetrics and Gynecology* 156 (6 pt 1):1678-1683.

83. Avery, M.D., and Rossi, M.A. 1994. Gestational diabetes. *Journal of Nurse-Midwifery* 39(2 Suppl):9S-19S.

84. Tremblay, A. 1992. Human obesity: A defect in lipid oxidation or in thermogenesis. *International Journal of Obesity* 16:953-957.

85. Metzger, B.E., and Freinkel, N. 1978. Effects of diabetes mellitus in the endocrinologic and the metabolic adaptation of gestation. *Seminars in Perinatology* 2:309-318.

86. Varney, H. 1996. *Varney's midwifery*, 3rd ed. New York: Jones & Barlett, p. 353.

87. Bung, P., Bung, C., Artal, R., Khodiguian, N., Fallenstein, F., and Spatling, L. 1993. Therapeutic exercise for insulin-requiring gestational diabetics—Results of a randomized prospective longitudinal study. *Journal of Perinatal Medicine* 21:125-137.

88. Jovanovic-Peterson, L., Durak, E.P., and Peterson, C.M. 1989. Randomized trial of diet versus diet plus cardiovascular conditioning on glucose levels in gestational diabetes. *American Journal of Obstetrics and Gynecology* 161:415.

89. Sandoval-Rodiriguez, T., Partida-Hernandez, C.G., and Arreola-Ortiz, F. 1997. Diabetes mellitus. Exercise and pregnancy [Spanish]. *Ginecologia Y Obstetricia de Mexico* 65:478-481.

90. Metzger, B.E. 1991. Summary and recommendations of the Third International Workshop-Conference on gestational diabetes mellitus. *Diabetes* 40:197-201.

91. Jovanovic-Peterson, L., and Peterson, C.M. 1996. Exercise and the nutritional management of diabetes during pregnancy. *Obstetrics and Gynecology Clinics of North America* 23(1):75-86.

92. Weller, K.A. 1996. Diagnosis and management of gestational diabetes. *American Family Physician* 53(6):2053-57, 61-62.

93. Bung, P., and Artal, A. 1996. Gestational diabetes and exercise: A survey. *Seminars in Perinatology* 20(4):328-333.

94. Bjorntorp, P., Fahlen, M., Grimby, G., Gustafson, A., Holm, J., Renstrom, P., and Schersten, T. 1972. The effects of physical training and acute physical work on plasma insulin in obesity. *European Journal of Clinical Investigation* 2:274-278.

95. Pederson, O., Beck-Nielson, H., and Heding, L. 1980. Increased insulin receptors after exercise in patients with diabetes mellitus. *New England Journal of Medicine* 302:886-892.

96. Burstein, R., Polychronakos, C., Toews, C.J., et al. 1985. Acute reversal of the enhanced insulin action in trained athletes. *Diabetes* 34:756-760.

97. DeFonzo, R.A., Sherwin, R.S., and Kraemer, N. 1987. Effect of physical training on insulin action in obesity. *Diabetes* 36:1379-1385.

98. Bogardus, C., Ravussin, E. Robbins, D.C., Wolfe, R.R., Horton, E.G., and Sims, E.A. 1984. Effects of physical training and diet therapy on carbohydrate metabolism in patients with glucose intolerance and non-insulin-dependent diabetes mellitus. *Diabetes* 33:311-318.

99. Magee, M.S., Walden, C.E., and Benedetti, T.J. 1993. Influence of diagnostic criteria on the incidence of gestational diabetes and perinatal morbidity. *Journal of the American Medical Association* 270:324.

100. Artal, R., Masaki, D.I., Khodiguian, N., Romem, H., Rutherford, S.E., and Wiswell, R.A. 1986. Exercise prescription in pregnancy: Weight bearing versus non weight bearing exercise. *American Journal of Obstetrics and Gynecology* 140:1464-1469.

101. Clapp, J.F. 3rd, and Little, K.D. 1995. Effect of recreational exercise on pregnancy weight gain and subcutaneous fat deposition. *Medicine and Science in Sports and Exercise* 27(2):170-177.

102. Hatch, M.C., Shu, X.O., McLean, D.E., Levin, B., Begg, M., Reuss, L., and Susser, M. 1993. Maternal exercise during pregnancy, physical fitness and fetal growth. *American Journal of Epidemiology* 137(10); 1105-1114.

103. Collings, C.A., Curet, L.B., and Mullin, J.P. 1983. Maternal and fetal responses to a maternal exercise program. *American Journal of Obstetrics and Gynecology* 145:702-707.

104. Kulpa, P.J., White, B.M., and Visscher, R. 1987. Aerobic exercise in pregnancy. *American Journal of Obstetrics and Gynecology* 156:1395-1403.

105. Clapp, J.F., and Kiess, W. 2000. Effects of pregnancy and exercise on concentrations of the metabolic markers tumor necrosis factor alpha and leptin. *American Journal of Obstetrics and Gynecology* 182(2):300-306.

106. Gutersohn, A., Naber, C., Muller, N., Erbel, R., and Siffert, W. 2000. G protein beta3 subunit 825 TT genotype and post-pregnancy weight retention [letter]. *Lancet* 355(9211):1240-1241.

107. Dye, T.D., Knox, K.L., Artal, R., Aubry, R.H., and Wojtowycs, M.A. 1997. Physical activity, obesity and diabetes in pregnancy. *American Journal of Epidemiology* 146(11); 961-965.

108. Briend, A. 1980. Maternal physical activity, birth weight and perinatal mortality. *Medical Hypotheses* 6:1157-1170.

109. Pinard, A. 1895. Note pour servir a l'historie dee la puericulture intrauterine. *Annales de Gynaecologiae et d'Ob* 44:417-422.

110. Letourneur, L. 1897. *De l'influence de la profession de la mere sur le poids de l'enfant.* These, Paris.

111. Peller, S. 1917. Langenewichtverhaltnis der neugeborenen und einfluss der schwangerenernahrung auf die entwicklung des foetus. *Deutsche Medizinische Wochenschrift* 43:847-848.

112. Erkkola, R. 1976. The physical work capacity of the expectant mother and its effect on pregnancy, labour and the newborn. *International Journal of Gynecology and Obstetrics* 14:153-159.

113. Hytten, F.E. 1991. Weight gain in pregnancy. In F. Hytten and G. Chamberlain (eds.), *Clinical physiology in obstetrics.* Oxford: Blackwell Scientific.

114. Durnin, J.V.G.A. 1987. Energy requirements of pregnancy: An integration of the longitudinal data from the five-country study. *Lancet* 2:1131-1133.

115. Naeye, R.L., and Peters, E.C. 1982. Working during pregnancy: Effects on the fetus. *Pediatrics* 69:724-727.

116. Hatch, M.C., Shu, X.O., McLean, D.E., Levin, B., Begg, M., Reuss, L. and Susser, M. 1993. Maternal exercise during pregnancy, physical fitness and fetal growth. *American Journal of Epidemiology* 137(10):1105-1114.

117. Hall, D.C., and Kaufmann, D.A. 1987. Effects of aerobic and strength conditioning on pregnancy outcomes. *American Journal of Obstetrics and Gynecology* 157:1199-1203.

118. Tafari, N., Naye, R.L., and Govezie, A. 1980. Effects of maternal undernutrition and heavy physical work during pregnancy on birth weight. *British Journal of Obstetrics and Gynecology* 87:222-226.

119. Felig, P. 1973. Maternal and fetal fuel homeostasis in human pregnancy. *The American Journal of Clinical Nutrition* 26:998-1005.

120. Felig, P., Kim Y.J., Lynch, V., and Hendler, R. 1972. Amino acid metabolism during starvation in human pregnancy. *Journal of Clinical Investigation* 51:1195-1202.

121. Tyson, J.E., Austin, K., Farinhot, J., and Fiedler, J. 1976. Endocrine-metabolic response to acute starvation in human gestation. *American Journal of Obstetrics and Gynecology* 125:1073-1084.

122. Kim, Y.J., and Felig, P. 1971. Plasma chorionic somatomammotripin levels during starvation in mid pregnancy. *Journal of Clinical Endocrinology* 32:864-867.

123. Battaglia, F.C., and Meschia, G. 1978. Principal substrates of fetal metabolism. *Physiological Reviews* 58:499-527.

124. Hull, D. 1975. Storage and supply of fatty acids before and after birth. *British Medical Bulletin* 31:32-36.

125. May, R. 1977. *The meaning of anxiety.* NY: Norton.

126. Jablenski, A. 1985. Approaches to the definition and classification of anxiety and related disorders in European psychiatry. In A.H. Tuma and J. Maser (eds.), *Anxiety and the anxiety disorders.* Hillsdale, NJ: Erlbaum.

127. Spielberger, C.D. 1972. Anxiety as an emotional state. In C.D. Spielberger (ed.), *Anxiety: Current trends in theory and research,* NY: Academic Press.

128. Willis, J.D., and Campbell, L.F. 1992. *Exercise psychology.* Champaign, IL: Human Kinetics, pp. 49-50.

129. Raglin, J.S., and Morgan, W.P. 1987. Influence of exercise and quiet rest on state anxiety and blood pressure. *Medicine and Science in Sports and Exercise* 19(5):456-463.

130. Raglin, J.S., and Morgan, W.P. 1985. Influence of vigorous exercise on mood states. *Behavior Therapist* 8(9):179-183.

131. Morgan, W.P. 1982. Psychological effects of exercise. *Behavioral Medicine Update* 4(1):25-30.

132. Bahrke, M.S., and Morgan, W.P. 1978. Anxiety reduction following exercise and meditation. *Cognitive Therapy and Research* 2(4):323-333.

133. Driscoll, R. 1976. Anxiety reduction using physical exertion and positive images. *Psychological Record* 26:87-94.

134. Morgan, W.P. 1973. Influence of acute physical activity on state anxiety. *Proceed National College PE Association for Men,* January 1973, pp. 114-121.

135. Sime, W.E. 1984. Psychological benefits of exercise training in the healthy individual. In J.D. Matarazzo (ed.), *Behavioral health: A handbook of health enhancement and disease prevention,* NY: Wiley.

136. Wood, D.T. 1977. The relationship between anxiety and acute physical activity. *American Corrective Therapy Journal* 31(3):67-69.

137. Morgan, W.P. (ed.). 1997. *Physical activity and mental health,* series in health psychology and behavioral medicine. Washington, DC: Taylor and Francis.

138. DaCosta, D., Brender, W., and Larouche, J. 1998. A prospective study of the impact of psychosocial and lifestyle variables on pregnancy complications. *Journal of Psychosomatic Obstetrics and Gynecology* 19(1):28-37.

139. Neter, E., Collins, N.L., Lobel, M., and Dunkel-Schetter, C. 1995. Psychosocial predictors of postpartum depressed mood in socioeconomically disadvantaged women. *Women & Health* 1(1): 51-75.

140. Herrara, J.A., Alvarado, J.P., and Restrepo, W. 1995. Prenatal biopsychosocial risk and preeclampsia (Spanish). *Atencion Primaria* 16(9):552-555.

141. Paarlberg, K.M., Vingerhoets, A.J., Passchier, J., Heinen, A.G., Dekker, G.A., and van Geijn, H.P. 1996. Psychosocial factors as predictors of maternal well-being and pregnancy-related complaints. *Journal of Psychosomatic Obstetrics and Gynecology* 17(2):93-102.

142. Copper, R.L., Goldenberg, R.L., Das, A., Elder, N., Swain, M., Norman, G., Ramsey, R., Cotroneo, P., Collins, B.A., Johnson, F., Jones, P., and Meier, A.M. 1996. The preterm prediction study: Maternal stress associated with spontaneous preterm birth at less than thirty-five weeks' gestation. National Institute of Child Health and Human Development Maternal-Fetal Medicine Units Network. *American Journal of Obstetrics and Gynecology* 175(5):1286-1292.

143. Hickey, C.A., Cliver, S.P., Goldenberg, R.L., McNeal, S.F., and Hoffman, H.J. 1995. Relationship of psychosocial status to low prenatal weight gain among nonobese black and white women delivering at term. *Obstetrics and Gynecology* 86(2):177-183.

144. Shiono, P.H., Rauh, V.A., Park, M., Lederman, S.A., and Zuskar, D. 1997. Ethnic differences in birthweight: The role of lifestyle and other factors. *American Journal of Public Health* 87(5):787-793.

145. Laatikainen, T.J. 1991. Corticotropin-releasing hormone and opioid peptides in reproduction and stress. *Annals of Medicine* 23(5):489-496.

146. Magiakou, M.A., Mastorakos, G., Webster, E., and Chrousos, G.P. 1997. The hypothalamic-pituitary-adrenal axis and the female reproductive system. *Annals New York Academy of Sciences* 816:42-56.

147. Rauramo, I., Andersson, B., and Laatikainen, T.J. 1982. Stress hormones and placental steroids in physical exercise during pregnancy. *British Journal of Obstetrics and Gynecology* 89:921-925.

148. Berkowitz, G.S., Kelwey, J.L., Holford, T.R., and Berkowitz, R.L. 1983. Physical activity and risk of spontaneous preterm delivery. *Journal of Reproductive Medicine* 28(90):581-588.

149. Bullock, L.F., Wells, J.E., Duff, G.B., and Hornblow, A.R. 1995. Telephone support for pregnant women: Outcome in late pregnancy. *New Zealand Medical Journal* 108(1012):4764-78.

150. Zimmer-Gembeck, M.J., and Helfand, M. 1996. Low birth weight in a public prenatal care program: Behavioral and psychosocial risk factors and psychosocial intervention. *Social Science and Medicine* 43(2):187-197.

151. Both unpublished data and anecdotal accounts covering 1982-93 held in the Dancing Thru Pregnancy, Inc. program evaluation files give clear indication of the importance of the group setting for prenatal exercise. More than 95% of clients responding to confidential evaluation forms and interviews report that being with other pregnant women was one of the most important parts of the program. As part of the same surveys, reports of complications, as measured by need for cesarean birth, were well below local and national percentages for all time periods surveyed.

152. Berger, B.G., and Owen, D.R. 1988. Stress reduction and mood enhancement in four modes: Swimming, body conditioning, Hatha yoga and fencing. *Research Quarterly for Exercise and Sport* 59(2):148-159.

153. Benson, H., Beary, J.F., and Carol, M.P. 1974. The relaxation response. *Psychiatry* 37:37-46.

154. Morgan, W.P. 1978. The mind of the marathoner. *Psychology Today* 11:38-40.

155. Odent, Michel. 1992. *The nature of birth and breastfeeding.* Westport, CT: Bergin and Garvey.

156. Varney, H. 1996. *Varney's midwifery,* 3rd ed. Boston: Jones & Bartlett.

157. National Research Council, Food and Nutrition Board, Commission on Life Sciences. 1989. *Recommended daily dietary allowances, 10th ed.: Report of the Subcommittee on the Tenth Edition of the R.D.As.* Washington, DC: National Academy Press.

158. ACOG. 1993. *Nutrition during pregnancy.* ACOG Technical Bulletin Number 179.

159. Burke, B.S., et al. 1943. Nutrition studies in pregnancy. *American Journal of Obstetrics and Gynecology* 25:38.

160. Brewer, G.S. with Brewer, T.H. 1983. *The Brewer Medical Diet for normal and high risk pregnancy.* NY: Simon & Schuster.

161. Ansar, A.S., Penhale, W.J., and Talal, N. 1985. Sex hormone, immune responses and autoimmune diseases. *American Journal of Pathology* 125:531-551.

162. Inman, R.D. 1978. Immunologic sex differences and the female preponderance in systemic lupus erythematosus. *Arthritis and Rheumatism* 21:480-484.

163. Spencer, M.J., Cherry, J.D., Powell, K.R., et al. 1977. Antibody responses following rubella immunisation analysed by HLA, and ABO types. *Immunogenetics* 4:365-372.

164. London, W.T., and Drew, J.R. 1977. Sex differences in response to hepatitis B infection among patients receiving chronic dialysis treatment. *Proceedings of the National Academy of Sciences USA* 74:2561-2564.

165. Paty, D.W., Furesz, J., Boucher, D.W., Rand, C.G., and Stiller, C.R. 1976. Measles antibodies as related to HL-A types in multiple sclerosis. *Neurology* 26:651-655.

166. Michaels, R.H., and Rogers, K.D. 1971. A sex difference in immunologic responsiveness. *Pediatrics* 47:120-123.

167. Rhodes, K., Scott, A., Markham, R.L., and Monk-Jones, M.E. 1969. Immunological sex differences. *Annals of the Rheumatic Diseases* 28:104-119.

168. Giguere, V., Yange, N., Segui, P., and Evans, R.M. 1988. Identification of a new class of steroid hormone receptors. *Nature* 331:91-94.

169. Vamvakopoulos, N.C., and Chrousos, G.P. 1993. Evidence of estrogenic regulation of human corticotropin-releasing hormone gene expression. *Journal of Clinical Investigation* 92:1896-1902.

170. Bateman, A., Singh, A., Kral, T., and Solomon, S. 1989. The immune-hypothalamic-pituitary-adrenal axis. *Endocrine Review* 10(1):92-112.

171. Kincade, P.W., Medina, K.L., and Smithson, G. 1994. Sex hormones as negative regulators of lymphopoiesis. *Immunological Reviews* 137:119-134.

172. Gabrilova, J., Zadjelovic, J., Osmak, M., Suchanek, E., Zupanovic, Z., and Boranic, M. 1988. NK cell activity and estrogen hormone levels during normal human pregnancy. *Gynecologic and Obstetric Investigations* 15:167-172.

173. Thong, Y.H., Steele, R.W., Vincet, M.M., Hensen, S.A., and Bellanti, J.A. 1973. Impaired in vitro cell-mediated immunity to rubella virus during pregnancy. *New England Journal of Medicine* 289:604-606.

174. Friedman, E.A., and Rutherford, J.W. 1956. Pregnancy and lupus erythematosus. *Obstetrics and Gynecology* 8:601-160.

175. Hench, P.S. 1938. The ameliorating effects of pregnancy on the chronic atrophic (infectious rheumatoid) arthritis, fibrositis and interior heat hydrarthrosis. *Mayo Clinic Proceedings* 13:161-168.

176. Wang, H.S., Kanzaki, H, Tokushige, M., Sato, S., Yoshida, M. and Takahide, M. 1988. Effect of ovarian steroids on the secretion of immunosuppressive factors from human endometrium. *American Journal of Obstetrics and Gynecology* 158:629-637.

177. Sulke, A.N., Jones, D.B., and Wood, P.J. 1985. Variation in natural killer activity in peripheral blood during the menstrual cycle. *British Medical Journal (Clinical Research Education)* 290:884-886.

178. Jaque-Fortunato, S.V., Wiswell, R.A., Khodiguian, N., and Artal, R. 1996. A comparison of the ventilatory responses to exercise in pregnant, postpartum, and nonpregnant women. *Seminars in Perinatology* 20(4):263-276.

179. Wolfe, L.A., Walker, R.M., Bonen, A., and McGrath, M.J. 1994. Effects of pregnancy and chronic exercise on respiratory responses to graded exercise. *Journal of Applied Physiology* 76(5):1928-1936.

180. Kemp, J.G., Greer, F.A., and Wolfe, L.A. 1997. Acid-base regulation after maximal exercise testing in late gestation. *Journal of Applied Physiology* 83(2):644-651.

181. Ohtake, P.J., and Wolfe, L.A. 1998. Physical conditioning attenuates respiratory responses to steady-state in late gestation. *Medicine and Science in Sports and Exercise* 30(1):17-27.

182. Bayliss, D.A., and Millhorn, D.E. 1992. Central neural mechanisms of progesterone action: Application to the respiratory system. *Journal of Applied Physiology* 73:393-404.

183. Clapp, J.F. 3rd. 1998. *Dose-effect of prenatal exercise,* presented at the Yale Conference on Women's Health and Fitness, Yale University/Yale-New Haven Hospital, May 2-3, New Haven, CT.

184. Ostgaard, H.C., Zetherstrom, G., Roos-Hansson, E., and Svanberg, B. 1994. Reduction of back and posterior pelvic pain in pregnancy. *Spine* 19(8):894-900.

185. McIntyre, I.N., and Broadhurst, N.A. 1996. Effective treatment of low back pain in pregnancy. *Australian Family Physician* 25(9 Suppl 2):S65-S67.

186. Andrews, C.M., and O'Neil, L.M. 1994. Use of pelvic tilt exercise for ligament pain relief. *Journal of Nurse Midwifery* 39(6):370-374.

187. Sweigard, L. 1974. *Human movement potential; Its ideokentic facilitation.* NY:UPA.

188. Bunker, L.K., Rotella R.J., and Reilly, A.S. 1985. *Sport psychology: Psychological considerations in maximizing sport performance.* London: Mouvement Pub, Inc.

189. Loehr, J.E. 1983. The ideal performance state. *Sci Period on Res Tech Sp,* Canada: Government of Canada BU-1, January.

190. Brynhildsen, J.O., Bjors, E., Skarsgard, C., and Hammar, M.L. 1998. Is hormone replacement therapy a risk factor for low back pain among postmenopausal women? *Spine* 23(7):809-813.

191. Vullo, U.J., Richardson, J.K., and Hurvitz, E.A. 1996. Hip, knee and foot pain during pregnancy and the postpartum period. *Journal of Family Practice* 43(1):63-68.

192. Dumas, G.A., and Reid, J.G. 1997. Laxity of knee cruciate ligaments during pregnancy. *The Journal of Orthopaedic and Sports Physical Therapy* 26(1):2-6.

193. Nygaard, I.E., Glowacki, C., and Saltzman, C.L. 1996. Relationship between foot flexibility and urinary incontinence in nulliparous varsity athletes. *Obstetrics and Gynecology* 87(6):1049-1051.

194. Wallace, K. 1994. Female pelvic floor functions, dysfunctions, and behavioral approaches to treatment. *Clinics in Sports Medicine* 13(2):459-480.

195. Bø, K. 1989. Female stress urinary incontinence and participation in different sports and social activities. *Scandinavian Journal of Sports Sciences* 11(3):117-121.

196. Mallet, V., and Frahm, J. 1992. Abdominal and pelvic floor muscle synergy in normal continent women. *Proceedings from the American Urogynecology Society Annual Meeting,* Boston.

197. Payne, C.K. 1998. Biofeedback for community-dwelling individuals with urinary incontinence. *Urology* 51(2A Suppl):35-39.

198. Delancey, J.O. 1996. Stress urinary incontinence: Where are we now, where should we go? *American Journal of Obstetrics and Gynecology* 175(2):311-319.

199. Sampselle, C.M. 1990. Changes in pelvic muscle strength and stress urinary incontinence associated with childbirth. *Journal of Obstetric, Gynecologic, and Neonatal Nursing* 19:371-377.

200. Sultan, A.H., Samm, M.A., and Hudson, C.N. 1994. Pudendal nerve damage during labour: Prospective study before and after childbirth. *British Journal of Obstetrics and Gynecology* 101(2):153-155.

201. Tancer, M.L., Lasser, D., and Rosenblum, N. 1991. Rectovaginal fistula or perineal and anal sphincter disruption or both, after vaginal delivery. *Surgery, Gynecology and Obstetrics* 171(1):43-46.

202. Wynne, J.M., Mules, J.L., Jones, I., Sapsford, R., Young R.E., and Hattam, A. 1997. Disturbed anal sphincter function following vaginal delivery. *Obstetrics and Gynecology Survey* 52(2):95.

203. Viktrup, L., and Lose, G. 1993. Epidural anesthesia during labor and stress incontinence after delivery. *Obstetrics and Gynecology* 82(6):984.

204. Schuessler, B., Hesse, U., Dimpfl, T., and Anthuber, C. 1988. Epidural anesthesia and avoidance of postpartum stress urinary incontinence. *Lancet* 1(8588):762.

205. Graham, I.D. 1997. *Episiotomy: Challenging obstetric intervention.* NY: Blackwell Scientific.

206. Klein, M.C., Janssen, P.A., MacWilliam, L., Kaczorowski, J., and Johnson, B. 1997. Determinants of vaginal-perineal integrity and pelvic floor function in childbirth. *American Journal of Obstetrics and Gynecology* 176(2):403-410.

207. Handa, V.L., Harris, T.A., and Ostergard, D.R. 1996. Protecting the pelvic floor: Obstetric management to prevent incontinence and pelvic organ prolapse. *Obstetrics and Gynecology* 88(3):470-478.

208. Sultan, A.H., et al. 1995. Obstetric perineal trauma: An audit of training. *Journal of Obstetrics and Gynecology* 15(1):19.

209. Wilson, P.D., Herbison, R.M., and Herbison, G.P. 1996. Obstetric practice and the prevalence of urinary incontinence three months after delivery. *British Journal of Obstetrics and Gynecology* 103(2):154-161.

210. Kegel, A. 1948. Progressive resistive exercise in the functional restoration of perineal muscles. *American Journal of Obstetrics and Gynecology* 56(2):238-248.

211. Cammu, H., and Van Nylen, M. 1997. Pelvic floor muscle exercises in genuine urinary stress incontinence. *International Urogynecology Journal and Pelvic Floor Dysfunction* 8(5):297-300.

212. Morkved, S., and Bø, K. 1996. The effect of postnatal exercise to strengthen pelvic floor muscles. *Acta Obstetricia et Gynecologica Scandinavica* 75(4):382-385.

213. Sampselle, C.M., Miller, J.M., Mims, B.L., DeLancey, J.O., Ashton-Miller, J.A., and Antonakos, C.L. 1998. Effect of pelvic muscle exercise on transient incontinence during pregnancy and after birth. *Obstetrics and Gynecology* 91(3):406-412.

214. Cammu, H., and Van Nylen, M. 1998. Pelvic floor exercises versus vaginal weight cones in genuine stress incontinence. *European Journal of Obstetrics, Gynecology, and Reproductive Biology* 77(1):89-93.

215. Blair, S.N., Kohl, H.W. 3rd, Paffenberger, R.S. Jr., Clark, D.G., Cooper, K.H., and Gibbens, L.W. 1989. Physical fitness and all-cause mortality: A prospective study of healthy men and women. *Journal of the American Medical Association* 162:2395-2401.

216. Bouchard, C., Shephard, R.J., Stephens, C., Sutton, J.R., and McPherson, B.D. (eds.). 1990. *Exercise, fitness and health: A consensus of current knowledge.* Champaign, IL: Human Kinetics.

217. North, T.C., McCullagh, P., and Tran, Z.V. 1990. Effect of exercise on depression. *Exercise in Sport Science Review* 18:379-415.

218. Jin, P. 1992. Efficacy of Tai Chi, brisk walking, meditation and reading on reducing mental and emotional stress. *Journal of Psychosomatic Research* 36:361.

219. Kennell, J., Klaus, M., McGrath, S., Robertson, S., and Hinckley, C. 1991. Continuous emotional support during labor in a US hospital. *Journal of the American Medical Association* 265(17):2197-2201.

220. Sosa, R., Kennell, J., Klaus, M., Robertson, S., and Urrutia, J. 1980. The effect of a supportive companion on perinatal problems, length of labor and mother-infant interaction. *New England Journal of Medicine* 303(11):597-600.

221. Seitz, V., and Apfel, N. 1993. Adolescent mothers and repeated childbearing: Effects of a school-based intervention program. *American Journal of Orthopsychiatry* 63:572.

222. Webb, K.A., Wolfe, L.A., and McGrath, M.J. 1994. Effects of acute and chronic maternal exercise on fetal heart rate. *Journal of Applied Physiology* 77:2207-2213.

223. Clapp, J.F. 3rd, Little, K.D., and Capeless, E.L. 1993. Fetal heart rate response to sustained recreational exercise. *American Journal of Obstetrics and Gynecology* 168:198-206.

224. Clapp, J.F., Rokey, R., Treadway, J.L., Carpenter, M.W., Artal, R.M., and Warrnes, C. 1992. Exercise in pregnancy. *Medicine and Science in Sports and Exercise* 24:S294-S300.

225. Bung, P., Huch, R., and Huch, A. 1991. Maternal and fetal heart rate patterns: A pregnant athlete during training and laboratory exercise tests: A case report. *European Journal of Obstetrics, Gynecology, and Reproductive Biology* 39:59-62.

226. Artal, R., Rutherford, S., Romen, Y., Kammula, R.K., Dorey, F.J., and Wiswell, R.A. 1986. Fetal heart rate response to maternal exercise. *American Journal of Obstetrics and Gynecology* 155:729-733.

227. Clapp, J.F. 3rd. 1985. Fetal heart rate response to running in mid-pregnancy and late pregnancy. *American Journal of Obstetrics and Gynecology* 153:251-252.

228. Hauth, J.C., Gilstrap, L.C., and Widmer, K. 1982. Fetal heart rate reactivity before and after maternal jogging during the third trimester. *American Journal of Obstetrics and Gynecology* 142:545-547.

229. Manders, M.A., Sonder, G.J., Mulder, E.J., and Visser, G.H. 1997. The effects of maternal exercise on fetal heart rate and movement patterns. *Early Human Development* 48(3):237-247.

230. Paolone, A.M., Shangold, M., Paul, D., Minnitti, J., and Weiner, S. 1987. Fetal heart rate measurement during maternal exercise—avoidance of artifact. *Medicine and Science in Sports and Exercise* 19(6):605-609.

231. Watson, W.J., Katz, V.L., Hackney, A.C., Gall, M.M., and McMurray, R.G. 1991. Fetal responses to maximal swimming and cycling exercise during pregnancy. *Obstetrics and Gynecology* 77(3):382-386.

232. Artal, R.M., and Posner, M.D. 1991. Fetal responses to maternal exercise. In R. Mittlemark, R. Wiswell, and B. Drinkwater (eds.), *Exercise in pregnancy,* 2nd ed. Baltimore: Williams & Wilkins.

233. Sjostrom, K., Valentin, L., Thelin, T., and Marsal, K. 1997. Maternal anxiety in late pregnancy and fetal hemodynamics. *European Journal of Obstetrics, Gynecology, and Reproductive Biology* 74(2):149-155.

234. Groome, L.J., Swiber, M.J., Bentz, L.S., Holland, S.B., and Atterbury, J.L. 1995. Maternal anxiety during pregnancy: Effect on fetal behavior at 38 to 40 weeks gestation. *Journal of Developmental and Behavioral Pediatrics* 16(6):391-396.

235. American College of Obstetricians and Gynecologists (ACOG). 1994. *Exercise during pregnancy and the postpartum period.* Technical bulletin no. 189.

236. Clapp, J.F. 3rd. 1994. The athletic woman: A clinical approach to exercise during pregnancy. *Clinics in Sports Medicine* 13(2):443-458.

237. Hatch, M.C., Shu, X.O., McLean, D.E., Levin, B., Begg, M., Reuss, L., Susser, M. 1993. Maternal exercise during pregnancy, physical fitness, and fetal growth. *American Journal of Epidemiology* 137(10):1105-1114.

238. McMurray, R.G., Mottola, M.F., Wolfe, L.A., Artal, R., Millar, L., and Pivarnik, J.M. 1993. Recent advances in understanding maternal and fetal response to exercise. *Medicine and Science in Sports and Exercise* 25(12):1305-1321.

239. Depken, D., and Zelasko, C.J. 1996. Exercise during pregnancy: Concerns for fitness professionals. *Strength & Conditioning* Oct 96:43-51.

240. Sternfeld, B. 1997. Physical activity and pregnancy outcome. Review and recommendations. *Sports Medicine* 23(1):33-47.

241. Clapp, J.F. 1989. The effects of maternal exercise on early pregnancy outcome. *American Journal of Obstetrics and Gynecology* 161(6):1453.

242. Clapp, J.F. 1994. Exercise in pregnancy and the postpartum period: Review of research findings on maternal and fetal outcomes. *Perinatal Health and Fitness Network Lecture Series,* Yale New Haven Hospital, June 25, 1994.

243. Pivarnik, J.M., Lee, W., and Miller, J.F. 1991. Physiological and perceptual responses to cycle and treadmill exercise during pregnancy. *Medicine and Science in Sports and Exercise* 23(4):470-475.

244. Pfeifer, W.A. 1951. Neuere unterscuchungen uber geburtsverlauf, fertilitat und konstitution bei spitzenkonnerinnen der leichtathletik. *Zentralblatt fur Gynaekologie* 73:17-23.

245. Pomerance, J.J., Gluck, L., and Lynch, V.A. 1974. Physical fitness in pregnancy: Its effect on pregnancy outcome. *American Journal of Obstetrics and Gynecology* 119:867-876.

246. Hall, D.C., and Kaufmann, D.A. 1987. Effects of aerobic and strength conditioning on pregnancy outcomes. *American Journal of Obstetrics and Gynecology* 157(5):1199-1203.

247. Clapp, J.F. 1990. The course of labor after endurance exercise during pregnancy. *American Journal of Obstetrics and Gynecology* 163(6):1799.

248. Botkin, C., and Driscoll, C.E. 1991. Maternal aerobic exercise: Newborn effects. *The Family Practice Research Journal* 11(4):387-393.

249. Kardel, K.R., and Kase, T. 1998. Training in pregnant women: Effects on fetal development and birth. *American Journal of Obstetrics and Gynecology* 178(2):280-286.

250. Goyert, G.L., Bottoms, S.F., Treadwell, M.C., and Nehra, P.C. 1990. The physician factor in cesarean birth rates. *New England Journal of Medicine* 320(11) 706-709.

251. Bungum, T.J., Peaslee, D.L., Jackson, A.W., and Perez, M.A. 2000. Exercise during pregnancy and type of delivery in nulliparae. *Journal of Obstetric, Gynecologic, and Neonatal Nursing* 29(3):258-264.

252. Clapp, J.F. 3rd, Little, K.D., and Capeless, E.L. 1993. Fetal heart rate response to various intensities of recreational exercise during mid and late pregnancy. *American Journal of Obstetrics and Gynecology* 168:198-206.

253. Clapp, J.F. 3rd, Little, K.D., Appleby-Wineberg, S.A., and Widness, J.A. 1995. The effect of regular exercise in late pregnancy on erythropoietin levels in amniotic fluid and cord blood. *American Journal of Obstetrics and Gynecology* 172:1445-51.

254. Berkowitz, G.S., Kelsey, J.L., Holford, T.R., and Berkowitz, R.L. 1983. Physical activity and the risk of spontaneous pre-term delivery. *Reproductive Medicine* 28:581-588.

255. Lokey, E.A., Tran, Z.V., Wells, C.L., Myers, B.C., and Tran, A.C. 1991. Effects of physical exercise on pregnancy outcomes: A meta-analytic review. *Medicine and Science in Sports and Exercise* 23(11):1234-1239.

256. Botkin, C., and Driscoll, C.E. 1991. Maternal aerobic exercise: Newborn effects. *The Family Practice Research Journal* 11(4):387-393.

257. Clapp, J.F. 3rd. 1990. Neonatal morphometrics after endurance exercise during pregnancy. *American Journal of Obstetrics and Gynecology* 163(6):1450

258. Clapp, J.F. 3rd, Simonian, S., Lopez, B., Appleby-Wineberg, S., and Harcar-Sevcik, R. 1998. The one-year morphometric and neurodevelopmental outcome of the offspring of women who continued to exercise regularly throughout pregnancy. *American Journal of Obstetrics and Gynecology* 178(3):594-599.

259. Clapp, J.F. 3rd. 1996. Morphometric and neurodevelopmental outcome at age five years of the offspring of women who continued to exercise regularly throughout pregnancy. *Journal of Pediatrics* 129(6):856-862.

260. Wolfe, L.A., Walker, R.M., Bonen, A., and McGrath, M.J. 1994. Effects of pregnancy and chronic exercise on respiratory responses to graded exercise. *Journal of Applied Physiology* 76(5):1928-1936.

261. Fuller, A.K., and Robinson, M.E. 1993. A test of exercise analgesia using signal detection theory and a within-subjects design. *Perceptual and Motor Skills* 76(3 Pt 2):1299-1310.

262. Guieu, R., Blin, O., Pouget, J., and Serratrice, G. 1992. Nociceptive threshold and physical activity. *The Canadian Journal of Neurological Sciences* 19:69-71.

263. Jessell, T.M., and Kelly, D.D. 1991. Pain and analgesia. In E.R. Kandell, J.H. Schwartz, and T.M. Jessell (eds.), *Principles of neural science,* 3rd ed. Norwalk, CT: Appleton & Lange, pp. 385-399.

264. Schwarz, L., and Kinderman, W. 1990. Beta-endorphin, adrenchorticotropic hormone, cortisol and catecholamines during aerobic and anaerobic exercise. *European Journal of Applied Physiology* 61:165.

265. Morgan, W.P. 1978. The mind of the marathoner. *Psychology Today* 11(11):38.

266. Kandel, E.R., Schwartz, J.H., and Jessell, T.M. 1991. *Principles of neural science.* 3rd. ed. Norwalk, CT: Appleton Lange, 1991, p. 681.

267. Annett, J. 1988. Imagery and skill acquisition. In M. Denis, J. Engelkamp, and J.T.E. Richardson (eds.), *Cognitive and neuropsychological approaches to mental imagery.* NY: Nijhoff, pp. 259-268.

268. Feldenkrais, M. 1977. *Awareness through movement.* NY: Harper & Row.

269. Savoyant, A. 1988. Mental practice: Image and mental rehearsal of motor action. In M. Denis, J. Engelkamp, and J.T.E. Richardson (eds.), *Cognitive and neuropsychological approaches to mental imagery.* NY: Nijhoff, pp. 251-257.

270. Salmon, P., Miller, R., and Drew, N.C. 1990. Women's anticipation and experience of childbirth: The independence of fulfillment, unpleasantness and pain. *British Journal of Medical Psychology* 63(3):255

CHAPTER 7

GOALS AND PRIORITIES OF PRENATAL FITNESS PROGRAMS

This chapter sets forth goals and priorities of a prenatal fitness program. Goals refer to the ends to which an effort is aimed, whereas priorities are the immediate concerns that help achieve goals. These concepts are discussed in chapter 3. In contrast to fitness for adolescent girls, with prenatal fitness there is a more specific body of research pointing the direction that goal setting should take. And pregnancy itself ends in birth, giving further direction to the task. This chapter begins with a discussion of the purposes of prenatal fitness and the ways in which these form both rationale and dilemma in the setting of goals and priorities. Then, it focuses on public health goals: promoting healthy mothers having healthy babies, developing skills for labor and birth, and facilitating a quick recovery. A final section of the chapter deals with the priorities needed to help ensure these goals: safety, effectiveness, and community.

THE RATIONALE AND THE DILEMMA: WHY ARE WE TRAINING PREGNANT WOMEN?

In setting meaningful public health goals, we are forced to look at a key issue: beyond the physical fitness concerns associated with identifying appropriate modes and an adequate level of physical activity to promote fitness and health, there are concerns about how maternal physical fitness might affect the practice of birth. Through research and practice, we have found that under certain conditions, exercise can affect labor and birth—labor by shortening the active phase, and birth by necessitating less medical intervention. The same benefits that promote the mother's health and the baby's development also prepare them for the rigors of birth. However, what we find when we begin to implement our prenatal fitness goals is a dilemma. The predominantly male model of birth in the United States sees the process as a struggle, in which the active application of technology to the maternal object makes the experience more pleasant. This model is innately unfriendly to the maternal empowerment provided by fitness. The dilemma we confront, then, is whether to limit the role of prenatal exercise to one of promoting fitness, general health, psychological well-being, coping, and healing, or whether to expect an impact on labor and birth outcomes, such as a lowering of the cesarean rate.

Fitness and Health

In pregnancy, as we have already seen, physiological parameters, biomechanics, and the psyche all undergo major changes. Some adaptations to exercise are minimized as a consequence of increased cardiovasculature, strengthened heart, and increased cardiac output. Other changes—weight increases and redistribution, respiratory and metabolic shifts—require more adjustment. Nonetheless, many aspects of exercise produce the same kinds of conditioning responses that occur in the general population. Therefore, as long as we pay attention to the peculiarities of this condition, and to the individuality that any personal situation demands, we can provide enhancements of endurance, strength, flexibility, and weight and stress management, as well as reduction of discomforts.

In addition, we know that babies whose mothers begin exercise early in pregnancy or continue exercise through pregnancy benefit from a large and healthy placenta. Of course, nutrition and hydration play integral parts in the enhancement of pregnancy when the mother is physically active. There is also sufficient evidence to tell us that physical activity during pregnancy—as in all periods of life—provides benefits in terms of bone, heart, metabolism, and mental health. By helping prevent the unwanted maternal weight gain that can occur in pregnancy, exercise acts as a means of forestalling obesity and related disorders. In the absence of uteroplacental insufficiency or other adverse conditions, activity at an appropriate level is clearly advantageous.

Birth

Birth is another matter. Birth may be like many things, but nothing else is quite like birth. An event for which women volunteer, it is also an event presenting demands that women are uniquely suited to. It involves an ultra-ultradistance, low- to moderate-intensity endurance component (labor), followed by a sprint (transition), then a strength test (pushing), and several years of sleep deprivation. The time periods of each of the stages vary from person to person and are unknowable at the outset. If difficulties occur, surgery may be employed. In the end, a new person comes into existence and the mother takes on an additional identity. This is a major life event. Who wouldn't want to be prepared for such challenges?

If prenatal exercise is effective, might we also expect to see a positive influence on birth outcomes? The answer relies not only on the ability of exercise professionals to develop activity interventions and studies that address this topic, but also on the incursion of these activities into the health care system that controls birth, as well as the popular culture from which pregnant women learn about the birth process. We have evidence, for example, that whether a given situation in labor results in surgical birth may depend on the particular physician, where she or he was trained, and her or his sex [1, 2]. Will increas-

ing the fitness level of pregnant women be a factor for change?

Profound psychological questions surround the birth process. Childbirth educators, health care practitioners, informal social networks, news media, and popular advertising all contribute to women's expectations concerning birth. Does the prenatal fitness specialist represent a new voice? Is the voice one that will reinforce or conflict with other images of pregnancy and birth that women carry? Birth is a phenomenon with a long history. The current style of birth in the United States, including high rates of surgery and drugs, is a recent development, concurrent with 20th-century changes surrounding the birth process, including its movement from a female-centered communal event to a male-centered technologically managed medical event. As we strive to attain our goals and priorities, it is necessary to confront the realization that the current style of birth has been strongly influenced by the desire of men to "help" women by acting on what they see as a situation requiring intervention.

SETTING GOALS AND PRIORITIES

The question whether or not widespread application of effective prenatal exercise programs will contribute to a change in birthing procedures or outcomes will be answered in the long run. In the meantime, the goals established for prenatal programs must derive from the motivations of childbearing women, their health, and most significantly, the health of their babies. In practice, through screening thousands of women from all parts of the United States, the author and her colleagues have been able to identify the following obtainable goals based on women's motivations for seeking assistance with prenatal exercise:

1. Being a healthy mother having a healthy baby
2. Developing skills for labor and birth
3. Having a quick recovery

In order to achieve goals, an instructor or trainer prioritizes activities within the exercise setting. In any setting, safety is always the highest priority. Being effective, that is, doing activities that promote health and that prepare women for labor and recovery, is the second priority. Fostering a supportive community is the third priority. The social nature of birth is sometimes a surprise to new instructors. Experience has taught us to prepare instructors and trainers to create a community around birth because this is productive for the health and well-being of the women, their infants, and programs.

FIRST GOAL: PROMOTE HEALTHY MOTHERS HAVING HEALTHY BABIES

Prior to pregnancy, an active woman's purpose for exercise may have been to be fit, to be healthy, to be attractive, or to be competitive. These women—as well as those who have not been involved in regular activity—may look to exercise as a way to avoid losing control of their bodies. Sometimes such women ask for advice by beginning a conversation with "I don't want my pregnancy to interfere with my exercise routine," "I really don't want to get fat," or "I want to have any easy labor." These are *mother-centered* motivations.

Another cadre of women may be primarily concerned with *healthy-baby* motivations. "If I keep doing what I'm doing will it be safe for my baby?" and "What should I do to have a healthy baby?" and "How can I prepare so my baby will tolerate labor?" are the kinds of question that these women may raise.

When a woman is committed to fitness and when circumstances allow, mother-centered motivation by itself may sustain her through pregnancy. Research findings tell us that the infants of women who exercise at high levels throughout pregnancy do well in the years that follow birth. It would seem that if the motivation is mother centered, the healthy-baby motivation is also served when circumstances allow.

But we need to keep in mind that most research results tell us about situations in which complicating factors are not present. What happens when circumstances do not allow a mother to continue exercising at the level she wants for herself? What happens to maternal and infant well-being when the pregnancy is labeled high risk, the mother develops an injury or disorder, or a change in family circumstances removes the support system? Although it is important for a mother to get the maximum benefit from her prenatal exercise program, some degree of skepticism is warranted when one is examining the mother-centered motive as the primary or only motivation.

In practice we find that by putting the healthy baby first in the mother's mind, we can positively affect the greatest number of women. Although *healthy baby first* might seem an obvious goal, the number of highly active first-time mothers who find this a startling concept is surprising. Taking this approach in no way negates the activity level of a woman whose situation allows her to work frequently at high intensities. In fact, encouraging all women to work as hard as they can clearly reaps benefits. But a woman who exercises often and intensely may be at high risk of dropping out altogether if she confronts difficulties and has no coping skills. When she can see her own health and fitness as a support system for a larger goal, she is free to be flexible.

SECOND GOAL: DEVELOP SKILLS FOR LABOR AND BIRTH

Women who are attended in birth by an experienced female support person have shorter active labors, require less intervention, and have fewer complications [3, 4]. The same may well be true for women who exercise hard nearly every day. Learning to work with one's body is a by-product of regular physical training. The mechanisms of this process were described at the end of the previous chapter. Instead of relying on coaching from an external source, learning to work effectively within oneself is akin to having an internal coach.

Perhaps the most valuable aspect of this phenomenon is the ability to improvise solutions, based on kinesthetic cues, in order to meet the objective of an event (such as getting to the finish line or getting a baby out). The ability to engage in strenuous physical activity without knowing ahead of time what will be required on that day, at that time, in order to accomplish the objective, may be the component of an effective prenatal exercise program that is most responsible for the positive outcomes we associate with highly fit women.

Rather than learning a specific set of do's and dont's, it may be that the capacity of a woman to figure out what she needs to do on the spot is the best measure of the effectiveness of prenatal training. If we take this principle back into the exercise group or one-on-one setting, it translates into an ability to improvise—to derive movement from one's own internal rhythm, feelings, or sensations. In dance, it is common knowledge that to teach improvisational skills, the first step is to create a highly structured movement setting in which only one or two elements are left to choice. For example, people might be told to walk back and forth in a room at a normal pace, but every now and then, at their own discretion, to walk faster or slower. Over time, increasing numbers of choices and motivations for choosing may be added—walking on tiptoes or very low to the ground, walking as if there were springs on one's feet or as if one's feet were made of cement, and so on. Eventually, people develop confidence in reading internal cues and allowing movement to come from this source.

Applying this technique to the preparation for labor, there is a vocabulary of movements that are useful in labor, and these can serve as one basis for choices within structured activity. In this text these movements are referred to as *special exercises* and are covered in the next chapter. Examples are strengthening and relaxing the pelvic floor (called *Kegel* exercises), getting into and out of a birth squat position, and rocking and tilting the pelvis. Of course, beyond these movements are unique, unspecified motions a woman may sense internally that she needs to make in order to get the baby out. These motions are accessible only if a woman can tap her inner-generated urges. Gaining the ability and confidence to do this requires a lot of practice. The person most likely to help a woman gain this ability is her prenatal exercise instructor or trainer.

THIRD GOAL: FACILITATE A QUICK RECOVERY

From a purely physiological perspective, the exercise-associated mechanisms that enable enhancement of the placenta, expansion of blood volume and vasculature, increases in heart strength, and improvements in metabolic function during pregnancy are available to speed tissue recovery in the weeks immediately following birth. Biomechanical and psychophysiological factors require their own rhythms, but may be enhanced as well in the postpartum period in women who are fit. To be sure, in practice we commonly see women returning to a regular exercise regimen within three to six weeks.

Regular physical activity clearly plays a critical role in preventing the birth process from being an illness or procedure. Although a percentage of births require procedural interventions, we know that highly fit women need this assistance in smaller numbers than the general population. In this way, fitness also contributes to recovery by preventing the stresses that intervention imposes.

When medical intervention is necessary, a woman who is strong and fit and who has stress management skills has more physiological and psychological resources than a woman without these advantages. This is not to say that being fit and bringing a strong psyche to labor and birth guarantee that all will be perfect and easy. But it is a realistic expectation that women who are physically fit and psychologically prepared for the rigors of birth will tolerate the process with equanimity or confidence.

FIRST PRIORITY: SAFETY

Above all else, safety must be accounted for. In addition to the safety issues concerning the physical environment that apply for any population, there are specific safety issues for pregnant women. Medical conditions that preclude exercise must be identified by the obstetrician or midwife. An appropriate starting point must be determined, based on prior experience and stage of pregnancy. Individual tolerances will affect the need to modify activity. General safety guidelines need to be kept in mind. Beyond these commonsense physical safety issues, women's need for psychological safety must be taken into consideration. These issues are reviewed briefly here and detailed in chapter 8.

When Medical Conditions Preclude Exercise

Women who have conditions for which exercise is contraindicated obviously must be discouraged from strenuous exertion. Some conditions allow for gentle activities that include centering, relaxation, and imagery, such as meditation, tai chi, or prenatal yoga. Others do not. When contraindications are present, it is critical to comply with the health care provider's instructions. Conditions that require assessment or monitoring—such as a low-lying placenta—may require patience early in the pregnancy on the part of the expectant mother, especially if she is used to a high level of activity. But safety is an acceptable issue to most women as a reason to be cautious. In the first trimester, fatigue or nausea may also slow women down. When a woman returns to exercise, a reminder about the effects of deconditioning is advisable, along with assistance in finding the appropriate level of exertion.

Some athletes feel reined in during their pregnancies. Two reminders are often helpful in allowing them to stop thinking of restrictions and think instead of the new possibilities that are opening in their lives. First, the physical restrictions will go away in time. Now is the time to be present in this body and discover the amazing things it can do. Making a healthy baby means that safety is goal number one. Second, such women need to take a lesson from children in their ability to create imaginative, awe-inspiring experiences out of the world as they find it. To see the possible rather than the impossible is a great coping skill. Pretending to play basketball, without the ball, the basket, or real opponents, for example, still provides the workout, but without the danger. Or, this may be the time to swim laps again . . . or take up belly dancing, which developed as a Middle Eastern birth preparation!

If the woman is enrolled in a special prenatal class that meets two or three times per week, the instructor is often the first to notice warning signs or symptoms that warrant immediate referral to the midwife or physician. A well-trained instructor will ask the client who shows up one day with edema of the fingers, hands, and face to refrain from class, go to her care provider, and have her blood pressure checked for possible pregnancy-induced hypertension.

Finding an Appropriate Starting Point

Research tells us that highly active women can continue their exercise regimen, with appropriate modifications, right into labor. Practice bears this out. With regular exercisers, when the body typically begins its dramatic shift in the center of gravity at midpregnancy, we see a need to alter the quality of movement (size, shape, speed, flow). This is more a redirection of effort than a change in intensity, or sometimes it is a change of mode.

For a woman starting a first-time regular exercise routine during the first or second trimester, it is particularly important to assess her capabilities, monitor her progress, and be aware of potential problems. An inactive woman should be discouraged from starting highly vigorous activities after 26 weeks. We know that the placenta adapts in the first and second trimester, so continuing higher-intensity activity is possible in the third trimester. However, in the third trimester, these placental adaptations cease. Beginning a strenuous program at this point may cause fetal hypoxia. Walking at a brisk but comfortable pace, and special prenatal exercises such as Kegels and pelvic rocks, are always suitable as long as no contraindications are present; but initiating a conditioning program aimed at achieving a high level of cardiovascular fitness is not advisable in the third trimester.

Individual Tolerances Affect Modification

As mentioned in the previous chapter, the need to modify exercises depends on individual tolerances. Modifications of ballistic or high-impact movements may be important, even for highly trained individuals. The meaning of "moderate aerobic intensity" will vary from individual to individual and day to day. Sports that require complicated equipment or a potentially hazardous environment may involve motions that are perfectly safe in themselves but become unsafe because of the situation, as with soccer or squash. A safe alternative for accomplished athletes or dancers is to execute the movements of the sport in a safe setting, without equipment or other players, or with a partner who is willing to be noncompetitive.

General Safety Guidelines

The following is a brief review of the safety issues arising from the interactions of pregnancy and exercise. It is a good idea to go over them with the expectant mother and keep a list somewhere visible—perhaps on the inside of the bathroom door in the office, gym, or home.

1. Don't work out so hard that you can't catch your breath or you feel you are burning up.
2. Don't exercise if you have a fever.
3. If you experience bleeding or a large amount of discharge, see your care provider.
4. If you are constantly light-headed, are seeing stars, or have an ongoing headache, see care provider.
5. If you have swelling in your face and hands, see care provider.
6. If you experience regular contractions or cramps that continue when you stop exercising, drink four glasses of water, void your bladder, and relax on your side; see care provider.
7. Avoid lying on your back after the third or fourth month; avoid standing still on your feet for more than 20 to 30 minutes; and do not suddenly change your position.
8. Avoid fatigue, overtraining, and binge exercise.
9. Avoid motions that produce discomfort or pain.
10. Eat often in small amounts, and include proteins (eggs, milk, nuts, seeds, fish, chicken, meat, soy, and beans and rice together).
11. Drink at least 8 cups of water a day and avoid hot, humid situations.
12. Wear good shoes, dress in layers, and make sure any equipment you use is in good condition.
13. Take a rest on your side during the day in the second and third trimesters.
14. Professional or competitive athletes or dancers and their fetuses should be carefully monitored by their care providers.

Women's Need for Psychological Safety

As with adolescence, pregnancy is a major life change that can easily prompt insecurity. The body changes so dramatically that even highly skilled athletes have periods of self-doubt. Association with other exercising pregnant women is a powerful way of meeting this psychological challenge. The exercise setting must be conducive to a positive sense of self through activities that foster mastery, cooperation, and companionship, rather than competition.

SECOND PRIORITY: EFFECTIVENESS

To determine what will constitute an effective program, one must take two factors into consideration. First, what types of exercise are effective in promoting the goals of being a healthy mom having a healthy baby, developing skills for birth, and being fit for a quick recovery? Second, each individual woman's nature affects her compliance. Such factors as motivation and personal goals, family and work influences, exercise and medical histories, genetic potential, age, lifestyle, and preferences have an effect on her activity level.

Effective Exercise Components

The types of exercise that predictably produce physical fitness, promote physical health (including fetal health), and affect a woman's physical tolerance for pregnancy, labor, and birth include cardiovascular or aerobic conditioning, strength or resistance training, and flexibility exercises. The types of exercise activities that relieve discomforts or develop special skills for labor and birth include special exercises aimed at specific areas of the body, such as the low back or pelvic floor. In addition, mind/body exercises promote the ability to focus on bodily sensations in a productive way during exertion. Each of these types of exercise is briefly described here and detailed in chapter 8.

Cardiovascular or Aerobic Conditioning

It is now well accepted that large, rhythmic, and repetitive movements using more than 50% of the body's muscle mass in a sustained manner—challenging the circulatory system and elevating the pulse—improve delivery of nutrients and oxygen, improve stamina, and are associated with positive birth outcomes. The development of creative programs that include sufficient amounts of cardiovascular conditioning to improve health, and that large numbers of women will enjoy, is a current challenge for the fitness industry.

Strength or Resistance Training

By contracting the skeletal muscles against resistance, using equipment or the body's own weight, the exerciser protects the skeleton and connective tissue, increases lean body mass, and raises resting metabolic rate. Strength exercises that target areas adversely affected by pregnancy can help women achieve a more normal alignment, which reduces the potential for damage to joint facets, nerves, and blood vessels.

Flexibility Exercises

Elongating the muscles in a controlled fashion—employing balanced alignment and static stretch—relieves discomfort, promotes kinesthesia and proprioception, and improves range of motion. We have found that when asked what they like most in a program that includes many exercise components, many women reply that stretching is their favorite part because it allows them to sense their body boundaries and thus control their movement.

Special Exercises

Activities designed particularly to relieve common discomforts of pregnancy, to prepare for birth, and to enhance recovery form a training-specific component of prenatal exercise. Such exercises include Kegels for the pelvic floor; specialized abdominal exercises to reduce strain on the linea alba and to prepare for pushing; birth squats to prepare for pushing and to strengthen the muscles of deep hip flexion; and stretches that relieve common discomforts such as carpal tunnel syndrome or sciatica.

Mind/Body Exercises

Learning to work with the body instead of struggling with it is a good skill to have in ultra-endurance events, as many minor movement adjustments produce efficiency and promote self-efficacy. The specific activities that we have found effective in this realm are centering, relaxation, and the use of imagery or mental rehearsal.

Centering. Balancing the body's bony levers and achieving the relaxation response is often done at the beginning of activities such as martial arts or dance to promote safe biomechanics and fluid movement, both of which are advantageous during pregnancy.

Relaxation. Resting in a comfortable position and achieving the relaxation response reduces stress and elicits feelings of well-being. The relaxation response is a physiologic state that promotes recovery from stress. Developing the capacity to relax effectively at will requires regular practice, as does any physical skill. Because early labor requires a state of relaxation to optimize the release of oxytocin, the hormone that induces uterine contraction, learning to relax is a critical skill.

Imagery or Mental Rehearsal. Once a person is relaxed, mentally watching or imagining herself doing something like properly swinging a tennis racket or pushing out a baby (without actually trying to do it) activates subcortical neural pathways that most efficiently pattern the action. The judicious use of imagery for birth allows women to develop an image of themselves giving birth. This way of *seeing in the mind's eye* helps the body prepare for the reality of the event. In practice, we often refer to this phenomenon as wrapping the mind around the idea of birth.

Individual Components

The effectiveness of any exercise regimen is tied to compliance. The gains are achieved in the actual practice. When practice is fun, meaningful, and rewarding, people find it easy to comply. If exercise is the means to the end (healthy baby, skills for labor, quick recovery) and if it can be viewed as fun, recreation, a game, or time to be with friends, it is enjoyable and becomes its own reward. A high level of compliance among a population probably reflects a good match between what happens in each session and the needs, concerns, and motivations of the individuals.

Clearly, if a woman is interested in being healthy, taking care of herself and her baby, and being prepared for the challenges ahead (labor, birth, and nursing) and if she has an active lifestyle, it will be easy to steer her toward a three- to five-times-a-week exercise regimen with activities that she enjoys and that will be effective.

For women whose commitment is less vigorous ("I know I should be exercising . . ."), ascertaining interests and previous experience is a key, as are support and positive reinforcement. Being a little active and enjoying it throughout the entire pregnancy is more beneficial than pushing early on, possibly being injured or becoming discouraged, and quitting. Being in a group class may also provide a social stimulus for regular attendance.

Women who have the mental stamina and exercise background to work hard throughout the pregnancy may require subtle encouragement to stay attentive to kinesthetic cues and fatigue. In general, women's instincts to protect themselves and their babies are keen. A schedule that provides a physical challenge on some days and puts the hard-working woman into a group of pregnant women on other days is an arrangement we have found important to keeping such women from extensive tapering or quitting during the last trimester.

THIRD PRIORITY: COMMUNITY

"The exercise was important, but the thing that really helped was the group," is one version of a comment often repeated on evaluation forms in the author's program. An added side benefit of group prenatal fitness classes is the community that is established among the participants. So striking has this feature been that we encourage our personal trainers and corporate fitness programmers to develop regular monthly or bimonthly get-togethers for individual clients, often with their spouses. A presentation by a midwife, physician, lactation consultant, or parenting educator may be the excuse, but one ulterior motive is group support.

In assessing why this phenomenon is so pronounced, we have come to the conclusion that we live in a time when many women give birth away from their extended families. In the past, the presence of mothers, sisters, female cousins, or aunts provided a community of knowledge and support that no longer exists for many women. A prenatal exercise group provides this community. There is evidence from a variety of sources that women benefit from female support, and this period of life is no exception.

PRACTICAL APPLICATION: TURNING RESEARCH FINDINGS INTO RELIABLE PROGRAMS

As evidence mounts attesting to the advantages of prenatal exercise and as women with little experience are drawn into the activity circle, it becomes increasingly important to establish goals and priorities aimed at positive outcomes. For those preparing to lead prenatal group exercise or one-on-one prenatal personal training, it is important to know how to structure a regimen to ensure compliance and a supportive environment. One also needs to know how to find the ideal balance of cardiovascular conditioning, strength, stretch, special exercises, and mind/body activities to assure health, to implement skills for labor and birth, and to contribute to a quick recovery. It is tremendously reassuring for a woman who wishes to continue high levels of fitness activity to know that—as long as the pregnancy is healthy and she pays attention to her bodily sensations—it will be safe to do so. It is likewise reassuring for a woman wishing to begin regular activity (or a care provider wishing to prescribe activity) in the first or second trimester to know that, as long as the activity is appropriate, she will do no harm and in fact will do some good. To ensure that the benefits of prenatal exercise occur, we keep focused on our goals—promoting healthy mothers having healthy babies, developing skills for labor and birth, and facilitating a quick recovery. Just as importantly, we keep focused on our priorities—safety, effectiveness, and community. In this way, it is possible to delineate principles of program design that meet these goals and priorities, the topic of the next chapter.

REFERENCES

1. Goyert, G.L., Bottoms, S.F., Treadwell, M.C., and Nehra, P.C. 1990. The physician factor in cesarean birth rates. *New England Journal of Medicine* 320(11):706-709.

2. Mitler, L.K., Rizzo, J.A., and Horwitz, S.M. 1998. Physician gender and cesarean sections, unpublished research. Yale University School of Medicine, Dept. of Epidemiology and Public Health.

3. Kennell, J., Klaus, M., McGrain, S., Robertson, S., and Hinckley, C. 1991. Continuous emotional support during labor in a US hospital. *Journal of the American Medical Association* 265(17):2197-2201.

4. Sosa, R., Kennell, J., Klaus, M., Robertson, S., and Urrutia, J. 1980. The effect of a supportive companion of perinatal problems, length of labor and mother-infant interaction. *New England Journal of Medicine* 303(11):597-600.

CHAPTER 8

PRENATAL PROGRAM DESIGN

This chapter covers procedures for designing, monitoring, and evaluating prenatal exercise programs. As so often happens in practice, these procedures have developed over time in response to research findings and as modifications of protocols borrowed from other health-related professions. The chapter begins with the intake process, then proceeds to descriptions of appropriate exercise components. The next section concerns making exercise prescriptions for individuals based on needs, screening, and familiarity with the individual woman. We then consider formatting group prenatal exercise programs, including sequencing activities and integrating physical activities with education and support. Following this is a review of program evaluation, and a final section of the chapter presents a brief discussion of physical activity for pregnant adolescents.

INTAKE PROCEDURES FOR PRENATAL EXERCISE

Because of the nature of pregnancy, it is critical to assess each individual woman's activity needs. Collection of data (including information about motivations, exercise history, and nutritional status), as well as medical screening, is the vital first step in assuring a meaningful and effective experience for every mother-to-be.

Data Collection for Needs Assessment

Collecting preliminary information helps the instructor or trainer bring each woman through a successful prenatal program. Such basic demographic information as age, number of previous pregnancies and children, and the name of the obstetrical care provider, along with (if appropriate) race, economic status, or other relevant information should be included in the registration process. If there are matters that concern liability or research, these should also be covered in the intake process. In addition, information concerning motivation, exercise history and classification, and nutritional status should be gathered.

Motivation

Women exercise during pregnancy for a number of reasons. An exercise habit, a desire to be with other pregnant women, wanting to have a healthy baby, and fear of losing control of one's body are common reasons pregnant women turn to exercise. To satisfactorily determine an appropriate exercise regimen for any individual, it is important to ascertain her motivation. Exercise—like pregnancy and parenting—requires a commitment; and unless she is involved in activity that engages her attention, a woman is likely to lose interest. For example, regardless of whether she is highly fit or just beginning, if a woman has a strong desire to be with other pregnant women, a prenatal group class is a good choice for her primary weekly activity. Even if the class includes participants at various fitness levels and varying stages of pregnancy, a prenatal fitness specialist can create a setting in which support and education occur informally, in addition to safe, effective, and enjoyable exercise routines that can be executed at several intensity levels at the same time. And a specialist can monitor participants' other activities to ensure that they are accumulating sufficient amounts of necessary fitness components to suit their fitness levels.

If a woman has acquired an exercise habit and is fearful of losing her sense of accomplishment with her regular routine, she may be encouraged to combine parts of her weekly routine with new, gentler activities that will provide a challenge without drawing attention to her new limitations. Or, she may benefit from joining a prenatal class where she can learn to modify her activities without fear of ridicule, bringing what she learns back to her regular exercise setting. A personal trainer qualified to deal with pregnancy might be a solution for a highly competitive or professional athlete or dancer. A woman who is new to exercise and feels self-conscious, or who has time constraints, might also find the services of a qualified personal trainer appropriate at this time.

Many women turn to exercise out of fear or worry that their bodies will become foreign to them or that they will lose control of themselves in some manner. This is not an ungrounded fear and should be treated seriously. Assurances can be given that activity will promote a woman's familiarity with her changing body and help limit weight gain. Being with a group for support can be helpful in this matter also. An exercise group or a support group, or a combination of the two, can be helpful. Other women—particularly if the group is mixed in regard to the number of pregnancies the members have experienced—are a great source of information and reassurance that these fears are normal and will pass.

Exercise History and Classification

It is important to gain as much information as possible about the type and quantity of exercise a woman has engaged in during the year or two prior to her pregnancy and during the first few weeks of gestation. Because we know that conditioning is specific and will vary depending on an individual's recent activities, it is critical to be at an accurate starting point. The most effective behavioral adaptations are made through small changes in the routine, and this is essential to keep in mind.

If a woman is a competitive athlete or a professional athlete or dancer who plans to continue working at a high level throughout her pregnancy, pre-pregnancy fitness testing is advisable. This should be done in conjunction with a member of the health care team trained in both exercise physiology and obstetrics. The woman's activities and fetal responses should be recorded and reviewed regularly throughout the pregnancy. If a study on exercise and pregnancy is being conducted in her area, she may wish to participate.

Most women who wish to exercise, however, present themselves after the fact of conception, often at 6 to 10 weeks gestation. Screening all women at this point is useful, to locate not only those who may have problems, but also those for whom it may be advantageous to be more active.

Taking an exercise history, using a form like "Exercise History (Prenatal)," is essential. Finding out whether or not the woman has a history of aerobic fitness, strength, or flexibility activities and whether she is familiar with relaxation or other calming regimens, as well as inquiring about her work and children, helps create a picture of how much of what type of activity she has as a base and how much guidance she may need as she progresses in her pregnancy. This type of exercise history combines the kinds of questions asked in various research models with more gender-specific questions to give a complete activity picture.

If a woman claims to get little exercise, but has a physically demanding job and a toddler at home whom she plays with several hours each day, she may not realize how much activity she is getting. Especially if work is stressful, she may need a recreational activity that permits her to slow down—perhaps a prenatal yoga class. On the other hand, if she was accustomed to doing regular vigorous aerobics classes, lifting weights, and swimming for the year prior to her pregnancy but has been ill and inactive for the last two months, she may need a group prenatal class or a prenatal personal trainer who will ensure that she is safely monitored and returns slowly to an appropriate level of fitness.

Women's impressions of their activity levels can be at odds with reality. Sometimes women claim to be highly active but in fact are highly stressed, getting very little activity that truly promotes health and fitness. Others—especially those with small children at home—may think they do very little exercise but actually are on the go for much of the day. Finding out as much specific information as possible is of great help in establishing an appropriate regimen for a given woman during a given pregnancy. Of course, if a woman is a continuing client, much of this information may already be on file.

After one has taken and reviewed a history, it is useful to classify a woman as to her activity level to help determine how much activity may be appropriate. If a woman is motivated by a desire to obtain the benefits of exercise in pregnancy, such as relief of discomforts, increased

Exercise History (Prenatal)

Name: _____ Date: _____ Due date: _____

1. For the year prior to your pregnancy, which of these things did you do regularly?

   ☐ *Aerobic exercise:* # of sessions/week: _____; approx. length of each session: _____.

   What was your target heart rate range? _____ bpm.

   What was your RPE (rate of perceived exertion) range? (Circle lowest intensity and highest intensity.)

   Very light   Light   Fairly light   Somewhat hard   Hard   Very hard   Very, very hard

   List your activities (running, aerobic dancing, etc.): _____

   _____

   ☐ *Strength activities (weightlifting, calisthenics, etc.):*

   # of sessions/week: _____ Hip and knee flexors/extensors and ab/adductors

   _____ Chest and back; shoulders and arms

   _____ Abdominals; spine (core strength)

   _____ Pelvic floor

   ☐ *Flexibility activities (yoga, stretching, dance, etc.)*

   # of sessions/week ____

   ☐ *Combination activities (advanced dance, martial arts, basketball, etc.):* # of sessions/week _____.

   List your activities: _____

   _____

   ☐ *Relaxation (progressive relaxation, autogenic training, hypnosis, etc.):* # of sessions/week _____

   ☐ *Centering (meditation, dance, tai chi, etc.):* # of sessions/week _____

2. Do you have one or more children in the 1- to 5-year-old range who are very active? ☐ Yes ☐ No
   If yes, how much time do you spend with her/him/them?

   _____

3. Do you have a physically demanding job? ☐ Yes ☐ No   Is it stressful? ☐ Yes ☐ No
   Are you on your feet a lot? ☐ Yes ☐ No

   Describe your work activities: _____

   _____

   _____

4. Describe your exercise and/or other physical activities since the start of this pregnancy: _____

   _____

   _____

stamina, help with her labor, and a quick postpartum recovery, being in the *active* category at a minimum is critical. If she is so motivated and is not very active, positive feedback about progress, encouragement, and rewards in the form of verbal praise are very important in assisting her to become sufficiently active to attain benefits.

The five practical classifications of activity level for purposes of designing a prenatal regimen [1] are as follows:

1. *Inactive or sedentary*—does no exercise; performs most activities of daily living, but not more strenuous tasks, such as moving furniture or mowing the lawn

2. *A little active*—accumulates one to three 30-minute activity sessions over the course of a week; these may involve walking, gardening, bicycling, badminton, or other recreational activity

3. *Active*—accumulates at least 30 minutes of activity or exercise almost daily, with at least three days involving 15 to 30 minutes of sustained moderate-intensity cardiovascular work; two days involving strength and stretch work; and some centering, relaxation/imagery, or other stress management

4. *Very active*—has five or more regular exercise days per week, involving moderate- to high-intensity aerobics, strength, stretch, relaxation, centering/imagery or other stress management

5. *Professional or competitive*—does exercise as a job or lifestyle, involving strenuous exercise daily and appropriate recovery work

Prenatal exercise research on the benefits of a prenatal exercise regimen has primarily concerned levels that would be considered active or very active. This encompasses a small portion of the population. As the beneficial relationship among exercise, fitness, and health becomes more evident for the entire population [2, 3], exercise prescription becomes increasingly important. As already mentioned, having a clear picture of the starting point is critical. Many of the standard measurements are not available when a client presents herself after becoming pregnant and maximal testing is inappropriate. Consequently, careful questioning regarding activity patterns is an essential source of information.

Nutritional Status

Also paramount is gathering information about a woman's nutritional status, including her hydration. Clearly, women who refuse to eat an adequate amount of food or drink enough water should not exercise. Those who do not make healthy choices about nutrition should

be persuaded to make what changes are possible. Nutrition, exercise, rest, and avoidance of drugs and alcohol form the bases of the healthy-mother-making-a-healthy-baby approach to childbearing.

For women who choose to be active in pregnancy, there are two major considerations in analyzing nutrition:

1. *Protein and hydration status.* Is the woman taking in sufficient quantities of usable protein and water to allow her to produce the additional blood volume required to sustain both fetal growth and her own muscle efficiency, and to grow a neurologically adequate fetus?

2. *Energy status.* Is the woman taking in sufficient quantities of carbohydrates (and especially complex carbohydrates) and high-quality fats to meet the energy requirements of her own body and her fetus?

A food diary is a useful tool for gathering information about a woman's nutritional status and helping educate her about her dietary needs as a mother-to-be. The diary illustrated in the form "Food Diary" elicits information needed to determine the adequacy of the daily food intake. After asking for a 24-hour food recall or having the woman keep a two- to three-day diary, a dietary specialist can review the list to determine calories and grams of protein as shown on the form "Protein Counter." A glance at the types of foods eaten also provides information about whether or not there is adequate intake of calcium, iron, folic acid, and other vitamins and minerals, as well as fluids and fiber. Reviewing the diary with the woman is helpful in adjusting a diet that has room for improvement.

Medical Screening

Assessment of medical conditions and physical signs and symptoms is an essential ongoing function of monitoring the prenatal exercise regimen, and screening is a fundamental first step in the assessment process. Adequate screening serves three very important functions: it protects the mother and baby, the health care provider, and the perinatal fitness specialist (group instructor, personal trainer, or program director).

The following categories should be evaluated:

1. Contraindications to exercise
2. Conditions for assessment
3. Conditions that may benefit from exercise
4. Warning signs and symptoms

Through a standardized screening procedure, the health care provider rules out clients with conditions that are contraindications to exercise, notes conditions that may benefit from exercise, and reviews conditions

Name: _____

Age: _____   Weight: _____   Gestational age in weeks: _____

1. How many 8-ounce glasses of water, juice, milk, or other non-caffeine, non-alcohol fluids do you drink each day? _____

2. How many times a day do you eat? _____

3. Approximately how many calories each time? _____

4. List foods eaten yesterday (or keep the diary for 2 to 3 days):

Time of day	Name of food(s)	Quantity	Calories*	Protein (gms)*

*These items can be filled in with your nutritionist, or you may refer to the form "Protein Counter" on page 142.

A.F. Cowlin, 2002, *Women's fitness program development* (Champaign, IL: Human Kinetics).

	Portion	Protein (gm)*
Dairy		
Cheese (most types)	1 oz.	7
Cocoa	1 oz.	12
Cottage cheese	1/2 c.	15-19
Eggnog	1 c.	12
Egg	1 med.	6
Ice milk	1 c.	9
Milk		
Evaporated	1 c.	16
Powdered, dry	1 c.	25
Skim	1 c.	9
Whole	1 c.	8
Yogurt	1 c.	8
Meat and poultry (cooked without bones or trimmings)		
Beef, chicken, turkey	4 oz.	23
Duck	4 oz.	13
Lamb	4 oz.	18
Liver	4 oz.	20
Pork, ham	4 oz.	16
Bacon	1 slice	2
Sausage	4 oz.	11
Seafood		
Clams, steamed	4 oz.	12
Cod, flounder, mackerel, mussels, perch, salmon, snapper, trout	4 oz.	22-24
Halibut, lobster, scallops, shrimp	4 oz.	16-19
Sardines	1 oz.	5
Tuna, canned	4 oz.	28
Vegetable sources (incomplete proteins, except for soy)		
Seeds and nuts		
Almonds, cashews, hazelnuts, walnuts	4 oz. = 1 c.	16-21
Peanuts, roasted	4 oz. = 1 c.	30
Peanut butter	1/3 c.	12
Pecans	4 oz.	10

	Portion	Protein (gm)*
Sesame seeds	2/3 c.	10
Sunflower seeds	4 oz. = 1 c.	26
Water chestnuts	4 oz.	2
Dried beans, cooked		
Chick peas	1 1/2 c.	23
Kidney beans	2 c.	23
Navy beans	1 1/2 c.	25
Soy beans (complete protein)	1 1/2 c.	38
Flours and grains, uncooked		
Bran 100%	2 oz. = 1 c.	9
Corn flakes	1 oz. = 1/4 c.	2
Rice, brown	1 c.	15
Rice, white	1/2 c. cooked	2
Pasta/noodles	1 c.	7
High protein pasta	2 oz.	12
Vegetables		
Broccoli, cooked	1 c.	5
Brussels sprouts	1 c.	6
Corn, cooked	1 c.	5
Lima beans	1 c.	8
Peas	1 c.	5
Popcorn (w/parmesan cheese)	1 c.	4
Tomato sauce	1 c.	5
Most other vegetables	1 c.	1-2

Fruits: Average portions of most fruits yield a trace to 2 grams of protein; fruits are most vital for vitamins, mincrals, trace elements, and roughage.

Combining incomplete proteins to increase the quality of protein intake:
The following combinations enhance the quality of protein intake of each element when consumed individually, as long as they are consumed within several hours of each other.

1. Nuts and wheat (e.g., peanut butter and whole wheat bread)
2. Beans and wheat (e.g., kidney beans and tortillas)
3. Rice and beans
4. Nuts and seeds
5. Add milk or other complete protein to any incomplete protein

---

*An active mother with one fetus requires 70 to 90 grams of protein per day.

© 1998 Women's Education Life Learning at Yale-New Haven-Hospital. Used by permission.

A.F. Cowlin, 2002, *Women's fitness program development* (Champaign, IL: Human Kinetics).

that may require ongoing assessment. The fitness specialist learns to pay attention to warning signs and symptoms. In this way, problems are most easily avoided and the chance of a positive outcome is maximized.

A perinatal fitness specialist requires completion of a screening form before taking a woman into a group class or as a one-on-one client. The screening form serves as an educational tool for the mother-to-be and gives the health care provider and fitness specialist an important means of ensuring that a woman is not engaged in inappropriate activities. Some fitness instructors prefer avoidance of information about a client's medical condition, but this has two drawbacks. First, it does not prevent lawsuits; and second, it does nothing to further knowledge and wisdom. "Medical Screening Form for Prenatal Exercise Participants" is an example of a useful screening form.

Medical Screening Form for Prenatal Exercise Participants

Name: _____

Signature of care provider: _____ Date: _____

To the care provider: Please review these conditions and indicate if any now exist or existed previously. Please make any notes you think may be helpful to the fitness instructor.

Contraindications for exercise

☐ Placenta previa

☐ Premature rupture of membranes (PROM)

☐ Incompetent cervix

☐ Chronic heart disease

☐ Premature labor

☐ Toxemia or PIH

☐ Tearing or separation of placenta (abruptio)

☐ Fever (or presence of infection)

☐ Acute and/or chronic life-threatening condition

Conditions that may benefit from exercise

☐ Diabetes

☐ Gestational diabetes

☐ Hyperinsulinemia

☐ Overweight

☐ Discomforts

☐ Depression

☐ Weakness

☐ Lack of stamina

Conditions for assessment

☐ Marginal or low-lying placenta

☐ History of IUGR

☐ Diabetes or hyperinsulinemia

☐ Irregular heartbeat or mitral valve prolapse

☐ Anemia

☐ Multiple gestations

☐ Thyroid disease

☐ 3 or more spontaneous abortions

☐ Excessive over- or underweight

☐ Extremely sedentary lifestyle

☐ Asthma

Warning signs or symptoms

☐ Edema of face and hands

☐ Severe headaches

☐ Hypertension

☐ Dizziness or disorientation

☐ Palpitations or chest pain

☐ Difficulty walking

☐ Nausea

☐ Bleeding or fluid discharge

☐ Regular strong contractions

☐ Cramps

☐ Fever

Contraindications for Exercise

Any condition in which physical exertion poses a threat to the life or quality of life of the infant or mother is considered a contraindication for exercise. In the conditions briefly defined in the following paragraphs, the demands placed on the circulatory system, vital organs, or the physical structure produce an untenable internal environment. Readers are referred to the major obstetrical texts for more detailed information on any of these conditions.

Placenta previa is a situation in which the placenta lies over the cervix, making exercise movements potentially damaging to the placenta and, in turn, the fetus. This condition warrants a cesarean birth, as the placement of the placenta prohibits normal descent and delivery.

Premature rupture of the membranes (PROM) is a situation in which the membranes rupture prior to active labor, leading to a loss of amniotic fluid. While the loss of fluid represents a dangerous situation in itself, the possibility that an infection is present (most commonly beta strep) is another significant danger and must be assessed. Occasionally, a woman experiences PROM in midpregnancy. If precautions are taken, the membranes may regrow and amniotic fluid volume increase sufficiently that the pregnancy continues normally. However, it is likely that an infection caused or contributed to the rupture. Under these conditions, it is highly unlikely that an individual will be permitted to resume exercise.

Incompetent cervix is a term applied to a situation in which the cervix will not stay closed. For a variety of reasons, the cervix begins to open—generally during the second trimester. In a first pregnancy, an incompetent cervix cannot be diagnosed in advance (although if there is a family history, clients may be alerted to the possibility), and usually a spontaneous abortion signals that a woman has the condition. Women with a history of this problem are likely to be placed on bed rest and in extreme cases may even be required to spend time with their upper bodies inclined downward in order to keep the baby inside the womb. A *cerclage,* or stitch to keep the cervix closed, may be employed; but even in this case, continuing exercise is contraindicated.

Chronic heart disease of any type (cardiac status Class II or higher) requires careful medical oversight during pregnancy. Detailed analysis of various medical conditions and their effects on pregnancy is beyond the scope of this text. However, it is clear that severe chronic heart conditions may preclude physical exertion. If the health care provider of a client determines that exercise is contraindicated, an exercise instructor or trainer is not in a position to question the decision. Such a situation is an opportunity to learn about a given condition and its effect on pregnancy.

Premature labor, or *preterm labor,* can occur for a variety of reasons. Many women experience Braxton-Hicks contractions (usually thought of as the uterus practicing for labor) from midpregnancy on. Distinguishing between these practice contractions and labor contractions that are actually causing dilation of the cervix is the critical issue. True labor contractions are not stopped by hydration, slowing down and relaxing, and emptying the bladder; these contractions' effect on cervical dilation cannot be halted. On the other hand, practice contractions are stopped by these actions. If a woman experiences increased contractile activity during exercise, it is important first to ascertain whether she is well hydrated, as dehydration itself can bring on preterm labor. If she is well hydrated, does emptying her bladder and slowing down or resting on her side reduce the frequency? If this contractile response occurs regularly, she should be checked to see if dilation is occurring. In practice, we find that most women who experience increased contractions during exercise are not dilating and are able to continue with their regimen. However, it is critical to distinguish who may be experiencing dilation.

Each hospital sets its own criteria and protocol for handling preterm labor. Yale-New Haven Hospital in Connecticut describes preterm labor as observed uterine behavior over a 1-hour period consisting of four or more labor contractions (as opposed to Braxton-Hicks contractions) that are unrelieved by drinking at least four 8-ounce glasses of fluid, resting on the left side, and emptying the bladder [4]. Similar definitions are common in most locales; four to five contractions are a threshold, and the amount of fluid required in locations with high heat, humidity, or altitude is more than four glasses.

Toxemia, pregnancy-induced hypertension (PIH), and *preeclampsia* are terms for various stages of hypertensive disorder of pregnancy involving systemic malfunction. Toxemia refers to the end-stage disorder in which there is massive organ failure accompanied by convulsions. Elevated blood pressure, edema of the hands and face, dizziness, and/or headaches are signs of PIH, which is a precursor of preeclampsia and toxemia. Preeclampsia is the development of elevated blood pressure with proteinuria of pregnancy.

Abruptio, or separation of the placenta from its bed (or any tearing of the placenta), clearly creates a situation in which the ability of oxygen and nutrients to be delivered to the fetus is compromised. The stress of exercise is therefore untenable. Any bleeding or fluid discharge should be addressed by the health care provider. Chronic dehydration, malnutrition, drug abuse, vigorous percussive actions, or blunt trauma to the abdomen all have the potential to cause tearing or separation.

Fever, or any indication of infection, requires that an individual refrain from any activity that may raise core body temperature. Although this contraindication is lifted when the cause is eliminated, the presence of an underlying disorder must be addressed first. Elevated core temperature may contribute to neural tube defects early in pregnancy (see chapter 6); and later, infection may cause PROM.

Acute or *chronic life-threatening conditions* are any and all situations in which the health care provider perceives that fetal or maternal well-being may be compromised. Health care providers come from varying educational and training backgrounds, have varying experiences, and have practices that handle a variety of pregnancies. Some providers may handle high-risk pregnancies only, whereas others are more diverse and still others have patients from a particular race or from high or low socioeconomic groups. Each situation produces a unique set of criteria on which a given provider relies in order to promote health and well-being among patients.

Conditions for Assessment

The advisability of continuing exercise or making alterations should be reviewed whenever conditions for assessment occur. The following conditions are associated with various stages of pregnancy and influence temporary or pregnancy-long changes in exercise prescription.

Marginal or *low-lying placenta* refers to a diagnosis of a placenta that is lying near the cervix. Early in pregnancy, it may be difficult to tell from an ultrasound whether such a placenta will become a placenta previa or remain low lying. (To characterize this situation, people commonly use the analogy of a balloon on which one has drawn a circle at the neck before blowing it up. When the balloon is fully inflated, the circle may be caught up in the knot or may appear to migrate upward, depending on exactly where it is located. If it is in the knot, it is akin to a previa; if it appears to migrate, it is low lying, but likely to be safe for moderate exercise.) If the placenta is considered marginal or low lying early in the pregnancy, a woman may be asked to refrain from exercise until a determination can be made of the exact location.

History of IUGR (intrauterine growth restriction) refers to a situation in which a pregnant woman has previously experienced one or more pregnancies in which the fetus was small for gestational age. For some reason (e.g., undernutrition, smoking, stress, genetics), previous offspring of this woman did not grow at an appropriate rate or were considered low birth weight or small size at birth. Even if there is no indication of this condition early in the pregnancy, the current pregnancy may be considered high risk and thus a woman may be asked to modify her activities in the direction of less intensity, duration, and frequency. If IUGR is suspected or diagnosed, she may be asked to cease activity altogether. On the other hand, if the pregnancy proceeds normally, she may be able to return to her prior level of activity or may not have to make any alterations as the pregnancy continues.

Diabetes and *hyperinsulinemia* are conditions in which it is generally preferable for nonpregnant people to exercise regularly, and so it is with pregnancy. However, it is always best to be clear with the physician or midwife who is providing prenatal care about the level of activity of such a client and to ascertain whether the care provider has any special instructions. Non-weight-bearing activities, such as swimming and stationary cycling, may be desirable elements of the exercise prescription because they burn a higher proportion of carbohydrates than weight-bearing activities.

Irregular heartbeat or *mitral valve prolapse* must be monitored for alterations. In practice, we have seen a large range of situations: women with mild mitral valve prolapses who had no symptoms and proceeded as normal through their pregnancies, as well as women with situations that were deemed mild before pregnancy but who developed a murmur and with whom we proceeded very cautiously. Irregular heartbeats are more common in women than in men; and because knowledge in this area is still not profound, it is always wise to proceed cautiously. Close consultation with the care provider is essential.

Anemia actually refers to many conditions, including *physiologic anemia* (discussed in chapter 6) and *pernicious anemias,* such as *sickle cell anemia* or deficiencies in iron, B12, or folic acid, that affect the ability of red blood cells to transport oxygen. Anemia is generally defined as a hemoglobin level below 12 grams per deciliter in the nonpregnant population and 10 grams per deciliter in the pregnant population [5]. This disorder reflects an underlying illness, and it is necessary to locate the source of the problem before making a determination about the consequences of physical activity. If a serious hemoglobin pathology is present, exertion is likely to be contraindicated. On the other hand, mild anemia that responds to iron taken in conjunction with vitamin C, or to B12 or folic acid, is not likely to require more than a temporary reduction of activities. It is important to note that hemoglobin levels in African Americans are generally about 1 gram per deciliter lower than for whites, regardless of socioeconomic group [6]. Sickle cell disease is prevalent in African Americans, as is glucose-6-phosphate dehydrogenase deficiency, which is also prevalent in persons of Mediterranean descent [5].

Multiple gestation, or a pregnancy with more than one fetus, represents the potential for one or more fetus to be at risk if its uteroplacental delivery system is not as well developed as that of the other(s). Once the diagnosis of multiple gestation is made (often around 12-16 weeks), the pregnancy is very carefully monitored to ensure that both/all fetuses are progressing normally. Any indication that one or more fetus is adversely affected, or the presence of uterine irritability, generally results in a woman's being restricted in her energy expenditure. Some twin and even triplet pregnancies progress well, and if women can maintain an adequate diet and there are no signs of premature labor, they continue to exercise with modifications right up to delivery. In practice, we have seen more than one set of 7- or 7 1/2-pound infants born at or very near term in women who continued regular moderate cardiovascular exercise, coupled with centering and relaxation, moderate strength training, and flexibility activities throughout pregnancy. On the other hand, we have also seen women who, at 20 to 24 weeks, were diagnosed as having one twin growing substantially slower than the other or showing signs that the uterus was becoming irritable as it stretched. In these cases, women were taken off their exercise regimen, although often allowed to proceed with stress management and special exercises such as Kegels.

Thyroid disease, either hyper- or hypothyroid disorders, can be affected by pregnancy. Because the thyroid is active in many physiological functions, it is important to be sure that there is no underlying condition that may adversely affect the pregnancy. Thyroid function can have so many effects in the body—from atrial fibrillation to immune responses—that it is important to work closely with the care provider to assure an appropriate regimen.

Three or more *spontaneous abortions* is an indication that a client is at risk to have another. If a client indicates that this is her history, she must present approval from her care provider before entering a program. If the client has a history of urinary tract infections, this is another indication that she is at risk of spontaneous abortion. In practice, we have been most successful with these clients by waiting until they are 16 or 18 weeks into the pregnancy before allowing them to join a moderate- to high-intensity exercise group or one-on-one program. They must adhere to guidelines for good nutrition and high intake of fluid, including cranberry juice on a regular basis. The term *miscarriage* is often associated with pregnancy loss; but technically, this term refers only to the loss of the corpus luteum of pregnancy prior to implantation. Spontaneous abortion is the term applied to the loss of the embryo or fetus after this period.

Excessive over- and *underweight* are conditions that must be carefully assessed before an exercise prescription can be made. Underlying causes come into play and must be taken into account. If there are no organic pathologies, a commitment to the process of becoming healthy and fit is essential, including pacing and diligence. Of course, eating disorders must be dealt with by qualified professionals.

Extremely sedentary lifestyle is an issue that arises with some frequency in this population. There are women who decide in their third trimester that this is the time to become physically active. A very careful screening of these women allows the fitness professional to determine who is actually sufficiently active to begin a simple low-intensity program and who should be encouraged merely to walk at a comfortable pace for 5 minutes at a time or move about gently in a pool. Inactive women who present themselves in the first or second trimester, on the other hand, can be incorporated into group fitness programs or work one-on-one with good results. The cutoff point of 26 weeks for joining a vigorous group program, if the client has not been active up to that time, is a wise guideline.

Asthma may continue, worsen, or improve in pregnancy. Consequently, as with all the conditions in this category, the etiology of a particular person's situation must be considered. Asthma is associated with increased perinatal mortality, hyperemesis gravidarum (excessive vomiting and weight loss), preterm delivery, chronic hypertension, low birth weight, and vaginal hemorrhage. Good asthma control can be key to limiting the incidence and severity of such outcomes.

Conditions That May Benefit From Exercise

As with the nonpregnant population, a number of conditions improve during pregnancy with regular, appropriate physical activity. Included in this category are various forms of *diabetes* (including *gestational diabetes*), *hyperinsulinemia (hypoglycemia), overweight, physical discomforts, depression, weakness,* and *lack of stamina.* We know from many research findings that because the body is designed for movement and work, lack of activity actually causes physiologic malfunction.

Warning Signs or Symptoms

The following are indications of potential or present dangerous conditions and require that the fitness professional refer the client to her health care provider. All of these signs must be evaluated or allowed to pass before the client can be allowed to continue.

Edema of the face and hands, severe headaches, hypertension, and *dizziness* or *disorientation* are all signs of PIH, a precursor to preeclampsia and toxemia. If a woman turns up one day with any one or a combination of these symptoms, the fitness professional must send her immediately to her care provider. Some generalized edema is common near term or in extremely humid weather; however, edema of the face and hands is an indication of a more extreme problem with not clearing fluid from the cells and is a marker that is easy to spot. Some women complain of "seeing stars" or lightheadedness. These symptoms must be evaluated by the care provider. In practice, we rarely see these symptoms in a well-run program that places emphasis on proper nutrition and prenatal care. However, even in the best situations, when women are taking excellent care of themselves, disorders such as PIH sometimes occur. Because the fitness instructor or trainer sees the client with greater frequency than any other practitioner, fitness professionals should be awake to these symptoms.

Palpitations or *chest pain* in pregnant women—as with any exercising individual—must be addressed by a qualified health care provider. If such symptoms occur, one should follow the same protocols as with any client who exhibits cardiovascular distress. In practice, we rarely see these signs, as screening allows for the elimination of potential problems in this area.

Difficulty walking may be a sign of separation of the pubis symphysis (the joining of the left and right pubic bones) and should be assessed. A sharp pain at the pubis may indicate that there is motion between the two sides. If this is the case, some situations require a reduction of weight-bearing activity, and some simply require a restriction of actions involving abduction of the legs or any wide stance. In practice, we have most commonly seen this condition in women who run or who participate in high-impact aerobics several times each week. The resolution of the condition following pregnancy varies depending on the severity of the problem and the individual's genetics and behavior.

Nausea may be an indication of a number of things, from early-pregnancy hormone shifts or immune reactions, to a midpregnancy bout with the flu, to later-pregnancy signs of labor. As a consequence, it should never be taken lightly. Early in pregnancy, some women find that exercise alleviates nausea. In practice, a number of cases of hyperemesis gravidarum (severe vomiting) have been referred to our exercise program as a last resort; and these women have done well, managing moderate weight gains and increased food consumption in conjunction with regular physical activity.

Bleeding or *fluid discharge* can signal a number of things, from torn membranes to infection to placenta previa. In any case, these are signs that must be evaluated by the care provider. Women who present with this situation should immediately contact their provider and should not exercise.

Regular strong contractions or *cramps* most often are Braxton-Hicks (practice contractions), but may be labor contractions. Labor contractions are generally much stronger than practice contractions, and the abdomen becomes a hard ball as the uterus contracts. Second-time mothers may be able to tell the difference, but first-time mothers will likely need a medical evaluation. Following the protocol for determination of preterm labor is wise: the woman should consume four glasses of water,

void her bladder, cool down, and rest on her side. Practice contractions will cease.

Fever of a temporary nature is a reason not to exercise on a given day. Generally, women with colds or the flu should not participate in an exercise session. If the fever continues, a more persistent infection may be present and the situation should be evaluated.

Developing Research Questions

Readers interested in developing research questions may wish to look at additional instruments that have been used to record information about childbearing women, concerning demographics [7-9], fitness testing [10, 11], pregnancy health status [12-19], pregnancy health beliefs and behaviors [20-25], psychosocial factors [26-36], commitment to pregnancy and motherhood [37-39], pregnancy and birth outcomes [40-46], fetal and neonatal outcomes [47-49], and adolescent pregnancy issues [50-53].

LIABILITY CONCERNS

Fitness professionals working with pregnant women can find themselves suddenly outside the scope of practice should a client have a medical development with which they are unfamiliar. To ensure that she or he will know when to contact a care provider, the fitness professional must obtain and maintain a solid education in the field and maintain a good relationship with the obstetrical health care providers in the community. Of equal importance is observing liability practices required by the state, including using a liability waiver during intake.

Education

It is important for fitness instructors or trainers to obtain adequate education and a certification in pre/postnatal health and fitness, to pursue continuing education in the field, and to tell local care providers about their qualifications. Awareness on the part of doctors and midwives that there is a knowledgeable, well-prepared instructor or trainer in their area is helpful and reassuring to them, as well as beneficial to the trainer or instructor and to the program.

Relationship With Health Care Providers

Years of practice have taught us that cooperation between fitness professionals and health care providers (obstetricians and midwives) is a key component in the success of prenatal exercise programs. There are four areas in which the fitness professional can interact with care providers for the benefit of both their clients and their programs:

1. Contact with the care providers themselves through meetings, calls, and brief letters
2. Inclusion of care providers on the advisory board for the program
3. Adequate public relations, including press releases, advertising, and contact with care providers' offices to make sure they have up-to-date brochures, flyers, business cards, or newsletters
4. Contact through screening forms these enable the provider to see that the fitness professional is knowledgeable and often serve to educate providers about which conditions alarm practitioners in the exercise field

Liability Forms

Requirements for liability forms vary from state to state. Forms that are effective for the general population are also used in many locations with no special alterations for pregnancy. Perhaps the most effective factor for limiting liability is to get across to each client that she must take responsibility for her body. A pregnant woman is usually willing to be "in touch with" or "listen to" her body, and this is her best tool for finding an appropriate path at any given time or in any given situation.

APPROPRIATE EXERCISE COMPONENTS

Chapter 7 outlined the exercise components that are effective in promoting the goals of healthy moms having healthy babies, skills for labor and birth, and quick recovery. These are cardiovascular or aerobic conditioning; strength or resistance training; flexibility exercises; special exercises; and mind/body exercises including centering, relaxation, and imagery. We now consider these components in more detail.

Cardiovascular or Aerobic Conditioning

Cardiovascular conditioning strengthens the lungs, heart, and circulation for delivery of oxygen and nutrients. It also improves and maintains stamina and contributes to a sense of well-being. Examples are walking, jogging, running, treadmill, stair stepper, bicycling, step aerobics, aerobic dancing, rowing, and swimming. From research presented in previous chapters we learned that a minimum of three sessions per week for a minimum of about 20 minutes (and maximum of about 45 minutes), at a perceived exertion in the 12 to 16 range (somewhat hard to hard), is a threshold for the level of conditioning that may have a positive effect on a woman's experience of labor.

Safe Activities for Pregnant Women

In addition to exercise history, when one is determining what is appropriate for a specific individual, it is helpful to take into account the inherent challenges of a given activity. Movement patterns (which parts of the body do which actions in what sequence), intensity, and effort/shapes (the way the energy takes form—for example, some actions are smooth gliding movements whereas others are ballistic slashing motions), as well as dangers from the equipment, other players, or the environment, affect safety. Obviously, more active women possess greater movement skills, and more activities are therefore reasonably appropriate for them. Nonetheless, if changes need to be made in a woman's typical activity for safety reasons, it is good to look at other similar activities that may be less risky. Doing more than one type of activity also has benefits. *Cross-training* helps prevent overuse injuries and avoids boredom.

Table 8.1 is a prenatal cardiovascular activity chart covering common recreational sport, exercise, and dance activities. It reviews various activities and their suitability for pregnant women at various stages of pregnancy and various fitness levels, grouping the activities by similarity of action. On the basis of movement patterns, intensity, effort/shapes, requirements for equipment, and special skills, the author has assessed the suitability of each activity during each trimester for women with various activity levels. Any individual woman must ultimately make her own decision about whether or not to participate in any given activity, but it is useful to have some guidance based on the difficulty of the activity and the experience of the participant.

Modifying Activities

If a woman has been participating in low-impact aerobics for many years prior to her pregnancy, she may simply need to adjust her intensity level on any given day if she feels like taking it easy. If she is skilled at the physical aspects of her regular activity but is feeling like a fish out of water, she may need to find a prenatal aerobics class where she can learn to make necessary modifications and also get the support of her peers. A well-designed and well-taught prenatal aerobics class takes into account the special needs of the pregnant body, for example by including gluteal/hamstring curls (to help balance shortened iliofemoral flexors) in the cardiochoreography, as shown

Table 8.1 Prenatal Cardiovascular Activity Chart

1 = first trimester 2 = second trimester 3 = third trimester; the activity is generally safe for the trimester listed, although the woman should constantly assess safety and appropriateness.

† = requires special skills and/or familiarity with equipment that should already be present and poses dangers because of demands of those skills or equipment.

* = is risky even with previous experience because of contraindicated effort/shape or lack of control in the environment, and becomes increasingly dangerous as pregnancy progresses.

Reminder: The appropriateness of any activity is ultimately a matter only the expectant mother herself can assess. An activity with no numbers is not recommended at this point in pregnancy.

Activity	Inactive	A little active	Active	Very active	Competitive or professional
Walking	1 2 3	1 2 3	1 2 3	1 2 3	1 2 3
Speedwalking		2 3	1 2 3	1 2 3	1 2 3
Jogging†			1 2	1 2 3	1 2 3
Running†			1 2	1 2	1 2 3
Track events†			1	1 2	1 2
Treadmill†		1 2	1 2 3	1 2 3	1 2 3
Stair machine†			1 2	1 2 3	1 2 3
Slide*†					
Glidewalker*†				1 2	1 2
Stationary cycling	1 2	1 2	1 2 3	1 2 3	1 2 3
Recreational cycling*†		1 2	1 2	1 2	1 2
Competitive cycling*†					1
Recreational swimming*†	1 2 3	1 2 3	1 2 3	1 2 3	1 2 3
Water aerobics	2	1 2 3	1 2 3	1 2 3	1 2 3
Lap swimming†			1 2 3	1 2 3	1 2 3
Competitive swimming*†				1 2	1 2
Snorkeling*†		1 2	1 2 3	1 2 3	1 2 3
Water skiing*†					
Scuba diving*†					
Surfing*†					
Day sailing*†			1 2	1 2	1 2 3
Sailboarding*†				1	1
Rowing or sculling, carefully*†				1 2	1 2 3
Ergometer rowing†			1 2	1 2 3	1 2 3
White-water canoeing, kayaking*†					
Prenatal aerobic/exercise class	1 2 3	1 2 3	1 2 3	1 2 3	1 2 3

	Inactive	A little active	Active	Very active	Competitive or professional
Low-impact/low-intensity aerobics	1 2	1 2 3	1 2 3	1 2 3	
Low-impact/high-intensity aerobics†			1 2	1 2 3	1 2 3
High-impact/high-intensity aerobics*†					
Low step aerobics, beginning†		1 2	1 2 3	1 2 3	1 2 3
Low step aerobics, advanced*†			1 2	1 2 3	1 2 3
High step aerobics, advanced*†				1	1
Modern dance, beginning	1 2	1 2	1 2 3	1 2 3	1 2 3
Modern dance, advanced†			1 2	1 2 3	1 2 3
African/Caribbean dance, beginning		1 2	1 2 3	1 2 3	1 2 3
African/Caribbean dance, advanced			1	1 2	1 2
Mideastern (belly) dance	1 2	1 2 3	1 2 3	1 2 3	1 2 3
Ballet, beginning†		1 2	1 2 3	1 2 3	1 2 3
Ballet, advanced†			1 2	1 2	1 2 3
Jazz dance, beginning†		1 2	1 2	1 2	
Jazz dance, advanced*†		1	1 2	1 2	
Ballroom dance, beginning	1 2	1 2 3	1 2 3	1 2 3	1 2 3
Ballroom dance, advanced*†			1 2	1 2	1 2 3
Contra dance		1 2	1 2 3	1 2 3	1 2 3
Gymnastics*†				1	1
Prenatal yoga	1 2 3	1 2 3	1 2 3	1 2 3	1 2 3
Yoga, beginning†			1	1 2	1 2
Yoga, advanced†			1	1	1
Tai chi	1 2	1 2 3	1 2 3	1 2 3	1 2 3
Karate, beginning†			1	1	1 2
Karate, advanced†					
Judo, beginning†			1	1	1 2
Judo, advanced†					

Friendly games of:

	Inactive	A little active	Active	Very active	Competitive or professional
Badminton†	1 2	1 2 3	1 2 3	1 2 3	1 2 3
Basketball*†			1	1 2	1 2
Frisbee*†	1	1 2	1 2	1 2	1 2
Golf†		1	1 2	1 2	1 2
Handball*†					
Ping-pong†		1	1 2	1 2	1 2
Racquetball*†			1	1	1

(continued)

Table 8.1 *(continued)*

	Inactive	A little active	Active	Very active	Competitive or professional
Soccer*†			1	1	1
Softball*†			1	1	1
Squash*†					
Tennis*†			1 2	1 2	1 2 3
Volleyball*†			1	1 2	1 2
Cross-country skiing*†			1 2	1 2	1 2
Ski machine*†			1	1	1
Downhill skiing*†					
Snow- or skateboarding*†					
Roller skating or blading*†			1	1 2	1 2
Ice skating*†			1 2	1 2	1 2 3
Rock climbing*†				1	1
Skydiving*†					

Cowlin, unpublished data

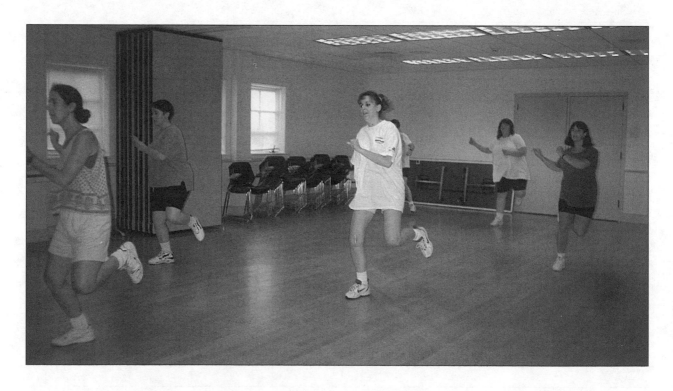

Figure 8.1 Prenatal aerobic session. A prenatal cardiovascular workout should incorporate movements that are helpful to the pregnant body in establishing balance and mobility, such as gluteal/hamstrings leg curls.

in figure 8.1. The instructor also demonstrates movements at several levels of intensity by altering the size or speed of movements, allowing individuals to choose a comfortable level for themselves.

Some serious athletes participate in activities that they can continue doing with minor modifications for comfort and safety. The 38-weeks-pregnant swimmer shown in figure 8.2 continued swimming freestyle and backstroke laps right up to delivery, although she found breaststroke too uncomfortable to continue on a regular basis. On the other hand, those whose sports involve uncontrollable environmental dangers may need help finding something else that is challenging but safe. A professional downhill skier might want to try an African dance class. While skills in both these activities require an ability to carry one's weight down into the legs, the new aspects of the dance class provide new challenges. As an anonymous beginner the skier might feel she has plenty of small learning moments ahead of her that will be rewarding.

Water Exercise

Immersion in water affects hemodynamics, metabolism, and endocrine function, driving fluid from cells into the

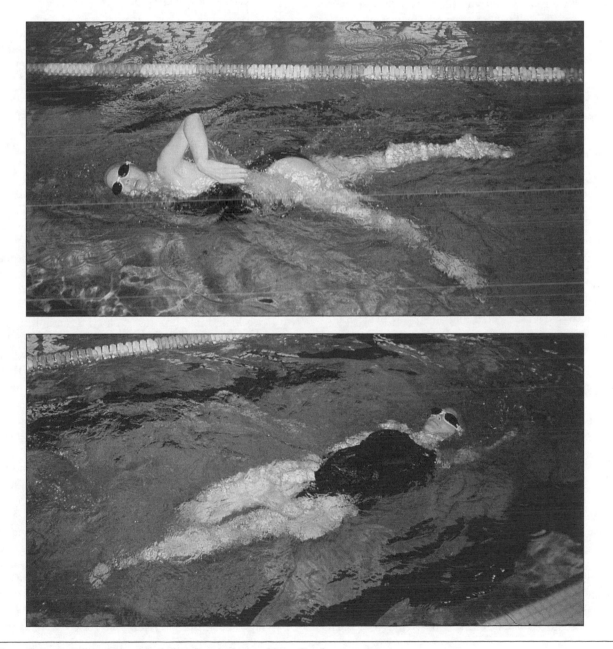

Figure 8.2 Swimming freestyle and backstroke laps at 38 weeks of pregnancy.

central blood volume [54-59; also see chapter 6, references 28-33]. These effects, as well as buoyancy and cooling, make water exercise ideal for women who are heavier or those who need to improve circulation [60]. Moving a land class into water during the summer months is one way to avoid problems with hot, humid weather and its negative effect on maternal cooling. Whether people are doing lap swimming, water jogging, or water aerobics, a good warm-up and thorough cool-down are essential. Reduction of blood pressure includes lowered pressure in the brain; and without a proper cool-down, participants may experience light-headedness or faintness when emerging from the water. Land choreography does not translate literally to the water, because of the particular effects of water pressure on movement—slowing down motion and requiring greater stabilization for many movements. Intensity can be controlled by increased range, first, and increased speed, second. Keeping a set tempo for all participants may not be realistic. Rather, demonstrating a movement and allowing participants to work at their own pace or make smaller or larger motions ensures safety and allows individuals to assume responsibility for their workouts.

Sedentary Women

A sedentary woman who may have biomechanical or medical health risks because she does not work with her body can offer a great challenge. Unless she is highly motivated, she will likely require much education and support, even if a simple walking program is all she can do. Whether this client needs a personal trainer, a group situation, or merely a friend who will walk with her on a regular basis, it is essential for someone with the appropriate training to assess her physical capabilities and motivational requirements.

Strength Conditioning

Although scientific studies concerning the effects of strength training on pregnancy are few, there is no evidence in the literature of serious damage to the mother or fetus among women who do moderate, well-supervised strength training. There are three generally accepted strictures in regard to resistance or strength training in pregnancy. One is to avoid the Valsalva maneuver because of downward, expulsive pressure on the abdominal contents and pelvic floor when holding one's breath during exertion. Exhaling on the effort—a standard of practice in any case—is essential in pregnancy. Secondly, as the center of gravity makes its dramatic shift in later pregnancy, it is advisable to work with machines at low resistance; to use bands, tubes, or the body's own weight

---

> ### Restrictions for Strength Training During Pregnancy
>
> - Avoid the Valsalva maneuver. Exhale through the sticking point—generally the most difficult part of the exercise—and inhale during the less stressful phase of the exercise.
> - Avoid free weights after midpregnancy. Use machines at low resistance, bands, tubes, or the body's own weight while seated.
> - Avoid the supine position after the first trimester. Use only for learning the hiss/compress and testing for diastasis recti.

---

while seated on the floor rather than standing; and to avoid free weights. Providing a closed kinetic chain or removing the stress of standing minimizes abnormal joint motion. Thirdly, women should avoid the supine position after the first trimester, and especially in later pregnancy. Sometimes, as when a woman is learning the hiss/compress or testing for diastasis recti, the supine position is the most productive. However, one does not perform exercises regularly in this position.

In practice, there have been many thousands of women actively involved in strength training over the course of their pregnancies. Their experiences shape the practice of this activity as information is passed through women's networks. Commonsense guidelines aid in the formatting of resistance programs, and the biomechanics of pregnancy (see chapters 5 and 6) guides the design of individual exercises.

If we look at the process of carrying and birthing a baby in terms of the strength demands, two things become immediately apparent. First, there is a slow but steady body weight increase and a change in plumb. These changes are great enough that even our most athletic women are affected to some degree. Second, the events for which women are training (pregnancy, birth, and recovery) require strength endurance. Women must carry the extra weight of pregnancy 24 hours a day. In birth, contractions are repeated over and over for many hours. And, although the baby is relatively light in weight at birth, the posture of constantly holding the baby is a new one and requires adaptation.

These two phenomena—changing body weight and the need for strength endurance—characterize the type of strength activity that will be most useful. As body weight increases, it is logical to gradually reduce resistance into the lower ranges but to keep the number of repetitions high. To prevent damage to joints whose bones may be moving in abnormal configurations, lower weights provide safety. To prevent long-term fatigue but also allow a maximum number of repetitions, we often suggest that women do fewer repetitions within sets, but more sets. If, for example, they were accustomed to doing three sets of 15 repetitions, they might switch to four sets of 12. In this way they will still get a large total, but if they feel fatigued on a particular day they can forego part or all of the final set or some of the reps in each set.

Group instructors who are accustomed to choreographing their workouts may find it useful to distribute sets throughout the course of an hour session. Functional motions and actions taken from daily living can be analyzed for their components and utilized as part of the strength conditioning process at several times during the workout. For example, the instructor might use the action of pulling a seatbelt to the side and latching it to strengthen the latissimus dorsi muscles. With advanced exercisers, this action could be coordinated as an oppositional arm movement during a traveling grapevine step.

While strengthening all major muscle groups remains a goal, the shifts in alignment that occur particularize the strains placed on the body. Specifically, as discussed in preceding chapters, the following areas need a focus on strength in order to help maintain alignment and function in as healthy a manner as possible: abdominals and pelvic floor, gluteals and hamstrings, and upper back and thoracic spine. These are discussed in the pages that follow.

In addition, the hip flexors (iliopsoas, pectineus, and rectus femoris) and knee extensors (quadriceps) are challenged by many activities of daily living—getting out of bed, sitting down and standing up, walking upstairs, and bending to pick up things. Ideally, all the leg muscles are involved in a global interplay when standing activities involve resistance to gravity, but the psoas and quadriceps seem to dominate the action. And, in pregnancy, because of the changing center of gravity, this situation is pronounced. Consequently, another essential area of strength training is whole-leg flexion and extension, or squats, also discussed in this section.

Abdominal and Pelvic Floor Strength

As one might suspect, core body strength is a key element of prenatal strength training. Focusing on the deep abdominal muscle—the transverse abdominal—not only provides a basis for postural health, but also prepares a woman for the expulsion stage of birth (pushing) and for the recovery of her torso and abdomen from the stresses of pregnancy. By focusing on the pelvic floor, the woman learns to control the tightness and relaxation of the muscle group that must support her viscera but still stretch enough to let a baby out.

Abdominals. The transverse abdominal muscle has three critical features:

1. It is a large, deep (slow twitch, endurance) bilateral muscle.
2. Its fibers run horizontally, so that its action pulls the edges of the abdomen toward the center, resulting in slight posterior rotation of the pelvis, downward rotation of the ribs, and slight flexion of the lumbar spine.
3. It provides anterior support and compresses the viscera.

Anatomically speaking, each side (left and right) of the transverse abdominal muscle attaches to the lumbar fascia, inner surface of the cartilage of the lower six ribs, inner rim of the iliac crest, the lateral third of the inguinal ligament, the iliopectineal eminence, and the crest of the pubis; it inserts into the linea alba, where it joins its fellow from the other side [61]. A good image of this muscle is of two large hands with splayed fingers that wrap around the deep midsection of the torso from the sides of the low back, along the lower edges of the ribs and the top and front of the pelvis toward the center line of the torso. When contracted, the muscles act as an internal girdle. Aside from the psoas, this is the deepest abdominal muscle; it lies underneath the obliques and recti abdominal muscles (see figure 8.3). In some people, the lowest fibers interdict with the internal obliques [62].

The function of the transverse abdominal is to compress the contents of the abdomen (and thus support the lumbar spine) and assist with urination, defecation, emesis (vomiting), parturition (the expulsion or pushing stage of birth), and forced exhalation [62]. Its influence on bone movement is greatly enhanced by its integration with other abdominal muscles.

The action to strengthen the transverse muscle (see figure 8.4) consists of hissing or blowing air out through the mouth while compressing the abdomen. We commonly call this action *hiss/compress.* As a by-product, the back of the waist presses out, reducing the curve (lumbar spine flexes slightly).

When the other abdominals assist, a deeper curve results; this is commonly called a *C-Curve* (see figure 8.5). Developing hiss/compress and C-Curve strength before pregnancy or as early in pregnancy as possible, and continuing throughout pregnancy, is requisite for avoiding or limiting damage to the abdominal muscles.

Abdominal exercises can be executed in a variety of ways that do not require the supine position. In the seated position, one can also do curl-downs, being sure after 20 weeks to splint the abdomen with the hands (described later). Other positions for abdominal exercises include

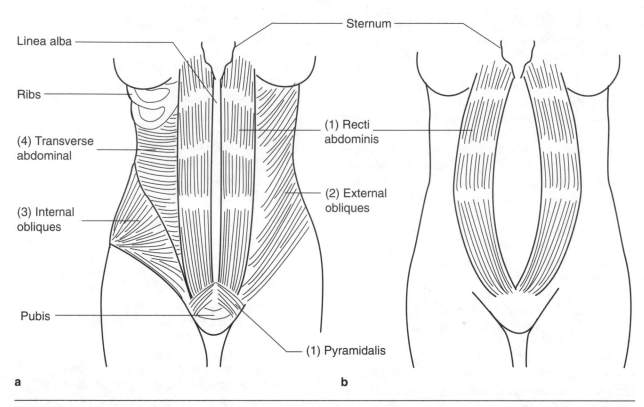

Figure 8.3 Abdominal muscles: *(a)* pre-pregnancy, 1 = top or most superficial muscle layer. 4 = deepest muscle layer; and *(b)* diastasis recti postpartum.

the crawling position on hands and knees (see figure 8.6) and side-lying (see figure 8.7).

• *Diastasis Recti in Pregnancy.* Pregnancy-related stretching of the abdominal muscles often results in a separation that is called *diastasis recti* (see figure 8.3*b*). The reason for the name is that the separation is most commonly assessed by palpation of the linea alba between the recti abdominal muscles during a curl-up. The condition is associated with a pulling away of the abdominal muscles from the linea alba, similar to the pulling that creates shinsplints. In pregnancy, tearing results in a bulging of soft tissue through the space between the recti during execution of a curl-up, shown in figure 8.8. It is difficult to determine the depth of the tearing until a woman has given birth. This needs to be assessed in the postpartum period and is discussed later (see "Course of Labor, Birth, and the Immediate Recovery" in chapter 11). In any case, the hissing/compressing or C-Curve action should be continued through the pregnancy, and abdominal curl-downs should be started by the hissing/compressing or C-Curve action and continued with a splinting of the abdominal area.

• *Splinting the Abdomen.* We commonly recommend that all women splint their abdomens during abdominal exercises after 20 weeks, or midpregnancy. It is easy to

do. Women can place their hands on the sides of the abdomen and push toward the center line, or cross the arms over the belly and pull toward the center (see figure 8.9), or place a towel around the back and pull the ends across the center in the front.

Pelvic Floor Exercises (Kegels). Strength exercises for the pelvic floor muscles include closing and opening the pelvic outlet, lifting and lowering and the preparation for pushing, and sphincter exercises. The descriptions of these actions (see below) refer to muscles described in figure 5.3 in chapter 5. It is important to note that it is necessary not only to contract these muscles, but also to release them. In order to prepare the pelvic outlet to stretch so that the baby can be released from the body, these muscles must learn to relax on cue. The bulbocavernous muscle, which surrounds the vagina, must stretch maximally as the baby leaves the body in a vaginal birth.

• *Closing and Opening the Pelvic Outlet.* We use three specific exercises to isolate and train the pelvic floor. The first is the superficial closing and opening of the pelvic outlet. When one contracts the ischiocavernous, transverse perineal, and gluteal muscles, the pelvic outlet is made smaller as the

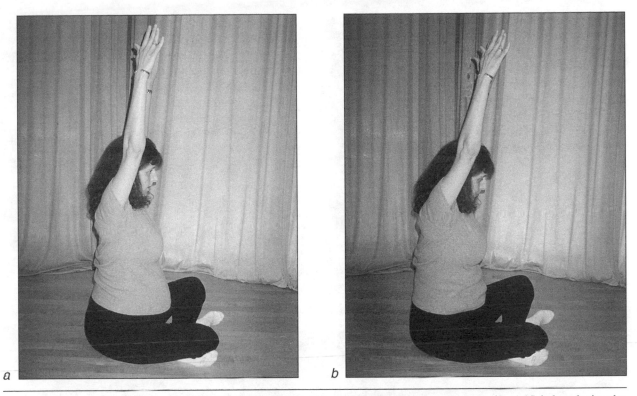

a   *b*

Figure 8.4   Training the transverse abdominal muscle during pregnancy with the hiss/compress exercise. *(a)* Inhale, relaxing the abdomen. *(b)* Exhale by hissing or blowing through the mouth while compressing the abdomen.

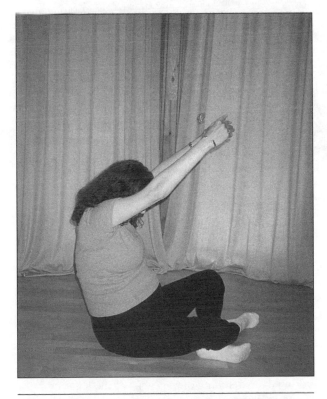

Figure 8.5   The C-Curve begins in the same way as the hiss/compress. When exhaling, enlarge the actions of the transverse abdominal muscle and include the recti abdominal muscles, creating the shape of the letter *C*.

sitsbones, pubis, and coccyx are pulled together. Relaxing these muscles allows the outlet to be stretched. Although this exercise is not traditionally taught as part of Kegel exercises, we have found it effective because when nervous or scared, many women tense these muscles. Learning where the muscles are by tensing and releasing them helps develop the control to relax them.

• *Lifting and Lowering and Preparation for Pushing.* The second exercise is lifting and lowering the pelvic floor, sometimes referred to as *elevator Kegels*. Through contraction of the bulbocavernous, ischiocavernous, urogenital diaphragm, and levator ani muscles, the pelvic floor is lifted, maintaining the internal organs in position. If these muscles atrophy, the uterus and bladder may fall through the vagina. Contracting them supports the viscera. The exercise involving these muscles that serves as a preparation for pushing entails relaxing these muscles and actually pressing them outward slightly (bearing down). To do this, one should drop the jaw, exhale audibly, and compress the transverse muscle. The effort of the diaphragm in exhaling is repelled off the transverse muscle and directed toward the vaginal opening. Women can gently practice this coordination once a month during a relaxation session, but should not do this pushing action regularly or with any force until pushing in labor.

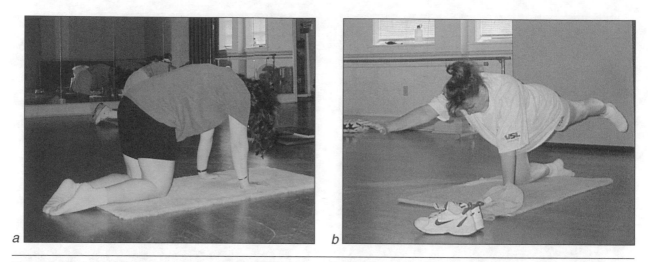

Figure 8.6 Abdominal exercises in the crawling position. *(a)* In the crawling position, the hiss/compress is highly effective. *(b)* For the obliques, the opposing arm and leg extension can be done. When executing the opposing arm and leg exercise, exhale on the extension and inhale returning to the crawling position.

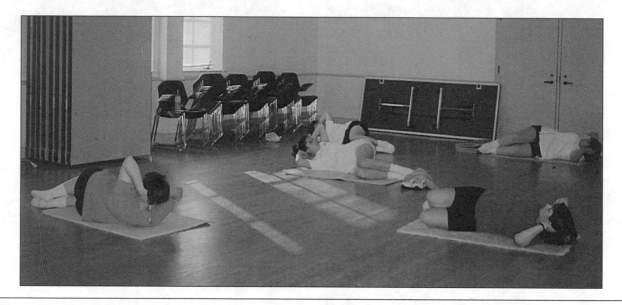

Figure 8.7 Abdominal exercises in the side-lying position. In the side-lying position, many abdominal exercises can be accomplished nearly as effectively as in the supine position. Exercises should be repeated on both sides.

• *Sphincter Exercises.* The third exercise women can do to train the pelvic floor involves the sphincter muscles. Contracting the sphincter muscles—the bulbocavernous and sphincter ani muscles—results in closing of the orifices of the vagina and urethra, and the anus, respectively. Relaxing these muscles allows smooth muscle function to be activated and enhances emptying. To test the strength of the sphincter that controls the vaginal and urethral openings, urinate until the bladder is about two-thirds empty, then squeeze and stop the flow of urine. Hold for a few seconds, then relax and empty completely. Women should practice by squeezing and releasing these muscles not when urinating, but when working out! Improvements in strength can be evaluated periodically with

the urine test. Closing first the anus and then the vagina and urethra, and next releasing the vagina and urethra, followed by the anus, is sometimes called the *wave Kegel.*

Gluteal and Hamstring Strength

Because of hypertrophy and postural shortening of the psoas major and quadriceps muscles, as well as the resulting overstretching of the backs of the legs and hips, healthy alignment in pregnancy is greatly enhanced by strengthening the gluteals and the proximal fibers of the hamstrings. As long as one takes precautions, making sure flooring is level and equipment and starting positions are safe, pregnant women can do most standard

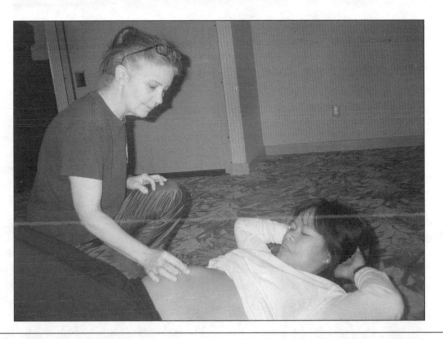

Figure 8.8 Checking for diastasis recti in a prenatal client. To check for diastasis recti during pregnancy, have the client exhale and execute a curl-up. The protrusion of soft tissue through the space between the two recti abdominis muscles indicates tearing of the muscles away from the linea alba. Here, the author palpates a small protrusion on a woman seven months pregnant, indicating only mild separation. Hiss/compress and splinting the abdomen should limit further separation.

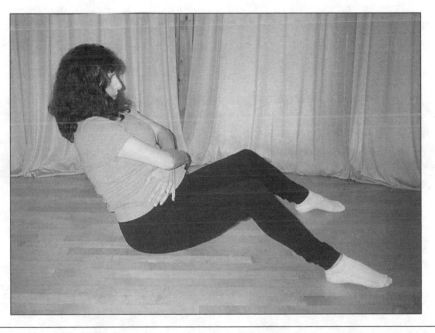

Figure 8.9 Splinting the pregnant abdomen after 20 weeks. Splinting the abdomen during abdominal exercises is commonly recommended after 20 weeks. Crossing the arms over the abdomen and pulling toward the center line during exertion is one often used method.

exercises for these muscles. A woman should not, for example, use a prone hamstring machine after the first trimester, although a seated hamstring machine would be safe.

Tubes and bands, placed around the feet or ankles, can be used in the standing position for both gluteal and hamstring strengthening actions. We don't recommend using such bands around the feet or ankles for abduction or adduction because of knee laxity in lateral motion (women should place them around the thighs for abduction or use one of the large, recreational balls for the adductors). However, with attention to line of pull in hip or knee flexion or extension, we have found the bands safe. Standing on one foot (using a wall or bar for support if needed), extending one leg back will challenge the gluteals on that leg, and a leg curl will challenge the hamstrings. Moderate or slow-paced, controlled motions are essential. Similar actions can be integrated into aerobic choreography, as well. The pelvic tilt, which is commonly used to strengthen the gluteals and upper fibers of the hamstrings, is described in the section "Special Exercises for Pregnancy."

Upper Back and Thoracic Spine Strength

The combination of increased spinal curves and added breast weight can cause increased kyphosis in pregnancy. A variety of equipment can be used to execute the essential exercises for increasing strength in this area. Among such exercises are the following:

1. Scapula retraction and depression
2. Horizontal extension of the arms (rowing with elbows horizontal to shoulders, slightly bent)
3. Extension of the thoracic spine

Machines, bands, and hand weights, when properly positioned, all provide resistance work for this area. In addition, seated exercises with partners are an excellent way to combine a social component with the strengthening element.

One can also use the body as its own resistance mechanism. Figure 8.10 shows women ready to begin shoulder retraction and depression. By imagining they are pulling back and down on a heavy object, they use their own antagonist muscles to create a resistance. Movement analysts call this type of controlled motion *bound movement*. One reason it is useful to work in this manner is that it is slow and purposive, and helps women to be mentally associative (paying attention to the sensations involved or being kinesthetically tuned in) while pulling the shoulder blades back and down. Equipment is not required. A similar process can be used to bring the elbows back in horizontal arm extension, or to lift the chest in thoracic extension.

An exercise we term the *back-up* (as opposed to curl-up) is practical for strengthening the erector muscles governing the thoracic spine. People can do this either on the knees or sitting on a chair; in the starting position, knees are apart and the torso is forward over the knees. In the crouched position, hands are on the floor under the shoulders; in the seated position, hands are on the knees. Start by looking forward, then toward the ceiling, extending the thoracic spine by contracting the upper fibers of the erector spinae muscles. Be sure to limit the arching of the spine to the area above the waist and exhale. The hands on the floor or knees provide some support for the low back. Slowly return to the starting position, inhaling, and curl the chin toward the chest at the end. The back-up is shown in figure 8.11.

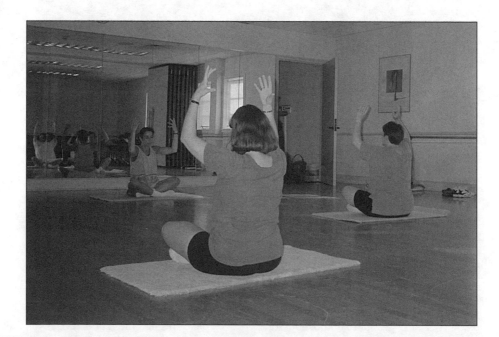

Figure 8.10   Using the body as its own resistance in upper back strength training. Scapular retraction and depression, and extension of the thoracic spine take on increased importance in pregnancy, when changes in the center of gravity can cause the spine to develop increased kyphosis. Beginning as shown—with arms bent, slightly forward and up, and scapula forward and up—pull scapula down and back for retraction and depression. Then, bring elbows back for horizontal arm extension. Lift chest and face toward the ceiling for thoracic extension.

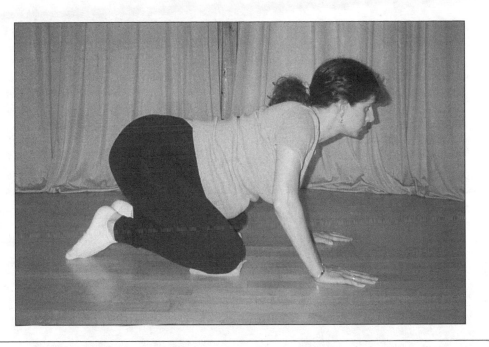

Figure 8.11 Back-ups. To increase strength in the erector spinae of the thoracic spine, the back-up starts in a crouched position, with chin tucked. Then, as shown, the woman looks forward and extends her upper spine.

Squats

To strengthen the whole leg, squats are an excellent choice. The basic fitness squat for women begins standing with weight centered, in the parallel-leg position (feet 6 to 8 inches apart, no internal or external femoral rotation). Bend the legs, with pronounced iliofemoral flexion and upper body pitched slight forward. Then, "push up" with all the leg muscles on the extension phase. A useful image is of the floor being pushed down by the effort. The depth of the squat depends on the strength and stability of the individual woman. Squeeze the gluteals and pelvic floor at the top of the action.

To help prepare for the birth squat (see special exercises), wide, outwardly rotated leg squats—or *plies* in *second position*, to borrow from ballet—are useful. Paying attention to the knees to keep them over the center of the foot is critical, as is initiation of the movement from the outward rotation of the femur by the six deep lateral rotators, including the piriformis. Limit the depth of the squat, or plie, to a horizontal line of the thighs. To include lower legs and feet in these leg squats, one can take a small squat and then push up onto the balls of the feet (not the toes) as the legs extend.

Strength Training for Other Major Muscle Groups

The question of parameters for strength or resistance training in pregnancy is unresolved. There are, however, many practices that have evolved through trial and error over the past 20 to 30 years. Research in this area is seriously needed. As noted earlier, we have found that training for strength endurance during pregnancy seems to be the most helpful approach. The use of low to moderate resistance, medium to high repetitions, and many sets, sometimes spread out or in a circuit training technique, most closely mimics the physical demands of pregnancy and birth. Women need to be sure to use good form and exhale on the effort. If a woman cannot compress the transverse abdominal muscle during effort, she should modify the exercise so she can, or not do that exercise.

If time and energy permit, other important but nonessential strength exercises include the following:

- Overhead press
- Lat pull-downs or rows
- Internal and external rotator cuff exercises
- Chest—modified push-ups, wall push-ups or flys (do not lie on the back after the first trimester; after 20 weeks, do not use an incline for flys—use bands or a partner, in a seated position)
- Biceps and triceps exercises
- Hip adduction and abduction (bands or resistance above the knees only)

Standard strength work for the chest, shoulders, and arms—including free weights, machines, or tubing—is helpful for maintaining and developing the strength for lifting and carrying the baby upon arrival. Attention to alignment, breathing, fatigue, and discomfort is critical. Fatigue is of greater concern in pregnancy than at other times because of the metabolic shifts in insulin production and decreased availability of glucose. With joints at risk due to changing plumb and laxity, fatigue can translate into unhealthy joint motion. As with all strength work, pain or discomfort is a danger signal and must be assessed. A practice-based schedule for strength training by trimester and experience is shown in figure 8.12.

First trimester
Experienced exerciser

Day	1	2	3	4	5	6	7
	x		x		x		
Or	x			x			

2 to 3 sets, 8 to 12 repetitions, 50% to 70% 1RM*
Machines, bands, tubes, partners, and free weights

Beginning exerciser

Day	1	2	3	4	5	6	7
	x			x			

Start: 1 set, 8 reps, 20% to 50% 1RM
Progress to: 2 to 3 sets, 8 to 12 reps, 40% to 60%
Machines, bands, tubes, or partners
In the first trimester, if nauseous or tired, modify or reduce schedule.

Second trimester
Experienced exerciser: Continue with first-trimester schedule, but reduce resistance 40% to 60%, do not lie on back, and stop using free weights or inclines around 20 weeks.
Beginning exerciser: Follow first-trimester recommendations.

Third trimester
Experienced exerciser: Continue, but reduce resistance to 30% to 50%.
Beginning exerciser: Do exercises seated or standing with no resistance.
Note: *If there is no opportunity to determine 1 repetition maximum (1RM), to figure out how much resistance to use, have the woman estimate how much is 1/4, 1/3, 1/2, and 2/3 of what she feels she could lift or resist at maximum effort, for each exercise. Use the following guidelines:

Experienced exerciser's effort

First trimester	Second trimester	Third trimester
1/2 to 2/3	1/3 to 2/3	1/3 to 1/2

Beginning exerciser's effort

First trimester	Second trimester	Third trimester
Start: 1/4 to 1/2	1/4 to 1/2 (no progress)	Work without resistance
Progress to: 1/3 to 2/3		

Figure 8.12   Schedule for strength training by trimester and experience.

Flexibility

In the author's practice, internal surveys taken over a 20-year period have taught us that pregnant women almost universally enjoy and prefer flexibility exercises. Two types of flexibility exercises are in play here. One is range of motion exercises. These involve locating the edges of controlled motion, then safely increasing them. Leaning forward and back, shifting side to side, making gentle but ever larger flexion/extension or circular motions of the limbs, and taking larger and larger steps help establish a kinesthetic awareness of the outline of safe movement or locomotion. This appeals to pregnant women as a way of sensing their body boundaries through proprioception.

The second type of exercise for flexibility is static stretching. We think this activity is satisfying to pregnant women largely because it serves to relieve discomforts, especially in the areas of the body where muscles are shortened as a result of pregnancy-induced alignment changes:

- Lumbar spine and low back
- Chest and anterior shoulders
- Iliofemoral joint (psoas major)
- Back of the neck
- Quadriceps
- Anterior portion of the lower leg (shin)

In addition, the calf muscles (gastrocnemius and soleus), hamstrings, and deep lateral rotators of the femur (including piriformis) are highly active in maintaining upright and seem to benefit from stretching.

Yoga-based prenatal exercise programs provide this type of stretching, as well as isometric strengthening and mind/body activities. Stretching can be incorporated into a general exercise program for pregnancy by alternating strength and stretch exercises, on the schedule for strength training outlined earlier.

Special Exercises for Pregnancy

The following movements—including C-Curves, pelvic tilts, Kegels, the deeply folded position, birth squat, carpal tunnel release, piriformis release, and side-lying rest position—performed regularly for many months prior to birth are useful for relief of pregnancy discomforts, as preparation for labor, or both. Gathered through trial and error, pilot studies, and application of research findings, these are essential training-specific exercises that have shown themselves to be beneficial for many women. A schedule for special exercises and mind/body techniques is included at the end of the next section, "Mind/Body Exercises."

Cautions for Stretching While Pregnant

Because of joint laxity and the potential for damage, several cautions for stretching are wise:

- Move slowly and use good form, identifying the line of stretch.
- Stretch muscle and Golgi bodies, not joint capsules. Limit the sense of stretch to the belly of the muscles and the area near but not within the joint.
- Stretch along the line of stretch, anchoring one or both ends with stabilizing muscles—the floor, a bar, or other stable object—in which case one pushes against the object(s). Pushing against the anchor, pull away from the anchor at the other end with the help of gravity or antagonist muscles.
- Breathe deeply, remain static for 15 to 30 seconds, and focus on lengthening the line of stretch and letting go of tension or tightness.

Spinal C-Curve©

Begin in seated, upright position. Inhale and relax the abdomen, then exhale (hiss/compress) and slightly flex the lumbar spine. *Emphasize transverse abdominal muscles and avoid tightening of the gluteals or pelvic floor* (see sidebar above). The exhaling, curving action will cause a slight rolling back and under toward the coccyx. The inhaling action will cause a return to upright on the sitsbones. Repeat 8 to 12 times, increasing the curve by innervating the rectus abdominal muscles at the end of the hiss/compress. Work at a moderate pace. This action is demonstrated in figure 8.5. It can also be executed standing. However, in this position the action is more difficult to execute without including the gluteals and pelvic floor.

Anterior-Posterior Pelvic Tilt

This action involves flexion and extension of both iliofemoral joints by alternately contracting the iliopsoas muscles, then releasing the iliopsoas and contracting the gluteals, proximal fibers of the hamstrings, and pelvic floor. Shown in figure 8.13, this exercise has three positions: anterior tilt, neutral, and posterior tilt. Particularly when combined with lateral pelvic tilts, explained next, the total motion of the anterior-posterior pelvic tilt produces changes in the shape of the space inside the pelvis, assisting the baby to find the path of least resistance.

Distinguishing the C-Curve Action

It is important that women can distinguish the C-Curve action separately from the action of the gluteals and pelvic floor, which will produce a pelvic tilt. During labor, achieving a C-Curve is useful in creating internal space in the pelvis so the baby is aided in traveling down the birth canal. If a woman cannot separate the action of the transverse abdominal muscles from the gluteals and pelvic floor, this creates a difficulty. While attempting to expel the baby (using the transverse muscle), the mother is pushing against a tightened outlet (gluteals and pelvic floor). It is critical that women learn to contract the abdominal muscles while relaxing the gluteals and pelvic floor to avoid this difficulty.

Lateral Pelvic Tilt

This action involves rotation of the pelvis around the vertical axis at the level of the lumbar spine, with accompanying iliofemoral extension and sacroiliac flexion on the forward side and the reverse on the other side. It is easy to accomplish this by lifting the iliac crest (the hip bone that protrudes on the side just below the waist) and bringing it slightly forward. The action is also accompanied by lateral flexion in the lumbar spine.

The combination of anterior tilt, right lateral tilt, posterior tilt, and left lateral tilt creates a circular motion of the pelvis on the spine and legs. This motion is particularly helpful to strengthen the muscles that control the female pelvis, mobilize the sacroiliac (SI) and iliofemoral joints, and alter the internal space within

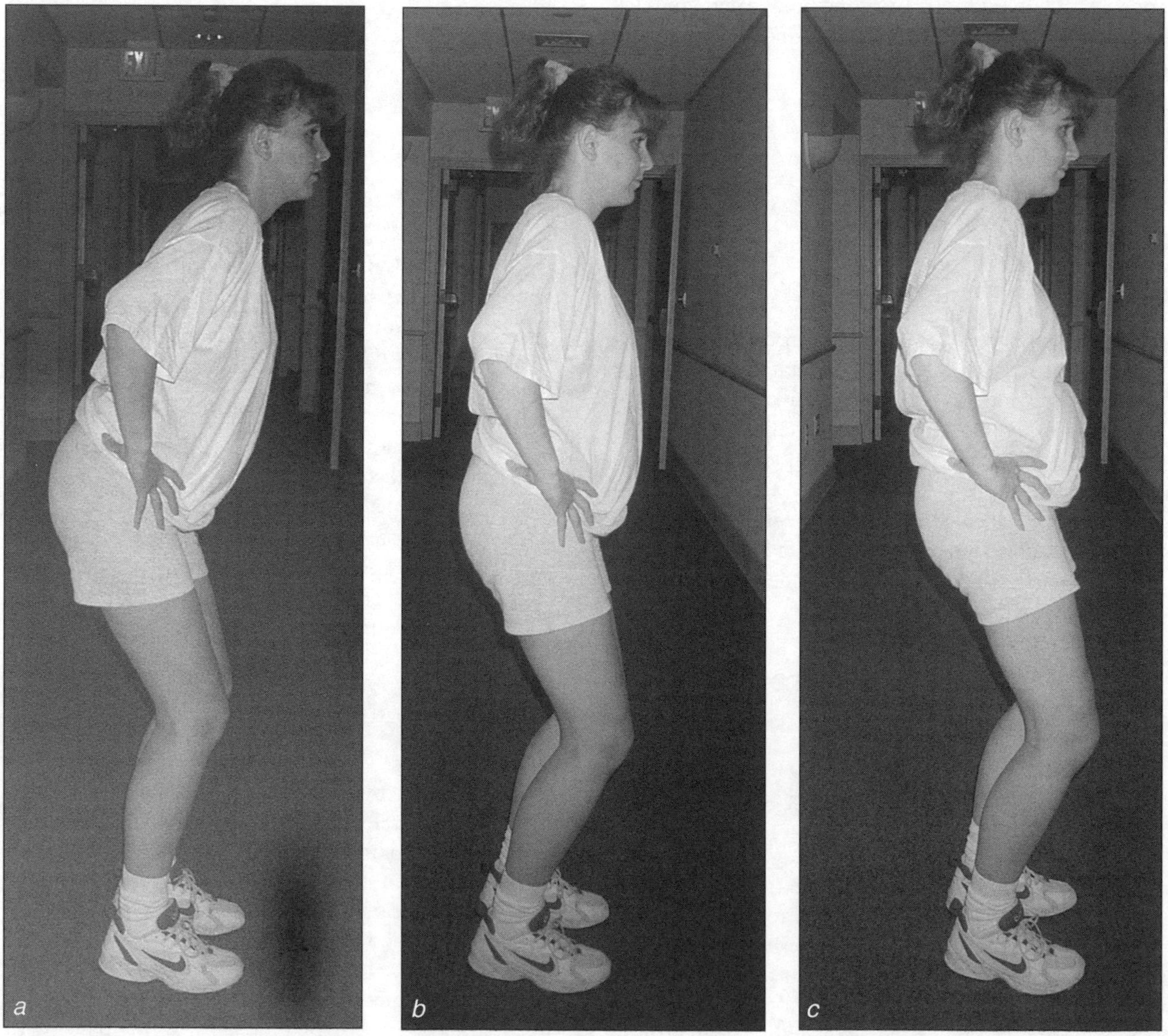

Figure 8.13 Pelvic tilt: (*a*) anterior tilt, (*b*) neutral stance, (c) posterior tilt.

the pelvis, assisting the baby in its descent during labor.

One can also achieve a lateral tilt by bringing one leg forward, lifting it several feet off the ground, and placing it on a stool or chair, or by lunging forward onto one foot very slowly while standing or kneeling. Trained dancers and athletes sometimes seek to counteract the natural tendency of the pelvis to twist when they are lifting the leg forward or lunging to the side, but they should be encouraged to allow this twisting to occur.

Kegels

Contracting and releasing muscles involved in support of the abdominal contents and opening of the pelvic out-

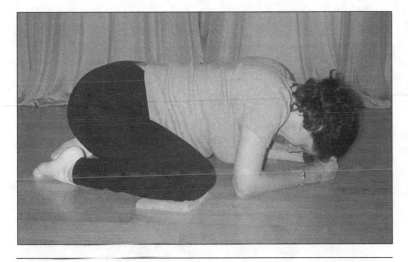

Figure 8.14 Deeply folded position. Resting in this position, with all major joints folded, provides an opportunity for muscles governing the spine and trunk to relax, and for the low back to stretch gently.

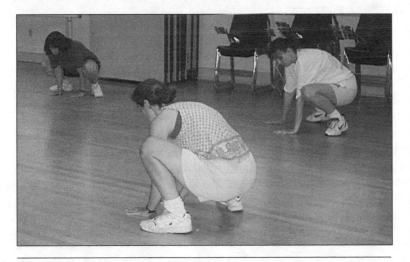

Figure 8.15 Birth squat. Working into the squatting position from sitting reduces much of the stress to the knees. Placing the elbows on the inside of the upper thigh helps to protect the medial meniscus. This position practiced often is helpful both as a preparation for delivery and as a labor position for helping the baby to descend.

lets are key exercises for women and were described earlier in this chapter.

Deeply Folded Position

The deeply folded position is one that many pregnant women find comfortable for stretching and relaxing the spine and muscles of the back. From a crawling position on hands and knees, pull the pelvis back and down over the feet, knees apart, and fold deeply in the iliofemoral and knee joints. Balance the spine by relaxing the head forward, as shown in figure 8.14. Breathe deeply and slowly. As the pregnancy progresses, a woman will find that opening the knees wider and wider creates more and more space for the baby.

Birth Squats

Many people are under the impression that squatting must be done from a standing position. This is not the case. Starting seated on the floor or on a bed may be easier for many women. Begin cross-legged and bring one knee toward the armpit, placing the foot on the floor. Lean forward or to the side on the hands until the other foot can be brought onto the floor. The squatting position is shown in figure 8.15. If both feet will not stay flat on the floor, lift one heel as high as possible and bring the pelvis over that foot; alternate sides.

Carpal Tunnel Syndrome Release Exercises

Edema in the hand and arm, tightening of the tendon encircling the wrist, increased breast tissue mass, and nerve impingement at the shoulder and neck during pregnancy can result in impingement of the nerves feeding the hand and can cause a great deal of discomfort. Several simple, noninvasive procedures may bring temporary relief. The first is at the wrist itself. Bringing the thumb side of the hand and the little-finger side toward each other and flexing slightly at the wrist can create a small space in the front of the wrist that permits nerves and blood vessels more space to enter the hand, thus improving circulation and relieving some discomfort.

At the shoulder and neck, changes in alignment and increased breast tissue can contribute to nerve compression as the radial and ulnar nerves exit the spine and pass through the shoulder. To open these areas,

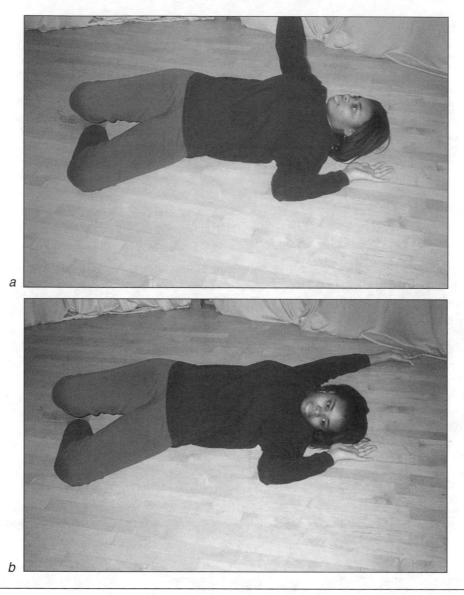

a

b

Figure 8.16   Relieving carpal tunnel syndrome by opening the shoulder and neck area. In this exercise, the shoulder blades should remain on the floor and the knees should move to the side only as much as is comfortable. The hand moves toward the floor on a diagonal away from the knees. Turn the head away from the extended arm, and breathe in and out several times. Gently return the arm toward the core of the body by folding first the hand, then the elbow, and last the shoulder.

women may lie on their back in constructive rest, allow their knees to fall gently and to a comfortable degree to one side, and position the scapula on the opposite side squarely on the floor. Do not strain this position. The arm on the scapula side then extends slowly toward the ceiling. Slowly and gently, allow the arm to fall to the upper diagonal, 180° away from the knees, as shown in figure 8.16. When the hand touches the floor, stretch the hand, lengthening the arm slightly and opening the shoulder. Breathe in and out. Turn the head away from the extended arm and breathe in and out a few more times.

To bring the hand and arm in, begin at the fingertips, curling them into the palm; then bend slightly at the wrist, then at the elbow, then at the shoulder. This keeps each lever arm short and reduces the risk of strain at the shoulder.

Piriformis Muscle Release for Sacroiliac Joint Discomfort or Mild Sciatica

In chapter 5, figure 5.2 illustrates how the piriformis muscle lies over the sciatic nerve as it exits the spine and moves under the sciatic notch toward the back and outside portions of the leg. In pregnancy, the piriformis muscle can impinge the sciatic nerve, causing discomfort. In addition, the SI joint can be pulled out of alignment when the piriformis is overly active in helping maintain upright—a situation that can easily occur in pregnancy with the added abdominal weight in front. As a first effort to relieve these problems, a two-step exercise can be helpful.

Beginning on all fours, determine which side is to be relieved first. Take the hand and locate the area of the piriformis (it is a deep muscle and hard to palpate directly—the instructor should simply indicate its location from the lower edges of the sacrum to the greater trochanter). To begin Step One, have the exerciser move her *other* leg to the diagonal in between the side and the back, tuck the toes under, then shift weight toward the heel of that toe as indicated in figure 8.17a. This decreases

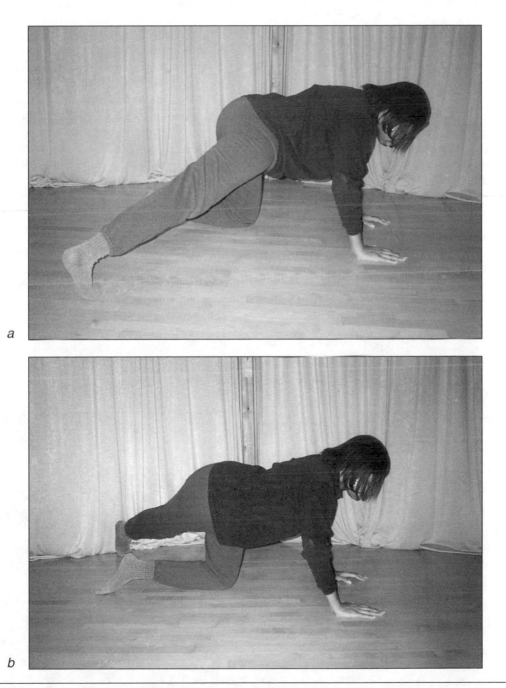

a

b

Figure 8.17   Relieving piriformis muscle tightness to reduce sacroiliac joint dysfunction and mild sciatica. *(a)* Step One involves shortening the piriformis muscle (in this case, the left hip); *(b)* Step Two involves stretching the piriformis muscle. Mobilizing the posterior aspect of the iliofemoral joint can relieve nerve discomfort in the low back and leg.

the distance between the attachments of the piriformis on the affected side and allows the muscle to calm down. The client should breathe deeply and slowly several times, and wait for a sense of the muscle calming, releasing, or ceasing to be tense, perhaps for 90 seconds. She should center the weight.

In the second step, the exerciser should bring her leg just used across the back of the affected leg to the other back-side diagonal, tuck the toes, and again shift weight into the heel, as indicated in figure 8.17*b*. This increases the distance between the attachments of the piriformis on the affected side and allows the muscle to stretch. Again, she should breathe deeply and slowly several times. After stretching, she should try the deeply folded position again and notice the change in the low back on the affected side. This exercise tends to release and mobilize the SI joint as well as taking some pressure off the sciatic nerve. If there is chronic pain or swelling in this area, these should be evaluated by a qualified care provider or physical therapist.

Rest in the Side-Lying Position

By incorporating even a brief 2- or 3-minute rest period into a prenatal exercise program, the instructor or trainer provides clients with two useful tools in one: a ritual method for practicing relaxation in preparation for birth, and a way of ensuring maximum blood flow so that both mother and baby can recoup from strenuous activities. The side-lying position, which is recommended for these purposes, is illustrated in figure 8.18.

Mind/Body Exercises

Increasingly, exercise and movement specialists recognize that exercise encompasses more than vigorous aerobic, strength-building, stretching, balance, and coordination activities. Coaches have long recognized that mental attention can be polished just as physical practice can and that this attention makes a difference in the physical outcome. Many coaches, athletes, and dancers have individual systems they use to focus attention prior to competition, performance, or practice. Systems abound, as the local gym, bookstore, and video store attest. But what are the underlying phenomena at work when a particular system is successful in improving outcome? These phenomena are relatively easy to identify, although they are often referred to in popular literature without any precise meaning and in ways that overlap. In this text, these activities—*centering, relaxation,* and *imagery* (or *mental rehearsal*)—have specific definitions as given in the following pages.

Centering

A number of disciplines use centering as a critical first step in conjunction with motor activity. Dance and the martial arts employ well-developed routines to achieve this important step, which requires anywhere from a few to 20 minutes, depending on the individual's skill. When a person brings the righting function into the center of the body, superficial muscles are free to move the body without the impedance of other superficial muscles that

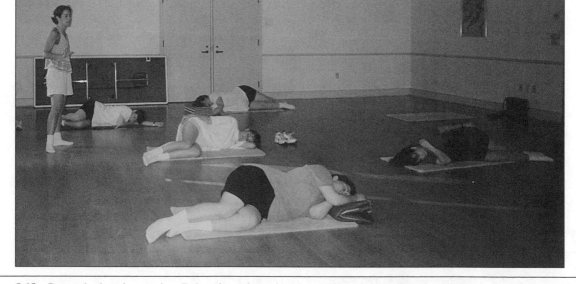

Figure 8.18 Prenatal relaxation session. Relaxation prior to intense cardiovascular or aerobic activities is a useful method of helping women learn to execute difficult work while remaining at ease, a skill that will come in handy during labor and delivery.

may be active in enforcing a mental concept of a static "proper" alignment.

Centering her body and mind at the start of an exercise session helps a pregnant woman achieve physical balance as her body changes, helps her relax and focus on her body in order to enhance concentration, and helps her to become more aware of her movements and thus helps prevent injury as she exercises. There are three elements of centering:

- Physical balance
- Deep abdominal breathing
- Mental focus

Physical Balance. One can achieve physical balance standing or sitting (see figure 8.19). In the standing position, place the feet about 6 to 8 inches apart (ankles directly below hip sockets), knees slightly bent and relaxed. Torso is erect. Relax the shoulders and neck. Head is balanced gently at the top of the spine. Check for balance by rocking slowly forward and back, then finding a middle ground. Check side to side the same way, mak-

ing sure the weight is even on the two feet. Balance the weight equally in all directions. (This balances your body around your central axis, or plumb line.) Centering can also be done seated on a chair or "tailor fashion" on the floor. Sit up tall on the sitsbones, torso erect and head, neck, and shoulders relaxed. Rock forward and back, then side to side, to center the weight on the sitsbones instead of the feet.

Deep Abdominal Breathing. Then, begin deep abdominal breathing exercises. Inhale, expanding the lungs and relaxing the abdomen. Exhale, letting the air out with a hiss, and compress the abdomen, pulling the belly button toward the back of the waist. Repeat a total of three times. This is the "hiss/compress" exercise also used to strengthen the transverse abdominal muscles (figure 8.4).

Mental Focus. Next, focus the mind by paying attention to the body. Notice any tightness in the muscles and let them relax. Make a mental note of how the body feels when balanced and relaxed. Carry this feeling into the exercise program. After practicing once or twice, women find it is easy to assume this centered posture, ready for

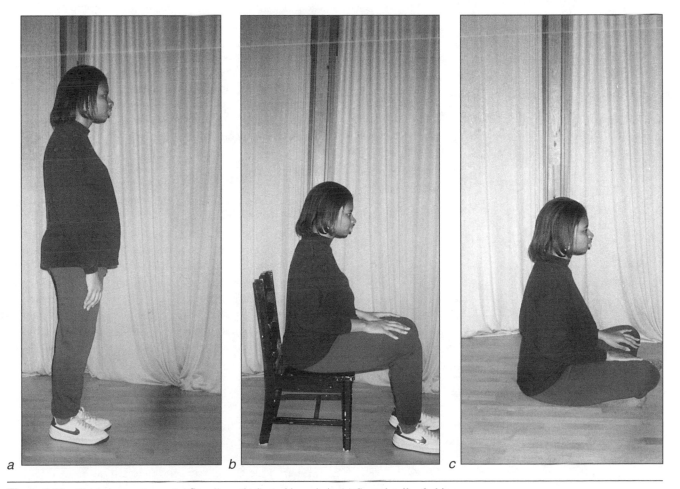

a   *b*   *c*

Figure 8.19 Centering postures. *(a)* Standing. *(b)* Seated in a chair. (c) Seated, tailor fashion.

movement. It is also helpful to use centering as a way to finish a workout session. This allows women to carry a conscious presence into their daily activities.

Relaxation

Learning to relax is as important as working the body. Relaxation reduces stress and helps a woman with labor by allowing the uterus to contract effectively. The term *relaxation* refers to elicitation of the relaxation response as outlined by Benson, who defines it as "the inborn capacity of the body to enter a special state characterized by lowered heart rate, decreased rate of breathing, lowered blood pressure, slower brain waves, and an overall reduction in the speed of metabolism" [63]. This state appears to function as a protective mechanism against overstress. As a phenomenon, it was first described by Hess (*Functional Organization of the Diencephalon*, 1957). The physiological term for this phenomenon is the *trophotropic* response, which opposes the *ergotropic* response (fight or flight). The trophotropic zone in the brain is located in the area of the anterior hypothalamus. It extends into the supra- and preoptic areas, septum, and inferior lateral thalamus. This area produces an alpha rhythm that dominates brain function during this response. The response is mediated by the parasympathetic nervous system and affects autonomic functions.

The actual practice of attaining the response is fairly simple (remember, it is an inborn response). The four prerequisites, as identified by Benson, are

- a quiet location (quiet refers to an environment with little interfering sensory stimuli that provides a safe feeling);
- conscious relaxation of skeletal muscles;
- a single mental device, such as a word, phrase, or image; and
- a passive attitude toward intrusive thoughts—that is, not blocking thoughts or trying to hold onto them [63].

The five physiological measures of having achieved the response are: achieving alpha brain waves, lowering the resting pulse, slowing respiration, lowering blood pressure, and lowering basal metabolism (decreased oxygen requirements) [63].

Simple directions for achieving this state are as follows:

1. Find an appropriate space and get comfortable.
2. In pregnancy, lie on the side; use pillows or clothing for comfort. Postpartum, lie on the back, knees bent up, feet flat on floor (see "Constructive Rest and Relaxation," chapter 11).
3. Breathe in and out from the abdomen.
4. Release skeletal muscles, using progression (e.g., feet to head) or image (e.g., leaking sandbag).
5. Mentally look inside the body.
6. Stay calm and check breathing (6-9 breaths per minute).
7. Practice for 3 to 20 minutes at a time.

Imagery or Mental Rehearsal

What is imagery and how is it useful in pregnancy? Most commonly, imagery is used during relaxation sessions to help women rehearse the process of birth. By focusing the mind on the physical process, women uncover gaps in their understanding of the stages of birth, which ideally leads to asking questions. In finding answers, women develop a greater understanding of the process; this in turn leads to less fear of the unknown. As the early childbirth educators noted (see chapter 5), fear is a key factor in the fear-tension-pain cycle that can sabotage labor. Imagery also has a positive effect through the impact on self-image of body experience during exercise. During nurturing physical activity, a woman develops confidence in her body. Thus, she gains not only the functional capacity to withstand labor, but also the attitude of self-efficacy.

While physical practice refines movement execution, imagery refines the intention of the action. Physical and mental aspects cannot be completely disconnected from each other, but focusing on one aspect enhances the entire process. Most human movement is composed of unconscious, subcortical reflex actions and rhythmic motor patterns. The cognitive contribution is seeing in the mind's eye and refining intention by ideation and sensory feedback. Beyond having a precise and accurate intention, there is little one can consciously do to govern movement execution.

The two predominant theories regarding the effectiveness of imagery in mental rehearsal of motor action are the psychoneuromuscular theory and the symbolic-perceptual theory. According to the first theory, what makes imagery effective is kinesthetic feedback (the sensations created when neuromuscular pathways fire at very low threshold as the mind reviews the action), leading to corrections in execution. According to the second theory, what makes imagery effective is the facilitation of planning and motor learning through improvements in the cognitive realm (i.e., perceiving movement in greater and greater detail).

According to Savoyant [64], these two theories may not be all that different—a matter of a shift of focus. The psychoneuromuscular theory relies heavily on the inflow aspects of the nervous system (the peripheral nervous system, kinesthesia, sensory function, afferent fiber), while the symbolic-perceptual theory relies on the outflow aspects (central nervous system, cognition, motor planning and execution, efferent fiber). Since sensation is always significant to the formation of an image of the movement, and since planning or intention is always present at some level, these two theories simply describe different portions of the arc on the circle of perception-behavior-perception-behavior.

In the process of skill acquisition—be it in the workout or in labor—the only truly effective mental practice factor is the image of the desired action or goal [65]. *Imagery, mental rehearsal,* and *ideokinesis* are all terms applied to the use of visualizing or identifying in the mind the goal of an action while not actually trying to move. Todd [66] and Sweigard [67] have used this phenomenon to effect changes in bone alignment over time, improve flexibility, and lower impedance to movement patterns. Similar work has been shown to enhance the immune system's response to cancer [68].

How does one use imagery to improve physical skills? Here is an example, for improving your jump shot in basketball. Step One: Pretend to have a basketball and go through the motions of shooting it at the basket. Step Two: Close your eyes and watch yourself dribbling the ball, focusing on the basket, bringing the ball to the shooting position while centering, and preparing to shoot. Then watch while you bend your legs, then jump, pushing the ball into a clean arc, flicking the wrists just right. Watch the ball drop through the basket, swish into the net, and fall through. Next, repeat Step One, and notice the greater detail and ease of movement, as well as the sureness with which you can make the shot.

Every image we see in real life and in our mind's eye contributes to neuromotor patterning of actions. This is why demonstrations are most effective when we see a successful action. In teaching women to execute, we can achieve the best result by helping them to perceive the intention of a movement, and allowing each woman to develop her own execution. One of the best positive images for a woman who is 10 weeks pregnant and has experienced a first trimester of nausea, vomiting, and limited activity may be a 36-weeks-pregnant woman who is having a great time working out, sweating, drinking water, and laughing.

Regularly including pregnancy and birth imagery in the prenatal workout through charts, books, videos, and guided imagery during relaxation is one way instructors and trainers can help their clients. Taking the time to facilitate each woman's ability to perceive the intent of movements so that she becomes a graceful, efficient, and powerful mover is another way. A schedule for special exercises and mind/body techniques is shown in table 8.2.

EXERCISE PRESCRIPTION

Setting out a fitness prescription for a given pregnant woman depends on the result of the screening procedures outlined in the first part of this chapter and on supervision by the instructor, trainer, or program director. Some trainers may supervise all of their client's physical activity sessions—and may have done so for some time. In another situation, a group fitness instructor may see a client once or twice a week, while the client swims or gardens or jogs on her own, and may continue to do so through her pregnancy. A group prenatal fitness program instructor may meet a client for the first time at 10 or 12 weeks. A trainer at a commercial gym or health club may

Table 8.2 Schedule of Special Exercises and Mind/Body Techniques

Day	1	2	3	4	5	6	7
Centering*	Do this at start and finish of workout.						
C-Curves and pelvic tilts†	x	x	x	x	x		
Kegels†	x	x	x	x	x		
Birth squat*	x		x		x		
Relaxation in side-lying*	x	x	x	x	x	x	
Imagery*	x		x		x		
Deeply folded*	x		x		x		
Carpal tunnel and piriformis release	Do these when needed.						

*Do these just once or twice per session.
†Start with 1 set of 5, progress to 3 sets of 5, then 3 sets of 10 or 12.

see a client periodically, but infrequently. A program director may see a woman only at the initial interview. In all cases, fitness professionals who have contact with the pregnant client are well served by being aware of the entire activity program and screening results of each woman with whom they work.

In this part of the chapter, we review situations commonly encountered in the course of prescribing and modifying a client's prenatal exercise program. The fact that universal prescription is not a practical reality can be frustrating for the fitness professional beginning work in this area. A situation with a clear contraindication to all exercise can be easier to deal with than a condition requiring assessment. The latter situation means establishing communication with a health care provider and being sensitive to danger signs. Women desire to begin prenatal exercise regimens at many stages of pregnancy. They have many exercise histories, many motivations, and many medical histories. Gathering information is a critical skill in developing the capacity to ensure that a woman gets the most out of her program. Of course, experience is a great help.

Assessing a Starting Level

Because women who wish to exercise in pregnancy start at a variety of fitness levels, and because the relationship of the client to the fitness professional can vary, we divide the process of assessing starting level into five categories:

1. The instructor or trainer is familiar with the woman's exercise history, and the woman is fit.
2. The instructor or trainer is familiar with the woman's exercise history, and the woman is somewhat active or modestly fit.
3. The instructor or trainer is not familiar with the woman's exercise history, and the woman is fit.
4. The instructor or trainer is not familiar with the woman's exercise history, and the woman is somewhat active or modestly fit.
5. The instructor or trainer is not familiar with the woman's exercise history, and the woman is inactive or unfit.

Familiar and Fit

In the simplest case, once the screening procedure has been completed and a woman pronounced healthy to continue her regimen, some women will experience very little alteration in their activity levels. Initially, adjusting to the increased hormone levels, changes in glucose/insulin balance, and increased metabolic demands barely phases some fit women. Others need to slow down for a period of time or on occasion, and are generally very good at assessing this situation.

Cardiovascular or aerobic activity is the only mode of exercise that has been consistently shown to affect birth outcomes. Although monitoring heart rate is somewhat useful in pregnancy, subjective evaluation of an appropriate level by the woman herself is the primary measurement tool we have found effective. If a familiar, fit woman finds the first trimester difficult, she may need to adjust her level of exertion downward until she finds a level she can tolerate. The difficulty is likely to be only temporary.

Occasionally, we see a woman in this category who has *superemesis gravidarum,* a condition in which a woman vomits so frequently that her health, and that of the fetus, are placed at risk. In this case, her care provider may prescribe a break from exercise. When women with this difficulty have been referred to our practice, we have found that they do well when we involve them initially in 15 to 20 minutes of low to moderate cardiovascular activity combined with mild weight training, flexibility activities, and stress management (centering, relaxation, and imagery).

Familiar and Somewhat Active

Sometimes clients are erratic exercisers or are new clients with a fairly low level of conditioning. Once they have been screened, continuing with their fitness program through the early stages of pregnancy is often helpful in keeping their attention on their well-being. Because we know that regular cardiovascular exercise—even at a low level—is important in the first half of pregnancy to establishing enhanced placental function, we strongly encourage these women to walk/jog 15 to 20 minutes three to five times a week, or enroll in a prenatal group exercise program that meets once or twice a week and walk one to three days a week. Continuing with other components of prenatal fitness is also important. Our primary focus in these areas is often on centering to help women get in touch with, become familiar with, and feel safe about the sensations of pregnancy.

Unfamiliar and Fit

One of the groups the author's practice deals with most often is women who are fit and are looking for guidance or companionship in their activities during pregnancy but are unfamiliar to the instructor. They often come to us at anywhere from 8 weeks to 20 weeks. Once they are screened and assessed, we put them into a group class and monitor their outside activities. These women generally thrive on a combination of all the prenatal exercise components, but often in proportions that depend on their individual preferences. For example, some women swim, run, ride stationary bikes, use elliptical transports or step machines, or take high-intensity aerobics classes on days they are not participating in our group class. Others continue to lift weights, take ballet, or do martial arts with modifications on alternate days. Only women who are currently fit are taken into the program after 26 weeks.

If unfamiliar, fit women arrive with clear knowledge of appropriate intensity levels, we generally allow them to work at the pace they find comfortable on any given day. We monitor for obvious signs of distress—extremely labored breathing, anguished face, lack of adequate fluid intake, faintness, and so on—as well as evaluating perceived exertion and pulse.

If a woman who is used to working at a high intensity slacks off for a period of time, it is important to inquire about her other activities. She may be trying too hard to stay abreast in a nonpregnant class, exhausting herself, and having difficulty keeping up with the rest of her life. On the other hand, she may have become discouraged, dropped out of other activities, and become depressed about her performance level. This behavior can signal that changes in the center of gravity—which tend to create biomechanical disadvantages—have become extreme enough to profoundly affect the woman's ability to perform movement with speed and precision. Depending on a woman's height and proportions, it is common to see these problems arise at 20 to 30 weeks. One sign of a well-run prenatal program is its ability to help women work at appropriate levels throughout their pregnancies. A woman who is in touch with her body is able to recognize low, moderate, and high levels of exertion by internal cues. She is not derailed by the need to change the size, shape, or speed of movements in order to maintain balance and safety.

Unfamiliar and Somewhat Active

Women who present themselves for prenatal exercise and have an erratic or low level of activity require careful attention to their screening procedures. Providing there are no medical contraindications, one of the first priorities is to establish a pattern of activity that is regular and does not involve binge exercise. If the woman presents herself early in her pregnancy, involving her in a group program allows her to interact with other pregnant women and may stimulate her to commit to a regular schedule. If she is reinforced by the contact with a "tribe" of her own kind, the social motivation can serve to protect her physical well-being.

During activity sessions, such women should be encouraged to assess their sensations at frequent intervals, during a variety of types of activities. Working *somewhat hard* to *hard* during cardiovascular portions is critical to learning what it feels like to work at a moderate pace. Strength training, stretch, centering, and relaxation are all essential components in a well-rounded prenatal program. If the client is familiar with these elements, formalizing or ritualizing these activities so that she gains mastery of them may help her to maintain a commitment to a regular regimen. If she is not familiar with these elements, it is helpful to introduce them in a manner that stimulates curiosity and provides a series of small challenges.

Unfamiliar and Unfit

The client whose exercise history is unfamiliar to the instructor and who is inactive or unfit presents an interesting challenge. Of course, screening is critical. Being with a community of other pregnant women can take on added importance in this case. Having a sense of belonging may allow a woman to experience exercise for the first time as a means to self-knowledge and enhanced living. Feeling comfortable and supported—that is, noncompetitive—within the group is important for helping such women develop values around the experience of physical activity. Placing these women in group programs allows them to see people working out at a variety of intensities at the same time. In individual cases in which the client has a specific problem (e.g., lower back pain or profound shyness), or in corporate fitness programs where trainers work with women on an individual basis only, a good prenatal trainer can take on some of the role of the support system.

Methods to Monitor Activity

In any case, once information about the client has been collected and reviewed, it is helpful to establish word descriptions for moderate activity, as well as the upper limits of exertion for each client. "You should be breathing hard but regularly and be able to answer my questions, not laboring for breath," is one common way of determining that a new client is working appropriately in cardiovascular exercise. "On a scale of discomfort from 1 to 10, this stretch should only be a 2 or 3" is another such method, suitable for establishing how aggressively to stretch. "Muscles will feel warm and a little tired, but not burning," is a way to describe resistance or strength work. It is important that the client has operative words delineating both what an appropriate sense of effort is and how to know when the upper limit has been crossed.

When clients have their monthly prenatal checkups, suggest that they review their exercise activities with their health care provider. This keeps the provider abreast of how a woman is progressing in her program and gives the provider an opportunity to advise any changes that might be necessary. The conversation also serves the functions of enriching the provider's knowledge of what is available to women in her area and preparing a line of communication for use if a problem arises.

Having the expectant mother maintain an exercise log, including the day, time of day, activity, components of exercise included (centering, aerobics, strength, stretch, relaxation, imagery, special exercises such as Kegels, tilts, etc.), and how she felt (before, during, and after the session), provides a good tool for evaluation, should the need to modify arise. Precise information about activity type, intensity, frequency, duration, and response makes it possible to identify which elements may be problematic. Adjustments toward improved fetal well-being are always the bottom line.

If a woman is enjoying her activities, is feeling good, is healthy, and feels she is benefiting from her program, and if her baby is growing properly, this is obviously a successful situation. If she is unhappy, complaining of discomfort, or not healthy, it is important to determine whether something in her program is detrimental or whether she is unable to comply with a safe program. Clearly, if conditions requiring assessment, contraindications, or warning signs appear, it is necessary to make adjustments. These may include modification of activities. Modification generally takes place in one of two areas:

1. Reduction in intensity or cessation of cardiovascular or aerobic components
2. Changes that reduce biomechanical stresses

Dealing With Clients When Expectations Change

As is clear by now, the process of pregnancy and birth involves massive physical, emotional, and identity changes. Often as the process unfolds it forces women to revise their earlier expectations about pregnancy. For example, some women have not realized how different their body would become; others cannot remain as active as they expected to; still others learn that they need to develop an activity habit for the first time. In all cases, the instructor or trainer needs to work from a supportive or nurturing perspective.

When a woman has invested a great deal of energy and ego in the creation of an ideal body, pregnancy can be disturbing. If she should also need to reduce or cease her physical activity because of medical considerations, she may need a great deal of support. In extreme cases, it may be necessary to refer her to a professional who is prepared to deal with the psychological fallout of lost expectations. It is a good idea to have one or more psychologists as advisors.

In such cases, if the instructor or trainer commiserates about how pregnancy is debilitating to the body, she or he does a great disservice to women. This attitude lends support to the idea that a woman's body is an object that has value only when it looks or acts a certain way. What about the value of a body that produces a healthy child? Although fitness in pregnancy helps the body maintain tone and form, the first goal is always health. For each of the many phases that a woman's body goes through over the course of a lifetime, there is an optimal state. Learning to live in the body that functions best in the present phase is a skill that the wise instructor or trainer will imbue in her clients.

At the other end of the spectrum is the woman who has never exercised, carries excess weight, and comes to a program because her physician or midwife has told her that she must become physically active. Fortunately, women in this category are often easier to deal with than active clients who must alter their activity regimens. An inactive woman who is brought into a supportive prenatal exercise group or who receives a good grounding in fitness basics is gaining something of value in her life. A woman who feels restricted by her pregnancy may feel that something is being taken away. A good instructor will be able to identify the positive components of any woman's experience and help to bring those factors into play in developing an effective exercise prescription for that woman.

Of course, most of the time, instructors and trainers are dealing with milder changes of expectation than those just outlined. A short woman may love step aerobics but find that she is having knee or sciatic nerve problems deriving from biomechanical disadvantage; she will need to figure out that by eliminating some or all of the step height she uses, she can reduce these problems. Even if she is spoon-fed information that will help her reach this conclusion, once she realizes the solution and can act on her realization, she is a successful problem-solver. This is very different, and much more productive, than if she is forced to think of herself as a wimp because her instructor says, "Just take the step away if you can't keep up."

Pregnant women will soon be required to nurture a new human being's development, much as the instructor or trainer is helping them develop. Much of the work of both instructor or trainer and mother involves facilitating psychomotor skills. An instructor or trainer who is a frequent influence in the life of a mother-to-be is a role model. Creating a setting where becoming a mother is a valued task is meaningful work. A good instructor or trainer provides a setting in which women feel comfortable if they need to change their expectations, and in which appropriate physical activity can lead to discovery and enlargement of self.

Twins and Other Multiple Pregnancies

Twins or other multiple pregnancies are either *identical* or *fraternal*. If two or four individuals are created because the embryo split at an early stage, these individuals are identical as they have the same DNA. If separate eggs have been fertilized by separate sperm, the individuals are fraternal. In the case of a split, the exact stage of development when the split occurs determines the arrangement of placenta and membranes. In any case, it is possible for one or both twins to be disadvantaged by the arrangement or attachment.

Twin pregnancies are often diagnosed at the end of the first trimester or the beginning of the second, as it becomes apparent that the uterus is growing faster than expected or as two heartbeats are heard. Sometimes the mother is unusually fatigued. The presence of more than one fetus means added stress on the mother's body and competition for nutrients between fetuses. If maternal nutrition or lifestyle habits are poor, this will have a profoundly negative effect on the pregnancy. The importance of protein and fluid intake increases with multiple gestation. The appropriateness of exercise depends on the size and development of the placenta(s), the mother's health, uterine irritability, and other factors. In the case of multiple pregnancies, maintaining good communication with the mother and care provider helps prevent surprises.

There is a great deal of variation in outcomes with multiple pregnancies. Over time, the author has seen a number of clients who have exercised moderately throughout twin pregnancies and delivered healthy identical or fraternal twins weighing 7 pounds or more each. In 20 years, she has seen only one triplet pregnancy during which the mother continued exercise past 30 weeks. This woman delivered healthy babies. The most common reasons for restriction of activity in multiple pregnancies are that one or more of the fetuses is small for gestational age and that restriction will help prevent preterm labor or preeclampsia.

Gestational Diabetes

Most cases of gestational diabetes can be controlled with diet [69]. As discussed in chapter 6, today's standard of care involves proper diet and exercise as part of an ideal method of treatment. Because gestational diabetes is rarely diagnosed early in the pregnancy, most exercising clients are well into their prenatal fitness program when this condition is determined. It rarely means a change in activity. However, extra attention should be devoted to making sure that the client is eating properly and regularly. Health care practitioners will provide diet guidelines, and it is useful to inquire into cultural customs in this area, so it is possible to be supportive.

Risk factors for gestational diabetes, other than genetics, include prepregnancy weight greater than 180 pounds and poor sugar metabolism. Typical screening includes fasting blood sugar level, the 1- or 2-hour glucose challenge test, and the longer glucose tolerance test. If the fasting blood sugar level is positive but the glucose challenge is negative, or vice versa, it is necessary to do a glucose tolerance test. If both the fasting level and glucose challenge are positive, the assumption is that the woman has gestational diabetes and thus the glucose tolerance test is not necessary, although it is still sometimes done. If both the fasting level and glucose challenge are negative, a glucose tolerance test is not needed, as the woman shows no signs of diabetes. However, women with risk factors are often rescreened at 34 to 36 weeks.

Issues for the baby with a diabetic mother include the potential for *macrosomia* (large body). These infants may develop hypoglycemia following birth. Also, because of the increased size of the baby, there is a higher incidence of *shoulder dystocia* (difficulty of the shoulders fitting through the birth canal) [69] than among nondiabetic mothers. *Polyhydramnios* (enlarged head and extra spinal fluid) is also a risk for this population. The risk of perinatal mortality does not increase except when there is a history of stillbirth or complications due to hypertension.

FORMATTING GROUP FITNESS INSTRUCTION

How much of which exercise components in what sequence is effective? What is an ideal setting? And what skills do I need to build a successful program when there is 100% attrition? These are frequent questions among new prenatal group fitness instructors. Traditional approaches to group exercise involve a brief warm-up, a cardiovascular component, then strength and stretch activities, and—if time allows—relaxation. Or, alternatively, the strength component leads off, followed by cardiovascular work, stretch, and relaxation, time permitting. Systems like this are often seen in masculine facilities, led by individuals whose main focus is developing charismatic leadership. But for the special needs of pregnancy and birth, they have rarely proved satisfactory.

Sequencing Group Classes

Because of certain factors (increased body weight and the changing center of gravity; the goal of acquiring skills for labor; and the priorities of safety, effectiveness, and community), a well-designed prenatal exercise program needs its own format. Included are a ritual start that allows each woman to be at ease in her body as it is on that particular day; opportunities to address individual discomforts, muscular weakness, or tightness; and aerobic activities that bring the group together to enhance preparation for labor and produce a supportive tribal effect. The sidebar below outlines a prenatal exercise group program format that meets these needs.

How much of each component depends on the focus of the session and time allowance. It is possible to focus on differing elements by expanding and contracting the length of various elements. Figure 8.20 outlines the steps one takes to format 1-hour sessions and gives three examples of such sessions, each with its own focus.

Setting: Physical and Emotional Safety

While the sequence can be tailored to each individual type of program, this is seldom the case with the setting, which often must be shared. But exercise settings are not neutral. Physical characteristics of the space—size, shape, light, flooring, temperature, color, smell, cleanliness, safety, and whatever else appeals to the senses—affect the client's response. Certain features of an exercise environment seem to have importance for pregnant women. A room where the doors can be closed, allowing the women to feel protected and sociable is necessary. The floor should be forgiving (resilient or soft); and a bathroom should be nearby so that women may use it with only minor interruptions in their workout.

It is also important to be in a place—a club, gym, hos-

pital, community center, church—where the administration or the larger group is respectful. In practice, many of the most successful programs are in places associated with organizations that are proud to sponsor such a program because it is a commitment to the well-being of women and children. This has been the case less frequently in clubs and gyms and more frequently in hospitals, community centers, and churches. As the fitness industry becomes more accepting of such activities as a means to attract female clients, this is changing.

An instructor who fosters interpersonal or group dynamics also affects client response. In a group situation where an instructor makes an effort to introduce newcomers, for example, class members may help a new participant overcome her resistance to new activities by providing peer leadership. When a woman who is further along in pregnancy, but clearly enjoying an exercise, helps new participants learn an action, this *peer leader* is a valuable asset in developing group cohesion. It is desirable that newcomers feel they are safe and supported. More information follows in the section "Interpersonal Instructor Skills."

As fitness programs are reaching more diverse populations than ever before, instructors must be prepared to work in more diverse locations and situations. Increasingly, through medical clinics, community projects, and schools, opportunities for inner-city and disadvantaged women to participate in health and fitness programs are becoming available. Programs are also seeing increasing numbers of women who speak English as a second language. And shelters for battered and abused women are providing activity programs in more and more locations. Among the important considerations for instructors working with these populations are the need to address women at an appropriate educational level and in some cases the need for skills in communicating with second-language speakers of English. There may be social and emotional issues—such as drugs or abuse—that come up in the course of a program. Instructors should be prepared to work with special groups, make sure that the situation has physical and psychological backup, and be aware of the resources available in the setting. Working with women from diverse backgrounds can be tremendously rewarding but understanding what constitutes physical and emotional safety for a given group of individuals is essential.

Interpersonal Instructor Skills

The commitment of the instructor or trainer to developing a cohesive group has a tremendous effect on the experience of the participant. There are skills an instructor can acquire that will help the group form a sense of unity or identity. This will, in turn, attract women looking for

---

General Outline for an Effective Prenatal Exercise Group Program

Centering

Combination of strength, stretch, and special exercises*

Relaxation and imagery

Warm-up

Sustained cardiovascular component†

Cool-down and strength work to drive blood back toward the torso

Whole-body stretch

Centering

---

* = Encourage questions.

---

† = Encourage verbal and nonverbal interaction.

Steps

1. Determine the focus of each 1-hour session.
2. Emphasize the associated fitness components.
3. Expand and contract time units for all components to reflect focus of the session.

Examples

1. Focus: Cardiovascular

3 min: Centering, seated on floor or chair

2 min: Slow, full ROM actions, seated

3 min: Special exercises: C-Curves, Kegels

3 min: Upper back strength exercises using Xertubes or bands

1 min: Deeply folded position, then slow transition to standing

5 min: Aerobic warm-up movement (walking, grapevines, slow cycling, etc.)

30 min: Sustained aerobic activities (make sure women are drinking water and visit ladies' room as needed)

5 min: Cool-down movement

3 min: Modified squats

5 min: Slow standing stretches

2. Focus: Mind/Body (Centering, Relaxation, Imagery, Special Exercises)

3 min: Centering

10 min: Special exercises (C-Curves, Kegels, squat from seated position, pelvic tilts, others as needed)

5 min: Strength work (upper back, shoulders, modified push-ups, side-lying curl-ups, hamstrings)

3 min: Static stretching (chest, psoas, quads)

7 min: Relaxation/imagery

2 min: Fill and spill (drink water and visit ladies' room)

5 min: Aerobic warm-up

15-20 min: Sustained aerobic work

5-10 min: Cool-down, modified squats, slow ROM actions

3. Focus: Strength

3 min: Centering

5 min: Special exercises

15 min: Upper-body strength

5 min: Relaxation

2 min: Fill and spill

5 min: Aerobic warm-up

15 min: Sustained aerobic work

10 min: Cool-down, modified squats, lower-body strength, slow ROM actions

---

Figure 8.20 Examples of prenatal fitness session formats.

the security and support of an ongoing group. Among such skills are increasing cohesiveness and interaction, responding to group needs, averting problems, personalizing class, ensuring supervision, and having professional accountability.

Increasing Cohesiveness and Interaction

Methods of facilitating interaction include both nonverbal and verbal techniques. Examples of nonverbal methods include the use of equalizing spatial structures such as circles, cooperative floor patterns like those used in square dancing, and physical interaction (e.g., by dividing groups into partners, trios). One way to stimulate verbal interaction is to initiate joint conversations. For example, if a woman confides that she is going to have amniocentesis and another woman has recently had the procedure, the instructor can ask the second woman to come over and share her experience with the first woman. Another method is to share information—for example, by telling the group when a class member has a baby, or letting them know about an upcoming speaker on a topic they may be interested in.

Responding to Group Needs

At the start of a class, it is important to scan the group, making eye contact and noticing whether there are signs that something unusual is happening. One develops the flexibility to adjust to group needs through the practice of two techniques, one of which is assessment. For example, on a particularly hot, humid day or on a snow day, the energy level of the class may vary and necessitate adjustment. Or, if a news item has been distressing, the group may need to talk a little more than usual. Another technique is creative response, both in actions (when half the group decides to go left instead of right, one adds this to the choreography) and administratively (when a woman who enjoys and benefits from the group needs to pay in installments instead of a lump sum, every effort is made to accommodate her).

Averting Problems

Successful programs integrate incoming clients by helping them feel welcome and giving them the sense that they are in the right place at this moment in their lives. There are a number of ways to avert attrition:

- Easing the way for new clients
- Meeting participant expectations (remember to find out about motivations . . . and don't forget about them!)
- Recognizing anxieties (if a woman is a new exerciser, reassure her that each person does what she can and be sure to explain terms and customs to her)

- Being nice to latecomers and helping them get going
- Identifying potential dropouts and gently trying to get a grasp of the situation
- Not playing favorites (if your best friend is also in your class and you have a lot to chat about, do it at lunch instead of during class)

Personalizing Class

Most instructors begin teaching prenatal programs after going through a training course or when taking over another instructor's program; most frequently, they initially adopt the style of the person from whom they have learned. At some point, often gradually, it is desirable to put one's own stamp on the class. Two ways instructors can do this are by adapting some of their special trademark choreography for pregnancy and using special music that helps them relax. Encouraging clients to bring in music and using music from children's animated films are two great ways to personalize a class. It is also very helpful to encourage a new mom to return and talk about her birth experiences.

Supervision

Nothing builds confidence among participants more than a professional attitude about the work. Ensuring safety and effectiveness through proper supervision of a program is critical. Methods to do this include screening, monitoring of heart rate and perceived exertion, paying attention to alignment, providing information, knowing warning signs and symptoms, and paying attention to hydration and nutrition.

Professional Accountability

Instructors working with groups soon realize there will always be new fads in style or equipment. Working with pre/postnatal clients requires taking a very careful look at new ideas and determining which are old ideas repackaged, which are new and useful ideas, and which are new and dangerous ideas for this population. Because the class members rotate regularly and pregnancy itself is a revelation, there is less need to come up with new material year after year than in other teaching situations. Instead, the need is to provide motion that is satisfying and effective. In practice, we find that instructors do well with the prenatal population when they expand their knowledge and experience in the usual ways: attending workshops and educational courses related to the field, reading professional literature, taking movement classes, exchanging information with other professionals in the field, and maintaining professional certification and update in pre/postnatal fitness.

Integrating Education and Support Into Fitness

Opportunities to take advantage of interactive learning and "teachable moments" often present themselves in the course of prenatal exercise sessions. Providing a nurturing environment in which to exercise, grow a healthy fetus, and prepare mentally and emotionally for birth and parenting through group activities is an important characteristic of an effective program.

Education

One of the great surprises for many fitness professionals who instruct or train pre/postnatal clients is the discovery that clients depend on them for educational information about the nature and course of pregnancy, for advice on how to deal with minor discomforts, and for help in selecting products ranging from bottles to care providers. For some reason—perhaps societal changes such that fewer women have extended families as sources of information—pregnant and postpartum women who join exercise programs see the program as the source of all the information they cannot find easily in the surrounding culture. Despite the abundance of books, Internet sites, and videos, pregnant women have a voracious appetite for more knowledge. For this reason, an instructor or trainer who wishes to do well with these clients seeks information from childbirth educators, midwives, physicians, doulas, and others involved in the health and well-being of pregnant and postpartum women and their offspring.

A number of practices allow the instructor, trainer, or program director to provide educational materials for clients. Bringing research articles, reputable popular writing, charts, or learning aids to class or to clients is one method. A group instructor can display materials in one part of the room and allow time for women to look over them before or after participating in activities. Organizing educational talks by local birth educators, medical professionals, lactation consultants, and parenting experts is another excellent procedure. The "teachable moment" is one of the best methods for fostering knowledge and growth. With time, those who persevere as teachers develop the ability to recognize when a question is an opening for a discussion or a mini-lecture on a hot topic. Grooming peer leaders is another excellent method of helping knowledge permeate a group program.

Support

In this text, the nature of women as network builders continually comes to the surface. Women have brains that permit them to multitask. They seek each other's counsel. They nurture. They are great connectors and suppliers. Being this way means that attention in any situation can go to the highest priority, the person with the greatest need, or whatever must happen next in order to get things done. Less attention goes to who's in control or whether people get their way. The focus is on success for as many as possible, not on winning and losing. For the instructor, creating support is mostly a matter of simply bringing women together. Such networks are self-organizing, and only a light hand is needed.

PROGRAM EVALUATION

For readers wishing to ensure safety and participant satisfaction, it is a good idea to use participant evaluations employing Likert-type scales to assess the perceived value of exercise components and program format. Comparing a woman's original motivations for exercise with her feelings regarding the contribution of exercise to her pregnancy and birth experience is an important means of evaluating the success of the exercise program on a personal level.

It is also advisable to keep track of birth outcomes to make sure that no adverse outcomes are resulting from the program. Statistics can be compared with overall figures from local hospitals and/or obstetrical practices. An example of a tool that can be used for in-house record keeping is the form "Birth Outcome Evaluation." This information should be recorded as soon after birth as possible.

Birth outcome information can be recorded on a self-evaluation report by the participant or can be gathered directly from her medical practice or hospital records. One can collect data for research purposes through a medical practice or hospital only by following certain procedures, including approval by a human subjects committee and informed consent from participants. Although getting the approval of a human subjects committee may not be practical or even necessary for in-house record keeping, it is still advisable to obtain informed consent from participants. Even at the in-house level of information gathering, confidentiality needs to be protected and women must feel that they are participating with full awareness of how the information may be used (see the form "Informed Consent" as an example of this type of form).

Another aspect of record keeping is attendance, participation, or workout records. Maintaining records of women's activities during pregnancy enables one to quantify dose effect, if there are findings regarding outcomes.

Birth Outcome Evaluation

Location: _____

Contact: _____

Birth of child: Year: _____ Quarter: ____*

Item: _____ id #	Example
Today's date	9-28-1998
Due date	9-27-1998
Delivery date	9-24-1998
Times	
Hours in hospital	46.5
Active labor (4-10 cm) – minutes	240
Pushing – minutes	45
Delivery	
Spontaneous vaginal	1
Forceps	0
Vacuum	0
Cesarean	0
Procedures	
Epidural	1
Painkiller, name:	0
Other, name:	0
Induced	0
Scalp pH	0
Episiotomy	0
Tear	1
Degree of tear	2
Outcomes	
Birth weight (gm or lb/oz)	3402 gm (7 lb 8 oz)
Length (cm or in.)	50.8 cm (20 inches)
Apgar 1	8
Apgar 5	9

Complications (list)

Notes

Epidemiological data

Mother's age at delivery (years)	20,5
Mother's race	Native American

Participation in program

First trimester	1
Second trimester	1
Third trimester	1
Notes	Active participant throughout pregnancy

*Quarters: **1** (January-February-March)   **2** (April-May-June)   **3** (July-August-September)   **4** (October-November-December)

A.F. Cowlin, 2002, *Women's fitness program development* (Champaign, IL: Human Kinetics).

181

In our efforts to make the program the best it can be, we are conducting a survey about the outcome of our participants' experiences. This information will be used only to determine statistical information and no names will be used. The data you provide will be placed on a Report Form that your instructor or program administrator maintains. When she collects this information, she will assign a number to your answers. Informed consent forms will be sent to our main office, kept in a locked file in the director's office and not made available to anyone. Data will also be sent to the main office, kept in a locked file and will be made available only to the survey statisticians.

This research will enable us to assess the value of our programs. It is possible that once enough data are collected some statistical information will be used for publication purposes. As we noted above, no personal identification will ever accompany any of the information. It will also assist us in determining ways to improve our program, and we welcome any comments you might wish to add.

The following information is requested:

Due date	Baby's birth weight
Delivery date	Baby's birth length
Hours in hospital	Did you have an episiotomy
Minutes in active labor (approx. 4-10 cm)	Did you tear and degree of tear
Minutes pushing	Baby's Apgar at 1 and 5 minutes
Type of delivery—spontaneous vaginal, forceps, vacuum, or C-section	Any complications
	Notes or comments
Whether you had an epidural	Trimesters of participation in the program
Whether you took painkiller(s) other than epidural	Your age
Whether you induced (Pitocin)	Your race
Whether the baby had a scalp pH	

There is no risk to you or your baby if you participate in this survey. If you have any questions, talk with your instructor or feel free to call our main office. You do not have to participate in the study.

Thank you for your consideration.

Informed Consent

I understand my rights as a study subject. I voluntarily consent to participate in this survey. I understand what the study is about and how and why it is being done. If I want a copy of this consent form, I will ask my instructor to supply me with a duplicate.

_____   _____

Participant's signature   Date

_____   _____

Witness' signature   Date

Developed by *Dancing Thru Pregnancy*®. Used by permission.

A.F. Cowlin, 2002, *Women's fitness program development* (Champaign, IL: Human Kinetics).

Professional Obligations

A program that yields fruitful evaluation data will bear the marks of professionalism. At the least, instructors will fulfill these professional obligations:

- Screen applicants for medical conditions and physical signs and symptoms.
- Require participants to sign a liability waiver.
- Require participants to sign an informed consent form.
- Maintain accurate records.
- Uphold the highest standards of confidentiality, both for written documents and verbal information.
- Lead a safe and effective program.
- Refrain from giving medical advice.

PROGRAM DESIGN FOR PREGNANT ADOLESCENTS

The significance of physical activity within the health care model for pregnant adolescents is almost an unknown. Very little information exists concerning such issues as how much activity and what type of activity are safe and appropriate. Moreover, those wishing to do research in this area in the United States face formidable barriers, foremost of which is societal schizophrenia surrounding Americans' perception of these girls.

Societal Considerations

While the rates of adolescent sexual activity are similar in all developed nations [70, 71], the rate of teenage pregnancy is far higher in the United States than in other Western nations, largely as a consequence of less U.S. public health education regarding safe sex and a more politicized landscape concerning sex education [71, 72]. Politicians and the media sometimes paint these girls as the cause of social ills and huge fiscal deficits, when in fact they are a very small portion of both the overall population and the population receiving social services and assistance. They are mostly minor children, who are protected by law and their families. As a result, reaching out to this population can require commitment, perseverance, and an ability to cut through stereotypes about who and where these girls are.

In the period from 1991 to 1996, the number of live births among adolescent girls declined [73, 74]. The smallest rate of decline in terms of age groups was in 10- to 14-year-olds (.02%); the largest rate of decline was among 15- to 17-year-olds (12%), with 18- to 19-year-olds having the next largest rate (8%). In terms of ethnic groups, the greatest rate of decline has been among African American girls (21%), and the smallest has been among Latinas (5%). In 2001, the Centers for Disease Control announced on its Web site a continuing reduction in the pregnancy rate among 15- to 19-year-olds, the rate in 1997 being comparable to that for 1976 [75]. Despite declining rates, nearly half a million children were born to adolescent mothers in the year 2000 [76].

Although information about declining numbers of live births to adolescent mothers has been widely reported, it has not been as often reported that the number of pregnancies is falling at a slower rate than the number of live births. It was also not widely reported that the decline in live births did not hold for poorer populations, particularly in places where health care services are less available. Sun Belt states have rates of adolescent pregnancy twice those of upper New England and of the upper-Midwest states, even controlling for ethnic population differences. Greater detail and state-by-state data are available on the Centers for Disease Control Web site [77].

For fitness instructors and personal trainers, this group does not represent a commercially viable clientele. However, as it becomes increasingly acceptable for pregnant teens to remain in school, and as more school-based programs come into existence, it is becoming easier to work with this population and be paid through school systems, universities, or grant-related programs. The National Organization on Adolescent Pregnancy, Parenting and Prevention [78] maintains a network of health care and social service professionals working with pregnant adolescents, enabling interested researchers and instructors to locate this population in their geographic area.

Health Care Needs

Adolescent pregnancy is a situation full of physical and psychological stresses. Pregnant adolescents are at increased risk for low-birth-weight infants and premature delivery. Younger pregnant girls are at risk of their own inhibited growth and development. Pregnant women under 20 are also at higher risk for disorders such as PIH. Prenatal care, begun in the first trimester, is key to ensuring positive outcomes for mother and infant. Adequate nutrition, a difficult issue for teens even outside of pregnancy, is all the more critical for a pregnant teen. Drinking, drugs, and smoking represent additional problems for this group, as they may not be aware of their pregnancy in the early stages.

These girls also face cognitive and psychological challenges. Despite becoming pregnant, they may have very little real understanding of their own sexuality, of sexual function, and of childbirth. They may be abused or may be living in dysfunctional family situations. Their pregnancies may be unplanned, representing serious threats to education or job plans. They almost always need to turn to family members for support and assistance, and they need negotiating skills. The extended family also absorbs the stress of the situation.

Physical Education and Birth Preparation

The only published study directly addressing exercise with pregnant adolescents examined the effects of a six-week aerobic exercise program. Results showed that the exercise group had a significant decrease in depressive symptoms over time and an increase in total self-esteem, while the nonexercising group reported a significant increase in physical discomforts associated with pregnancy [79]. The author concluded that aerobic activity should be viewed as an important aspect of prenatal self-care for healthy pregnant adolescents.

Another study looked at outcomes among adolescent mothers and infants; the findings showed that pregnant adolescents who sought prenatal health care in the first trimester and those who delayed prenatal care until the third trimester reported similar self-care knowledge and practices regarding diet, exercise, and other topics [80]. However, those who sought early prenatal care had significantly more positive outcomes [80], suggesting the need for combining early prenatal care with development of self-efficacy in the self-care practices of this population as a model for improving outcomes.

Practical examples of such a model exist, including the school-based center in New Haven, Connecticut. The Polly T. McCabe Center, which is part of the public school system, provides academic classes, childbirth preparation, postpartum and parenting programs, and life skills for pregnant and postpartum adolescent girls ranging in age from 12 to 19. Health education and physical activity are an integral part of the curriculum. Health care is provided through a number of venues, including area clinics. The school is the subject of a number of studies, including ongoing research, at Yale University. Results of these studies demonstrate a number of positive outcomes for students [81, 82].

The core elements of a physical education and birth preparation program for pregnant adolescents include the following:

1. Intake interview and health screening
2. Appropriate activities
3. Program evaluation

Intake Interview and Health Screening

When pregnant adolescents enter a special program, it is easy to gather demographic information, as well as information about their needs and interests, through informally structured interviews and class discussions. Effective screening is a cooperative effort between health care providers and the health and fitness specialists working with the girls. Some of the methods employed with adult pregnant women can be too cumbersome and can be ineffectual in a population that is somewhat tentative. Rather than obtaining forms and approvals prior to a girl's admission into the program, care providers should identify girls at risk and alert fitness instructors to the limitations on these girls.

Information that might be included on screening forms for adults can be adapted as class content. For example, an interactive session about foods and nutrition can precede filling out a food diary. The process of analyzing the nutritional content of the foods consumed can then become a project. The practical application of arithmetic helps to reinforce academic work and makes the point that what students learn in school has a real relationship to their lives. This topic can also be tied into the childbirth education component through a session on how nutrition gets to the baby.

Appropriate Activities

The following are some of the activities that an effective program for pregnant adolescents can include:

1. *Cardiovascular exercise.* Providing a practical learning experience about what makes the heart beat faster, how one counts the pulse, how one feels during exertion, and how exercise affects the baby forms the critical core of the content sessions. Fitness is the by-product.

2. *Special exercises.* Kegels, abdominal exercises, squatting, relaxation, and other preparatory exercises are practical skills the girls will need in labor and the postpartum period. Other strength and flexibility activities can be included, provided that diet is adequate. Centering and relaxation are also components that girls find useful. But, as with all fitness components, this population needs to uncover their significance through a combination of doing them and learning about them, that is, learning what various exercises do and why they are important.

3. *Self-care elements.* Topics of self-care for girls include personal hygiene, nutrition and exercise, preventing sexually transmitted diseases, getting to prenatal visits, techniques of stress management, and education as a means for survival.

4. *Childbirth education.* Integrating childbirth education into the school setting can greatly reduce barriers to

this information for these girls and can improve health behaviors [83]. Interactive learning units can be created around major topics, including pregnancy, nutrition, labor and delivery, birth control, and preventing sexually transmitted diseases.

Program Evaluation

A final exam covering topics of pregnancy, birth, and fitness can be used to assess students' learning and evaluate program results. An academic exam such as this as a way of measuring learning is familiar to students. By including questions concerning what they liked, learned, or wished was different about the program, the instructor can also assess the effectiveness of her teaching. The rewards of working with pregnant adolescents are many. Even when a girl has a supportive family situation, she needs support in the other areas of her life, which school-based programs can provide. Making the positive effects of physical activity and self-care available to this population is a project that needs attention. The possibilities for research and policy development in this area are enormous.

LOOKING AHEAD

In the late 1970s and early 1980s, because of serious concerns based on early research suggesting that fetal well-being would be adversely affected, health care providers were very reticent about encouraging women to exercise. Fortunately, through continuing research, the perseverance of exercising women, and the work of instructors who have cautiously expanded the repertoire of safe prenatal programs since the mid-1980s, a different picture has emerged. It has become clear that, as long as there is no uteroplacental insufficiency or underlying medical problem and the mother maintains a healthy lifestyle, exercise is not detrimental to the fetus. But what is more startling is the revelation that many of the powerful adaptations of pregnancy and exercise are feto-protective. In coming years, fitness professionals will have exciting opportunities to harness the benefits of prenatal exercise to help women achieve the goals of promoting healthy mothers having healthy babies, developing skills for labor and delivery, and having a quick recovery. They will also have opportunities to bring appropriate prenatal programs to underserved populations. In the next section of the text, we consider the postpartum period. One of the most complex challenges women face, the period that follows birth entails both immediate and longer-term adjustments that can be greatly aided by attention to the mother's physical state and social support.

REFERENCES

1. Cowlin, A.F. 1996. *Dancing Thru Pregnancy and AfterDance Perinatal Health and Fitness Instructor's Manual.* Stony Creek, CT: DTP, Inc.
2. Blair, S.N., Kohl, H.W., Paffenbarger, R.S., Clark, D.G., Cooper, K.H., and Gibbons, L.W. 1989. Physical fitness and all-cause mortality: A prospective study of healthy men and women. *Journal of the American Medical Association* 262:2395-2401.
3. Bouchard, C., Shephard, R.J., Stephens, T., Sutton, J.R., and McPerson, B.D. (eds.). 1990. *Exercise, fitness and health.* Champaign, IL: Human Kinetics.
4. Women's Education Life Learning (WELL) program. New Haven, CT: Yale-New Haven Hospital.
5. Reedy, N.J., and Varney, H. 1996. Screening for and collaborative management of antepartal complications. In H. Varney (ed.), *Varney's midwifery,* Boston: Jones & Bartlett, pp. 327-377.
6. Payton, R.G., and White, P.J. 1995. Primary care for women: Assessment of hematologic disorders. *Journal of Nurse Midwifery.* 40(2):120-136.
7. Hart, K.J., Palmer, M.H., and Fitzgerals, S. 1999. Perceived causes of urinary incontinence and reporting. *Clinical Nursing Research* 9:84-92.
8. Ford-Gilboe, M. 1997. Family strengths, motivation, and resources as predictors of health promotion behavior in single-parent and two-parent families. *Research in Nursing & Health* 20:205-217.
9. Littieri, D.J., Nelson, J.E., and Sayers, M.A. (eds.). 1985. *NIAA Treatment Handbook Series 2: Alcoholism Treatment Assessment Research Instruments.* Rockville, MD: National Institute on Alcohol Abuse and Alcoholism.
10. Clapp, J.F., III 1998. *Exercising through your pregnancy.* Champaign, IL: Human Kinetics.
11. Khodiguian, N., Jaque-Fortunato, S.V., Wiswell, R., and Artal, R. 1996. A comparison of cross-sectional and longitudinal methods of assessing the influence of pregnancy on cardiac function during exercise. *Seminars in Perinatology* 20(4):232-241.
12. Freston, M.S., Young, S., Calhoun, S., Fredericksen, T., Salinger, L., Malchodi, C., and Egan, J.F. 1997. Responses of pregnant women to potential preterm labor symptoms. *Journal of Obstetric, Gynecologic, and Neonatal Nursing* 26:35-41.
13. Michalek, A.M., Buck, G.M., Nasca, P.C., Freedman, A.N., Baptiste, M.S., and Mahoney, M.C. 1996. Gravid health status, medication use, and risk of neuroblastoma. *American Journal of Epidemiology* 143:996-1001.
14. Patterson, E.T., Freese, M.P., and Goldenberg, R.L. 1990. Seeking safe passage: Utilizing health care during pregnancy. *Image: The Journal of Nursing Scholarship* 22(1):27-31.
15. Alley, N.M. 1984. Morning sickness. The client's perspective. *Journal of Obstetric, Gynecologic, and Neonatal Nursing* 13(3):185-189.
16. Purlfield, P., and Morin, K. 1995. Excessive weight gain in primigravidas with low-risk pregnancy: Selected obstetric consequences. *Journal of Obstetric, Gynecologic, and Neonatal Nursing* 24:434-439.
17. Horns, P.N., Ratcliffe, L.P., Leggett, J.C., and Swanson, M.S. 1996. Pregnancy outcomes among active and sedentary primiparous women. *Journal of Obstetric, Gynecologic, and Neonatal Nursing* 25:49-54.
18. Tulman, L., Higgins, K., Fawcett, J., Nunno, C., Vansickle, C., Haas, M.B., and Specca, M.M. 1991. The Inventory of Functional Status—Antepartum Period: Development and testing. *Journal of Nurse Midwifery* 36:117-123.
19. Allen, R.J., and Hyde, D.H. 1981. *Investigations in stress control.* Minneapolis, MN: Burgess.
20. Tiedje, L.B., Kingry, M.J., and Stommel, M. 1992. Patient attitudes concerning health behaviors during pregnancy: Initial

development of a questionnaire. *Health Education Quarterly* 19:481-493.

21. Pender, N.J., and Pender, A.R. 1986. Attitudes, subjective norms, and intentions to engage in health behaviors. *Nursing Research* 35:15-18.

22. Walker, S.N., Sechrist, K.R., and Pender, N.J. 1987. Health-Promoting Lifestyle Profile: Development and psychometric characteristics. *Nursing Research* 36:76-81.

23. Ahijevych, K., and Bernard, L. 1994. Health-promoting behaviors of African-American women. *Nursing Research* 43:86-89.

24. Brinton, L.A., Shairer, C., Haenszel, W., Stolley, P., Lehman, H.F., Levine, R., and Savitz, D.A. 1986. Cigarette smoking and invasive cervical cancer. *Journal of the American Medical Association* 255:3265-3269.

25. Baecke, J.A.H., Burema, J., and Frijters, J.E.R. 1982. A short questionnaire for the measurement of habitual physical activity in epidemiologic studies. *The American Journal of Clinical Nutrition* 36:936-942.

26. Strang, V.R., and Sullivan, P.L. 1985. Body image attitudes during pregnancy and the postpartum period. *Journal of Obstetric, Gynecologic, and Neonatal Nursing* 14:332-337.

27. O'Connell, M. 1983. Locus of control specific to pregnancy. *Journal of Obstetric, Gynecologic, and Neonatal Nursing* 3:161-164.

28. Palmer, J.L., Jennings, G.E., and Massey, L. 1985. Development of an assessment form: Attitude toward weight gain during pregnancy. *Journal of the American Dietetic Association* 85(8):946-949.

29. Cardenas, J., Gibbs, C.E., and Young, E.A. 1976. Nutritional beliefs and practices in primigravid Mexican-American women. *Journal of the American Dietetic Association* 69:262.

30. Taffel, S.M., and Keppel, K.G. 1986. Advice about weight gain during pregnancy and actual weight gain. *American Journal of Public Health* 76:1396.

31. Chalmers B.E. 1991. Changing childbirth customs. *Pre-PeriNatal Psychology* 5:221-232.

32. Chalmers, B. 1990. *African birth: Childbirth in cultural transition.* Sandton, South Africa: Berev.

33. Engle, P.L., Scrimshaw, S.C.M., Zambrana, R.E., Dunkel-Schetter, C. 1990. Prenatal and postnatal anxiety in Mexican woman giving birth in Los Angeles. *Health Psychology* 9:285-299.

34. Hedegaard, M., Henrikse, T.B., Sabroe, S., and Secher, N.J. 1993. Psychological distress in pregnancy and preterm delivery. *British Medical Journal (Clinical Research Education)* 307(6898):234-239.

35. Kanner, A.D., Coyne, J., Schaefer, C., Lazarus, R.S. 1981. Comparison of two modes of stress measurement: Daily hassles and uplifts versus major life events. *Journal of Behavioral Medicine* 4:1-39.

36. De Longis, A., Coyne, J.C., Dakof, G., Folkman, S. and Lazarus, R.S. 1982. Relationship of daily hassles, uplifts, and major life events to health status. *Health Psychology* 1:119-136.

37. Gerson, M.J. 1978. *Motivations for motherhood.* Dissertations Abstracts International 39:1954. NYU Microfilms no. 78, 18420.

38. Lydon, J., and Dunkel-Schetter, C. 1994. Seeing is committing: A longitudinal study of bolstering commitment in amniocentesis patients. *Personality and Social Psychology Bulletin* 20:218-227.

39. Williams, T.M., Joy, L.A., Travis, L., et al. 1987. Transition to motherhood: A longitudinal study. *Infant Mental Health Journal* 8:251-265.

40. Zambrana, R.E., Dunkel-Schetter, C., and Scrimshaw, S. 1991. Factors which influence use of prenatal care in low-income racial-ethnic women in Los Angeles County. *Journal of Community Health* 16:283-295.

41. Petrowski, D.D. 1981. Effectiveness of prenatal and postnatal instruction in postpartum care. *Journal of Obstetric, Gynecologic, and Neonatal Nursing* 10:386-389.

42. Stark, M.A. 1997. Psychosocial adjustment during pregnancy: The experience of mature gravidas. *Journal of Obstetric, Gynecologic, and Neonatal Nursing* 26:206-211.

43. Lederman, R.P., Lederman, E., Work, B.A., and McCann, D.S. 1979. Relationship of psychological factors in pregnancy to progress in labor. *Nursing Research* 28:94-97.

44. Lederman, R.P. 1984. *Psychosocial adaptation in pregnancy: Assessment of seven dimensions of maternal development.* Englewood Cliffs, N.J.: Prentice-Hall.

45. Schroeder, M.A. 1985. Development and testing of a scale to measure locus of control prior to and following childbirth. *Maternal-Child Nursing Journal* 14(2):111-121.

46. Goyert, G.L., Bottoms, S.F., Treadwell, M.C., and Nehra, P.C. 1990. The physician factor in cesarean birth rates. *New England Journal of Medicine* 320(11):706-709.

47. Brazelton, T.B. 1976. Neonatal behavioral assessment scale. In O.G. Johnson (ed.), *Tests and measurements in child development: Handbook II* (Vol. 1). San Francisco: Jossey-Bass.

48. Dauncy, M.J., Gand, G., and Gairdner, D. 1977. Assessment of total body fat in infancy from skinfold thickness measurements. *Archives of Disease in Childhood* 52:223-227.

49. McAllister, D.L., Kaplan, B.J., Edworthy, S.M., Martin, L., Crawford, S.G., Ramsey-Goldman, R., Manzi, S., Fries, J.F., and Sibley, J. 1997. The influence of systemic lupus erythematosus on fetal development: Cognitive, behavioral and health trends. *Journal of the International Neuropsychological Society* 3(4):370-376.

50. Koniak-Griffin, D. 1994. Aerobic exercise, psychological well-being and physical discomforts during adolescent pregnancy. *Research in Nursing & Health* 17:253-263.

51. Stevens, J.W. 1994. Adolescent development and adolescent pregnancy among late age African-American female adolescents. *Child and Adolescent Social Work Journal* 11:433-453.

52. Adeyemo, M.O.A., and Brieger, W.R. 1995. Dissemination of family life education to adolescents by their parents in suburban Ibadan, Nigeria. *International Quarterly of Community Health Education* 15:241-252.

53. Rhodes, J.E., and Woods, M. 1995. Comfort and conflict in the relationships of pregnancy, minority adolescents: Social support as a moderator of social strain. *Journal of Community Psychology* 23:74-84.

54. Norsk, P., Bonde-Petersen, F., and Christensen, N.J. 1990. Catecholamines, circulation and the kidney during water immersion in humans. *Journal of Applied Physiology* 69:479-484.

55. Connelly, T.P., Sheldahl, L.M., Tristani, F.E., Levandoski, S.G., Kalkhoff, R.K., Hoffman, M.D., and Kalbfleisch, J.H. 1990. Effect of increased central blood volume with water immersion on plasma catecholamines during exercise. *Journal of Applied Physiology* 69:651-656.

56. Epstein, M., Loutzenhiser, R., Friedland, E., Aceto, R.M., Camargo, M.J., and Atlas, S.A. 1987. Relationship of increased plasma atrial natriuretic factor and renal sodium handling during immersion-induced central hypervolemia in normal humans. *Journal of Clinical Investigation* 79:738-745.

57. Norsk, P., Bonde-Peterson, F., and Warber, J. 1986. Arginine vasopressim, circulation and kidney function during graded water immersion in humans. *Journal of Applied Physiology* 61:565-74.

58. O'Hare, J.P., Dalton, N., Roland, J.M., Gooding, J., Payne, B., Walters, G., and Corrall, R.J. 1986. Plasma catecholamine levels during water immersion in man. *Hormone and Metabolic Research* 18(10):713-716.

59. O'Hare, J.P., Watson, M., Penney, M.D., Hampton, D., Roland, J.M., Corrall, R.J. 1985. Urinary prostaglandin E and antidiuretic hormone during water immersion in man. *Clinical Science* 69:493-49 gd6.

60. Katz, V.L., Ryder, R.M., Cefalo, R.C., Carmichael, S.C., and Goolsby, R. 1990. A comparison of bed rest and immersion for

treating the edema of pregnancy. *Obstetrics and Gynecology* 75(2):147-151.

61. Thompson, C.W. 1969. *Manual of structural kinesiology*, 6th ed. St. Louis: Mosby.

62. *Gray's Anatomy*, 27th ed. 1959. NY: Lea & Febiger.

63. Benson, H., Beary, J.F., and Carol, M.P. 1974. The relaxation response. *Psychiatry* 37:37-46.

64. Savoyant, A. 1988. Mental practice: Image and mental rehearsal of motor action. In M. Denis, J. Engelkamp, and J.T.E. Richardson (eds.), *Cognitive and neuropsychological approaches to mental imagery*. NY: Nijhoff, pp. 251-257.

65. Annett, J. 1988. Imagery and skill acquisition. In M. Denis, J. Engelkamp, and J.T.E. Richardson (eds.), *Cognitive and neuropsychological approaches to mental imagery*. NY: Nijhoff, pp. 259-268.

66. Todd, M.E. 1937 (1968). *The thinking body*. Princeton: Dance Horizons.

67. Sweigard, L. 1974. *Human movement potential: Its ideokentic facilitation*. NY:UP.A.

68. Achterberg, J. 1985. *Imagery in healing*. Boston: New Science Library.

69. Varney, H. 1996. *Varney's midwifery*, 3rd ed. Boston: Jones & Barlett, p. 354.

70. Jones, E.F., Forrest, J.D., Henshaw, S.K., Silverman, J., and Torres, A. 1988. Unintended pregnancy, contraceptive practice and family planning services in developed countries. *Family Planning Perspectives* 20(2) 53-67.

71. Jones, E.F., Forrest, J.D., Goldman, N., et al. 1985. Teenage pregnancy in developed countries: Determinants and policy implications. *Family Planning Perspectives* 17(2):53-63.

72. Brooks-Gunn, J., and Paikoff, R.L. 1993. Sex is a gamble, kissing is a game: Adolescent sexuality, contraception, and pregnancy. In S.G. Millstein, A.C. Petersen, and E.O. Nightingale (eds.), *Promoting the health of adolescents: New directions for the twenty-first century*. NY: Oxford U. Press.

73. Donovan, P. 1998. Falling teen pregnancy, birthrates: What's behind the declines? *The Guttmacher Report of Public Policy* 1:6-9.

74. Ventura, S., Curtin, S., and Matthews, T. 1998. *Teenage births in the United States: National and state trends, 1990-1996*. National Vital Statistics System. Hyattsville, MD: National Center for Health Statistics.

75. http://www.cdc.gov/nchs/releases/01news/trendpreg.htm

76. Martin, J., Hamiliton, B., Ventura, S., et al. 2002. Births: Final data for 2000. *National Vital Statistics Reports* 50:1-31.

77. http://www.cdc.gov/nchs/births.htm; or http://www.cdc.gov/nchs/about/major/natality49_05-4.pdf

78. National Organization on Adolescent Pregnancy, Parenting and Prevention, Inc. 1319 F Street, NW, Suite 400, Washington, DC 20004. (202) 783-5770.

79. Koniak-Griffin, D. 1994. Aerobic exercise, psychological well-being and physical discomforts during adolescent pregnancy. *Research in Nursing & Health* 17(4):253-363.

80. Lee, S.H., and Grubbs, L.M. 1993. A comparison of self-reported self-care practices of pregnant adolescent. *Nursing Practice* 18(9):25-29.

81. Seitz, V., and Apfel, N. 1993. Adolescent mothers and repeated childbearing: Effects of a school based intervention program. *American Journal of Orthopsychiatry* 63:572-581

82. Seitz, V., and Apfel, N. 1994. Effects of a school for pregnant students on the incidence of low birthweight deliveries. *Child Development* 65:666-676.

83. Dieterich, L. 1997. Assessment and development of adolescent childbirth education (CBE) to improve health behaviors. *Journal of Perinatal Education* 6(1):25-33.

PART III

POSTPARTUM PERIOD

This part of the text covers background information, terminology, and concerns pertinent to the postpartum period; goals and priorities of postpartum exercise programs; and program design. In contrast to what happens in the prenatal period, when a woman's mental and emotional focus turns inward as her body grows outward, giving birth draws a woman's focus outward onto the infant while her body needs literally to be pulled inward, back toward center. Although pregnancy and the postpartum period are often considered together as the *pre/postnatal* or *perinatal* period, they really are two distinct phases of a woman's life.

Birth—the event separating these two life phases—is so dramatic that it sharply focuses attention onto the baby. And caring for an infant is very demanding. It can be difficult for a new mother to think about her own health and fitness concerns when this small creature has so many needs. Many cultures recognize this dilemma and provide support mechanisms to allow the new mother opportunities to care for herself. In the United States, the appearance of doulas—women who assist the mother during and following the birth—demonstrates acceptance of the realization that by helping mothers we help the entire family. The growth of postpartum group exercise programs bringing mothers and babies together is an indication that elements of the fitness culture recognize a need. By providing support and opportunities for mothers and babies to learn from each other, such programs not only are a smart marketing move, but also facilitate healthy mother-baby relations.

The extent to which postpartum women have been culturally devalued is made evident by a lack of realistic popular images and the dearth of research concerning the characteristics or the effects of a healthy lifestyle on this phase of life. More than at any other time, the period following birth inaugurates the vast difference between what life holds for a woman who fulfills her biological destiny and a man who does the same. As economics journalist Ann Crittenden notes, not only is caregiving not financially rewarded, it is penalized [1]. Yet this makes little sense, for worldwide we know that when women head the household economically, families eat more and more nutritiously, and are healthier, than in households where the male controls the money [1, pp. 118-127]. In Brazil, for example, $1 in the hands of a woman has the same result for a child's survival as $18 in the hands of a man [2].

The current state of affairs in the field of postpartum physical activity is similar to the situation for prenatal exercise in the late 1970s. Since then, evidence has shown that physically empowering women in preparation for birth actually affects the degree to which they control their own birth process, as reflected in the reduced need for medical intervention. What might be accomplished for new mothers if they develop physical prowess while focusing outwardly on the well-being of their families? Fitness programs for this population provide a tremendous potential not only for helping women in this phase of their life cycle but also for research in this area.

REFERENCES

1. Crittenden, A. 2001. *The price of motherhood.* New York: Henry Holt.
2. Thomas, D. 1990. Intra-household resource allocation. *Journal of Human Resources* 25(4):635.

CHAPTER 9

UNDERSTANDING THE POSTPARTUM PERIOD

This chapter begins with a very brief review of labor and birth, included because it is important for the fitness instructor or trainer to be conversant in the language of birth in somewhat the same way most cultures are attuned to the language of war stories. Next is a discussion of the physical changes a postpartum woman undergoes, including anatomy and physiology, as well as terminology used to describe this period. A final section of the chapter covers health concerns and psychosocial considerations, including the unique needs to be met in postpartum fitness programs.

LABOR AND BIRTH

The events leading up to the moment of birth are called *labor.* It is work; it is a toll; it brings a prize of unbelievable consequence. Out of this process, a new human being comes into existence and a new consciousness emerges within the mother. A postpartum fitness instructor or trainer needs to be aware of the accepted medical concepts that guide birthing practices. Many instructors are drawn to work with this population following their own birthing experiences. While one's own birthing experiences are key preparatory experiences, it is important not to generalize them to all women.

Pre-Labor Signs

Under normal conditions, as a woman approaches her due date, there may be a number of cues to alert her that her body is preparing for birth. It is hard to say which of the signs will occur for which women and in what order. But when they occur, they are signs of the body's preparation.

Lightening or Dropping

The baby "drops" into the pelvis. With a "normal" presentation, the head enters the space below the plane created by the line between the top of the pubic symphysis and the ischial spine, as a first move toward the plane created by the line between the bottom of the pubic symphysis and the coccyx (the *plane of outlet*). The greater the size of these planes, the more space for the baby to maneuver. When lightening occurs, breathing and eating may be easier, but often urinary frequency increases. There may be discomfort in the pelvis and thighs due to increased pressure on the perineum.

Loss of Mucus

The mucous plug may be released gradually or all at once. This serves to lubricate the birth canal as well as indicating a relaxation of the cervix. Sometimes women are aware of this process, but it can also happen gradually and perhaps not be noticed.

Changes in Energy and Sleep

Because of a decrease in progesterone production, some women experience an energy spurt. Some women may also have difficulty sleeping. Urinary frequency and difficulty getting comfortable also often affect the capacity to rest.

Braxton-Hicks Contractions

Practice contractions often increase and may become especially uncomfortable in the groin and abdomen. Still irregular, they do not increase in length, intensity, or frequency. They generally do not produce *dilation,* or opening, of the cervix (although they may play a part in the *effacement,* or thinning, of the cervix). They are often relieved if the woman rests on her side or takes a warm bath. Sometimes walking or simply changing position relieves them.

Increased Edema

With the weight of the fetus lower in the abdomen, venous return from the legs may be even more compromised than it has been up to now, resulting in increased edema.

Positive Signs of Labor

Strong, effective uterine contractions that are opening the cervix, and sustained downward pressure of the fetus on the cervix that indicates the descent of the baby, lead to the rupture of the membranes encasing the amniotic fluid. These two signs—regular, strong contractions and rupture of the membranes—are welcome signs that labor is progressing.

Regular Contractions

Productive labor contractions become regular, frequent, and intense. They continue to progress despite resting, a warm bath or shower, walking or changing positions, effleurage (massage of the abdomen), or sitting on a birth ball, although these techniques are comfort measures for the laboring mother and assist the progress of the labor. Strong labor contractions produce cervical effacement and dilation.

Effective labor contractions are usually felt in the lower abdomen and sometimes in the back. If the baby is *posterior,* that is, if the baby will exit the birth canal with its face toward the pubic bone instead of the coccyx, back discomfort may be quite pronounced. In this case, the curve of the baby's spine is in the opposite direction from the curve created by the sacral table at the plane of inlet, causing greater pressure in the mother's lumbar spine as the baby tries to navigate into the birth canal. The uterosacral ligaments, which are dramatically stretched in this process, are also a major source of discomfort. The C-Curve exercise done during standing can help relieve the discomfort, as can a warm shower with water flowing onto the low back. Sitting on a stool or squatting in the shower is also helpful.

Pain

The nature of pain in childbirth is complex, apparently more so than other types of pain. In a study of 278 Swedish women following birth, Waldenstrom et al. found that although 91% of the women reported high levels of pain, 28% also assessed the pain as more positive than negative, suggesting that coping with pain is rewarding for some women [3]. Further, there were unusual correlations between women's scores of pain intensity and pain attitude, leading the authors to consider that the pain of childbirth has a different character and meaning than the pain of disease [3].

These findings are interesting in light of the conflict between those who are pro-analgesia and those who believe that all sensations, including labor pains, serve an important purpose. Believing that avoidance of pain is always good, some promote the use of analgesics in labor to relieve pain. On the other hand, many people view labor pain as purposive: all sensations provide information about the body's response to its internal and external environment. Evolutionary biologists believe these sensations are derived from evolutionary adaptations for survival [4].

Research concerning the pain of childbirth has focused primarily on two areas: rating pain on a scale with other types of pain, and determining the best method for reducing pain intensity. On scales using Thurston's paired comparison methodology, such as the Morse Pain Stimulus Scale [5], participants rate various pairs of pain stimuli (including childbirth); the items are then ranked from most to least painful. Childbirth ranks at or near the top in such scales. In part, methodologies for relieving pain have focused on developing the most effective painkiller drug combinations, such as epidural opioids with local anesthetics during labor [6, 7] and drugs for cesarean surgery and recovery [8]. Other methodologies include relieving anxiety, as proposed originally by Dick-Read (see chapter 5), through a variety of distraction and comfort measures [9-11]. Anxiety induces increased catecholamine release, leading to decreased uterine and placental blood flow and then to decreased uterine contractions, increased duration of labor, and greater anxiety.

Morgan's work on pain perception, cognitive strategies, and the effects of exertion on anxiety [12-17] holds clues to how the sensations of labor might be examined so that a more productive concept of childbirth pain could be introduced. Morgan's work reinforces what Waldenstrom remarked on—that complex somatopsychic phenomena govern the perception and response to exertion (as opposed to disease), and that pain avoidance is not always the safest or most productive methodology for dealing with sensory responses. Research in this area is greatly needed, and one hopes that new generations of exercise scientists will look with some skepticism on the prevailing construct of pain. The idea that pain is a tool that assists us in birth has yet to be examined seriously.

Rupture of Membranes

The rupture of membranes, or "breaking the bag of waters," is caused by increased pressure against the membranes due to the effect of the contractions. The fluid may exit in a gush or a slow trickle. If it is slow, it is sometimes mistaken for urine. To check, the woman should perform a Kegel; if the flow ceases, the fluid is probably urine. Generally the rupture of membrane is painless and comes without warning.

Spontaneous rupture is usually indicative that labor will begin within 48 hours if it is not already under way. Sometimes the membranes are ruptured artificially in an attempt to speed up labor if it is under way but progressing slowly. Once membranes are ruptured, the protective barrier is removed, and the risk of infection increases after 24 hours. If labor does not begin or is still slow, the use of Pitocin—an artificial form of oxytocin—may be instigated to stimulate labor. In a variety of cases, if labor continues to be unproductive, a cesarean birth may be performed.

Technically, rupture is called premature rupture of membranes any time it occurs before the onset of labor. Methods for dealing with premature rupture vary. Research generally indicates that rapid induction does not produce more desirable outcomes than expectant management (waiting), although results vary somewhat [18-23].

If the amniotic fluid is greenish or foul smelling, this is a sign of *meconium,* or fetal bowel movement. This may be a sign of fetal distress, especially if there are also abnormalities in the pattern of the fetal heart. Occurring on its own, it may or may not be a sign of fetal distress; and it does not always occur in cases of fetal distress.

Stages of Labor

The normal labor ranges anywhere from 7 to 18 hours. Labors of first-time mothers average around 12.5 hours, and labors of second-time mothers average around 7.5 hours. The first stage of labor is what we normally call labor and is characterized by uterine contractions. The second stage is the birth of the baby, and the third stage is the detachment and delivery of the placenta.

First Stage

The onset of labor is rarely a sudden event in which the woman has a clear perception that labor has "begun." More often, there is simply a sustained transition between the Braxton-Hicks and the effective labor contractions. The membranes may or may not rupture, and the discomfort may or may not be severe. The first stage of labor—contractions—has three phases: latent, active, and transition. Each phase has its own characteristics.

Latent or Early Phase. The latent or early phase of labor is generally defined as the period in which the cervix *dilates,* or opens, from 0 to 3 or 4 centimeters. Most women are able to do simple tasks around the home in this period. Relaxing, continuing to take fluids, and maybe taking a walk or doing simple household chores are common activities. Keeping energy expenditure low, staying well hydrated, and maintaining electrolytes (sports drinks, bland carbohydrates) are important in this phase. Women may perceive early-phase labor merely as a backache or upset stomach. If the baby is posterior, low back discomfort is common and the crawling position can be helpful. If back labor ensues, crawling or hanging forward while sitting or standing may be useful.

Active Phase. During the active phase of the first stage of labor, contractions become more powerful and command more of a woman's attention. In this period, she may need to slow and deepen her breathing during contractions so that she does not waste energy, maintains a steady flow of oxygen, and stays mentally calm. Before labor begins, if the baby's head is down it usually descends into the pelvis below the *plane of inlet.* This is called *engagement* and simply means that the head is into the pelvis. Lightening is a sign that this is taking place. During the first stage of labor, the head usually descends lower into the pelvis (known as *descent*), and the baby's chin touches its chest as its neck flexes to assist this pattern (known as *flexion*). If necessary, the head will mold in this period and rotate to fit the internal shape of the pelvis.

Paying attention to the internal flow of sensations *(associative mental focus)* may be helpful during this period. Breathing fully and deeply, going with the wave of the contractions, and beginning to eliminate external cues are all signs that a woman is becoming involved in the active phase of the first stage of labor. Some women respond well to distractions *(dissociative mental focus)* at this time, so playing music or looking at favorite pictures may be helpful. This phase is generally considered to be the phase when cervical dilation progresses from 3 or 4 centimeters to 8 centimeters.

If this phase never really takes over, a number of factors can be affecting the process, including (but not limited to) a head that is too large to fit into the pelvis even if the baby's cranial plates mold to the birth canal *(cephalopelvic disproportion)*; dehydration and/or fatigue due to lack of plasma glucose, lack of muscle glycogen, or build-up of lactic acid; psychological fears that inhibit mother and baby from progressing; or lack of patience on the part of the birth support team (including the care provider, the partner, and/or support personnel).

In this phase, women frequently are unable to carry on a normal telephone conversation during contractions, may appear edgy and cranky, and will often complain and need to move about to relieve tension. In this phase it is often difficult for the support persons to determine how much to follow the mother's call to higher powers (including drugs), and how much to urge her to change position, continue with her fluid intake, breathe deeply, go with the flow, and simply do the job at hand. The mother's own pain threshold and tolerance often become factors in this phase. Movement always tends to release stress (it occupies the attention of the central nervous system, and time passes).

Transition. The transition is generally thought of as the period in which the cervix dilates from 8 to 10 centimeters (or whatever constitutes the full extent needed for the head to pass through the cervix and into the vagina or birth canal). Many women need to be distracted during this time, as the transition is very demanding. If a woman has had pain medication, it may be allowed to wane in this period in order for her to gain greater motor control in preparation for pushing in the second stage. This is a time when the support persons need to exercise great skill in helping a mother to pass through the final stage of dilation. Making eye contact, joining her in moaning, and pulling her attention away from her body can all be helpful during this time, despite her desire at this point to consign all persons to the netherworld.

Second Stage

During this stage of labor, the baby makes its way through the birth canal and leaves the mother's body. Once the head is through the cervix, the baby can work its way through the pelvis. If the baby is not head down, a different part of the body other than the head will be leading the descent through the pelvis. In this case, the skill and training of the care provider come into play. Some labors with some care providers result in an unusual but successful delivery no matter what the situation may be. Some labors require massive intervention no matter who is watching over the birth process. Most labors are a compromise among the baby's physiognomy, the mother, the support persons, and the care provider.

During this stage of labor, 60- to 90-second contractions alternate with breaks of 3 or 4 minutes. During the uterine contractions, the mother bears down on the perineum, assisting the contractions in expelling the baby. Some women experience a desire to push and others do not. *Pushing* should be done in a position that is most comfortable and productive for the mother. Two major methods of pushing are taught to women: slow and steady (Valsalva) pushing, and self-directed, active or spontaneous pushing.

Slow and steady pushing involves a continuous effort with each contraction, preceded by one or two deep, "cleansing" breaths at the onset, then a third inhale and hold. The holding is not prolonged; rather, two or three times during each contraction the woman exhales and takes in another deep breath. This technique was developed by a male.

Self-directed pushing involves breathing deeply in the contraction until the urge to push occurs. Then the woman breathes in and drops her jaw, and as she is exhaling she presses the pelvic floor muscles down and out with a strong, direct, sustained effort. Exhaling and letting go, she often makes a deep, low moaning sound. This technique has been developed by women. For most women, a combination of methods is productive.

Once the head is delivered, it may be necessary for the mother to pant while the baby's airways are cleared and the remainder of the body rotates for delivery. If pushing is not productive but the baby is low enough, forceps or a vacuum extraction process may be used.

Some babies start their journey higher in the pelvis. Often, women in this situation do not feel the urge to push. A protocol known as *laboring down* may be used, in which the contractions proceed but the mother does not attempt to push; instead she passively allows the body to open and adjust and the baby to descend in the process. Once the baby is low enough, pushing is begun.

Third Stage

Following the delivery of the baby, the placenta separates from the uterine lining and is delivered. This may take 5 or 10 minutes or slightly longer. Once the placenta is delivered, if there has been any tearing of the perineum or pelvic floor muscles or an *episiotomy* (surgical cutting of the perineum or pelvic floor muscles) during delivery, then sutures may be used to stitch up the perineum. During this period, the baby is evaluated at 1 and 5 minutes (Apgar scores), dried, wrapped, and, if all is well, given to the mother to hold. Some babies want to suck, but many babies just want to recover!

Types of Birth

Birth occurs either vaginally or via cesarean section (a surgical delivery). Except in the case of an elective surgical delivery, it is rarely possible to know for sure ahead of time what the exact outcome will be.

Vaginal Birth

Babies born vaginally without any surgical intervention are considered *spontaneous vaginal births*. There may be some tearing of the perineum, but it is rarely as severe as tearing that results when an *episiotomy,* or cutting of the perineum, also tears. Among the factors that contribute to the ability of the perineum to remain intact during birth are the mother's elasticity, the speed of delivery, and the skill of the care providers or other birth assistants. An episiotomy, forceps, or vacuum may be used if the delivery is stalled or the fetus is in distress.

Cesarean Birth

If it is clear that the continuation of labor will compromise the well-being of mother or infant, then a surgical birth (cesarean) is performed. Among major operations performed in the United States, the cesarean section is the most common. A surgical incision is made through the mother's abdominal wall and into the uterus so that the baby can be surgically removed.

PHYSICAL CHANGES FOR THE POSTPARTUM WOMAN

Once the birth process is over, the mother is confronted by her "third body." Before pregnancy, she lived in her first body. It went through changes, but mainly it had been growing and developing. If she delayed childbearing beyond her early 20s, she may even have felt that she had tamed her body. From reading and experience, she may have learned how to care for her physical self through nutrition, activity, and other lifestyle factors so that she was healthy and felt positive about herself. Her second body was the body she developed in her first pregnancy. While she may have had some discouraging periods during gestation, she probably tolerated problems in light of the fact that she was making a baby. But after the birth of her first baby, she does not return to her first body. Rather, she lives in a third body, one that reflects her experience. We could even say that she will have a fourth body with a second pregnancy, and a fifth following a second birth. Perimenopause, menopause, and postmenopause will increase the number. In any case, the point is that women's bodies are polymorphous, taking on forms that follow function. Because functions change for women, our forms change also.

What are the characteristics of this third (or fifth or seventh) body? Suddenly there's no longer a baby in the womb, but most of the compensatory effects of pregnancy are still present, creating a tremendous imbalance—both physically and mentally. The feet have enlarged, the knees and hips are stressed, the perineum is swollen, and perhaps the woman has hemorrhoids. She has lordosis, a soft abdomen, an aching upper back (and kyphosis), swollen breasts, and a forward head, and she's losing her hair. She may have varicosities, periods of heavy sweating, and skin blotches; she rarely gets enough sleep, and she'd like to lose weight! Time plus a good mother-baby program will do wonders.

But it is also important to recognize that the third body has its own potential. Hopefully the processes of gestation and birth have taught the new mother about strengths that she could not have imagined before becoming pregnant for the first time. The third body has its own best state, different from what was before. We have often worked with women who became interested in regular exercise for the first time during pregnancy or following birth. While at six months postpartum they attain the lowest body mass index and body fat percentage they have ever had, they sometimes find that their waists are larger than before, requiring alterations in their clothing. The most common reason for this is an outward expansion of the rib cage or the iliac crest of the pelvis, so that the underlying structure is simply larger in circumference. When these women understand that they are happier and healthier than before, it can be a revelation: whose value is it to have a smaller waist? Especially if the larger waist is also stronger and provides support for the low back?

The female body is polymorphous, taking on shape depending on the needs of the life cycle phase. Following birth, the instinctive imperative is for the mother to adequately provide her own body with the sustenance needed by the newborn. And today, when so many women live in an environment of plentiful food, it is easy to fall into a pattern of eating for comfort because it is providing for the baby. But doing so drives the new mother away from the cultural norms for beauty. An appropriate postpartum exercise setting may be the one place where this particular complex of physical and psychosocial needs can be dealt with.

POSTPARTUM ANATOMY

Technically, the *postpartum* period refers only to the first six weeks following birth, during which time the female reproductive tract returns to a nonpregnant condition (not a prepregnant, but a nonpregnant condition). Generally, a six-weeks postpartum visit is scheduled with the care provider in order to check this progress. This period is also called the *puerperium,* and the woman passing through this time is a *puerpera.*

Returning the body to a true nonpregnant state can take longer than six weeks. However, by this time, most healthy women are able to do vigorous activity if they were active during pregnancy and began their recovery exercises within a few days of birth.

The Uterus

The *involution* of the *uterus* is one of the primary events of the postpartum period. This refers to the shedding of the decidua and endometrium at the placental site, along with the shrinking of the uterine muscle and the cervix. The uterus is the size of a watermelon when the baby is born, but must shrink back to about the size of a pear. *After-birth pains* are caused by contraction and relaxation of the uterus as it shrinks. They are more common in breast-feeding mothers because contractions are mediated by oxytocin, which is released during breastfeeding. Emptying the bladder and lying prone with a pillow under the abdomen lead to relief, although when a woman first lies down, she may experience severe cramps. After a few minutes, however, she should experience relief.

The *lochia* is the discharge that results from the shedding process during the puerperium. Figure 9.1 reviews the mechanism of the placenta and the location of the separation and shedding process. The *lochia* passes through three periods: the lochia *rubra, serosa,* and *alba.* Lochia rubra is the first portion and is red because it contains a high proportion of blood. It lasts for two or three days. The next portion is the lochia serosa, which is mostly pink or yellowish. It continues for about seven or eight days and is composed of serous fluid, decidual tissue, leukocytes, and erythrocytes. The last portion, the lochia alba, is creamy white and contains leukocytes and decidual cells. This generally lasts about another week.

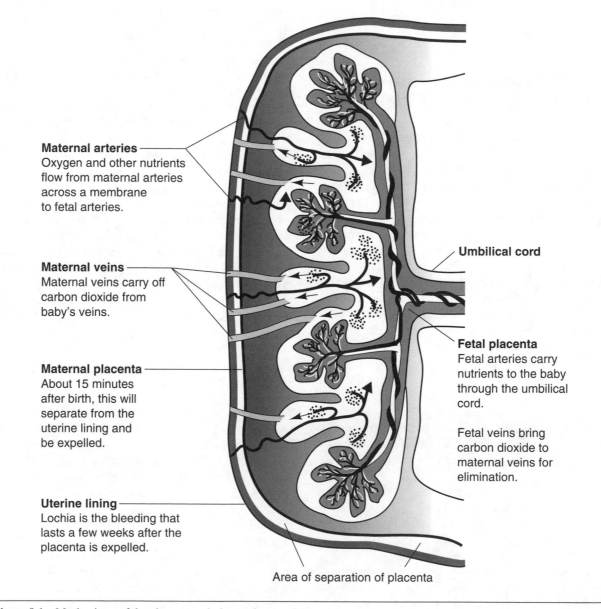

Maternal arteries
Oxygen and other nutrients flow from maternal arteries across a membrane to fetal arteries.

Maternal veins
Maternal veins carry off carbon dioxide from baby's veins.

Maternal placenta
About 15 minutes after birth, this will separate from the uterine lining and be expelled.

Uterine lining
Lochia is the bleeding that lasts a few weeks after the placenta is expelled.

Umbilical cord

Fetal placenta
Fetal arteries carry nutrients to the baby through the umbilical cord.

Fetal veins bring carbon dioxide to maternal veins for elimination.

Area of separation of placenta

Figure 9.1   Mechanisms of the placenta and placental separation.

The Pelvic Floor

The stretching of the vagina and perineum, as well as bruising and edema, is generally reduced by three to four weeks. Kegel exercises are important to the return of muscle tone and improved circulation in this area. A cold pack also helps reduce discomfort.

The Bladder

Changes in the renal system, including the bladder, ureter, and urethra, occur during the first four weeks postpartum. Following birth, the bladder is swollen, congested, and hypotonic. This can contribute to *incomplete voiding.* Women should be encouraged to completely void their bladders periodically, even if they do not feel the necessity, to help ensure that they will not develop a urinary tract infection. Diuresis in the first week following delivery is considerable, as the body rids itself of extra interstitial fluid. Increased urine output and excessive perspiration are the two major methods of releasing this fluid.

Constipation

Constipation may also be a problem in the first few days. Swelling, discomfort, or fear of tearing sutures can cause a new mother to hold back. She should be encouraged to eat and to drink fluids in adequate amounts to meet her energy needs and to relax and allow her body to function.

The Breasts

Lactation, or the production and release of breast milk, is a natural occurrence. Milk production occurs unless the mother receives a lactation suppressant. But the ongoing release of milk, called the *letdown reflex,* requires the baby's sucking action and is mediated by oxytocin. The dramatic fall in estrogen and progesterone levels at the time of the delivery of the placenta permits increases in the production of *prolactin,* a hormone that is essential for lactation.

There are two stages in the production of breast milk. In the first stage, late in pregnancy, the breasts prepare to synthesize milk. Evidence of this is the *colostrum,* or immature milk, which has a high protein and mineral content and provides immunological benefits. The *coming-in* of milk, or second stage, includes the transition to mature milk and involves the balancing of nutrients and growth factors.

Whether breastfeeding or using formula, when sitting upright the woman should use pillows or blankets to support the baby. This relieves the weight at the shoulders, reducing the pull on the upper back. It also frees the hands for handling the baby.

Breast engorgement is another common discomfort. Unless the instructor or trainer is also a lactation consultant, we recommend referring women to a midwife, pediatric nurse practitioner, certified lactation consultant, or the local La Leche League.

PHYSIOLOGICAL CHANGES POSTPARTUM

In the months following birth, changes occur in a number of physiological systems, including cardiovasculature, respiration, thermoregulation, metabolism, and biomechanics. Psychophysiological changes also occur; these we look at later in the section "Psychosocial Considerations."

Cardiovasculature

Some have challenged the concept of six weeks as the postpartum period by questioning whether the body truly attains a nonpregnant state during this time. Many women feel that they are truly postpartum for six months to a year, particularly if they are breastfeeding. In the area of cardiovascular changes, we know that physiological shifts due to pregnancy do not return to nonpregnant parameters in 6 weeks. Stroke volume and end-diastolic volume remain elevated over preconception values at 6 and at 12 weeks [24]. Systemic vascular resistance remains decreased at one year, and this change is additive with successive pregnancies [25].

Immediately following birth, some women experience puerperal bradycardia, with a pulse of 40 to 50 beats per minute. This is not considered indicative of disease, but rather a sign of well-being [26].

Respiration

Breathing returns to normal within a couple of months of birth. However, ribs may remain expanded for a year or more.

Thermoregulation

The amount of time it takes to return to normal thermoregulation varies among postpartum women. In many women, six weeks is adequate. For others, especially those who are breastfeeding, the return to normal thermoregulation may take longer.

Metabolism

The biochemistry of energy is also returning to a nonpregnant state. If the woman is not breastfeeding, the metabolic rate slows, reducing the need to eat as much or as often. If she is breastfeeding, it is generally thought she requires an additional 300 to 500 calories, so the need for food and fluids remains elevated during this time.

Biomechanics

A number of biomechanical shifts arise as a result of pregnancy and birth. The bone, nerve tract, and muscle alterations that result from movement of the center of gravity forward (outlined in chapter 5) are discussed in chapter 10 in terms of setting goals for return to a nonpregnant posture. These changes are further discussed in chapter 11 in relation to specific exercises that assist in accomplishing realignment.

Among the common structural conditions that result from the changing body dynamics of pregnancy and the demands of birth are *diastasis recti, separation of the symphysis pubis, broken coccyx, sacroiliac joint dysfunction, back pain,* and *lower limb problems.* Chapter 11 deals with these conditions in detail.

HEALTH CONCERNS

Serious complications or the sequellae of metabolic disorders or heart disease following childbirth are beyond the scope of this text. Instructors or trainers who feel that they have encountered severe conditions in a client must insist that the client contact her care provider. It is useful, however, to be aware of some of the more common situations that can arise so that, if necessary, instructors and trainers are prepared to describe what they have observed. Having accurate knowledge is also helpful in convincing an intractable client that she needs to secure appropriate professional assistance.

Fever and Other Signs of Infection

Infection can have any of a number of sources, from *mastitis* (inflammation of the breasts) to contamination during *internal procedures* done in labor. *Bacteremia*—bacterial infections—can come from the lower genital tract or bowel, or from the hands of attending personnel. Fever and elevated pulse are the common signs of infection. Infections include *infections of the perineum, endometritis, peritonitis,* and *septic thrombophlebitis.* Clearly, if a woman has a fever over 100.5° F or a racing pulse, or both, she must be persuaded to see her care provider and defer moderate or strenuous physical activity for the time being.

Other Biological Disorders

Thrombophlebitis, pulmonary embolism, hematoma, and *delayed postpartum hemorrhage* are circulatory problems that require medical attention [25]. Embolism and hemorrhage are life threatening. Thrombophlebitis is more common in women with varicosities; it can be superficial or deep and involves the veins in the lower extremities. Signs of superficial thrombophlebitis include slight temperature and pulse elevation, leg pain, and local heat, tenderness, and redness. Signs of deep thrombosis are more extreme; these include edema and pain. Women demonstrating any elevation of temperature over 100° F and leg discomfort or swelling should not exercise, and must seek advice from their health care provider. The great danger of deep thrombophlebitis is pulmonary embolism, the symptoms of which include sharp chest pain, dyspnea, tachycardia, and apprehensiveness.

Hematomas, which occur most frequently during delivery or shortly afterward, commonly involve the vulva, vagina, or broad ligaments and can result from procedures such as use of forceps, episiotomy, and repairs or rough handling of tissue [25]. Delayed hemorrhage is indicated by obvious external bleeding, signs and symptoms of shock, and signs and symptoms of anemia [25].

Subinvolution, the incomplete involution of the uterus, also needs attention. It is usually diagnosed at the six-week postpartum health care visit. The most common cause is retained placental fragments. All of the conditions mentioned in this section delay activity, the extent depending on the severity of the condition. Thyroid disease, consequences of diabetes, organ damage from toxemia, and other problems may also have a profound effect on exercise prescription.

Deconditioning Due to Bed Rest

One of the most common health and fitness challenges that instructors and trainers encounter is the client who is deconditioned and wishes to return to exercise. Continuing differences in cardiovascular parameters in the first few months postpartum affect the usual measurement procedures. As with pregnancy, in practice we have found that teaching women to recognize appropriate levels of exertion through the correlation of subjective terms and measured responses, such as heart rate and respiration, leads to the best long-term commitment to the process.

PSYCHOSOCIAL CONSIDERATIONS

Birth and the postpartum period are startling and complex experiences that have been studied in somewhat the same way that the blind men studied the elephant: some felt the ears, some the trunk, and some the tail, but none could describe the whole animal. The psychosocial events surrounding birth and the immediate postpartum period occur in settings that vary enormously around the globe. Sixty percent of the births worldwide take place unattended by care providers [27]. Social support for birthing and new mothers varies greatly from culture to culture. In developed nations, birth has been transformed into an event featuring medical technology. In the United States, birth became statistically safer for both mother and infant during the course of the 20th century. Yet the United States, with the highest level of birth technology in the world, also has a neonatal mortality rate higher than that of any other first-world nation, and an epidemic of maternal depression.

Psychophysiology

Postpartum blues is the term applied to a common "down" feeling, often occurring around the third to fifth day following birth. Rapid hormonal changes, the emotional and physiological letdown after a major athletic event, shifting attention of family and friends, and a sense of the loss of pregnancy with its particular intimacy may all contribute to a mild depressive state. Support, reassurance, positive reinforcement, physical activity, and caretaking from relatives can help minimize such effects. It is important to distinguish between the blues and true depression or psychosis.

Postpartum depression refers to an intense depression that starts later than the blues, often around three or four months, and that can be characterized by an inability to concentrate, loss of interest, lack of positive emotions, inability to control one's emotions, guilt and fear at thoughts of harming the baby, and thoughts of death [28]. Who will develop depression and to what extent has not been linked to a history of depression prior to birth [29]. If a woman demonstrates ongoing negative emotions, extreme fatigue, or an inability to focus on the exercises, or is unable to deal with her infant, efforts should be made to refer her to a mental health professional.

Even more serious is *postpartum psychosis,* in which the mother loses touch with reality. A number of very serious things can result, from maternal rejection to infanticide. *Maternal rejection* results from difficulties with bonding, or attachment. As with many functions that have traditionally been considered "woman's work," the behavior of *bonding* has been assumed to be immediately available to the new mother. But recent consideration of this phenomenon as culturally learned [30] has helped us see the necessity of assessing the inherent needs of the infant and the ways in which they are met by significant caregivers whom the infants become attached to. Attachment problems can result in infant *failure to thrive* or can manifest themselves in *child abuse.* Any indication of serious psychological difficulties, such as a detachment from the infant or a lack of social interaction with friends or other group fitness participants, should be referred to an appropriate professional.

Mood and *anxiety disorders* following birth are receiving increasing attention from mental health professionals. The role of physical activity in establishing feelings of well-being makes this an area in which future research can bear much fruit. In our experience, postpartum women report that their exercise group plays a significant role in their well-being [31]. There has been a small amount of research that helps us understand why this may be. Examining the psychological effects of an aerobic exercise session and a rest session on postpartum women, Koltyn and Schultes concluded that both factors resulted in decreased state anxiety and depression, and that the exercise was associated with significant decreases in total mood disturbance and significant increases in vigor [32]. Sampselle et al. [33] found that two markers of postpartum well-being were significantly improved in women who participated in self-reported vigorous physical activity by six weeks postpartum. In relation to the first marker, postpartum weight retention, women with higher levels of activity retained less weight than an inactive group. In relation to the second marker, Lederman's postpartum maternal adaptation questionnaire [34], vigorous exercisers had better scores on all adaptation subscales. When combined with the positive effects of group support and the health effects of regular physical activity, such findings suggest why postpartum group exercise produces positive psychological outcomes.

One area that warrants further study is the relationship of childbearing to the exacerbation of *obsessive-compulsive disorder* (OCD) [35]. Leckman and colleagues have observed that oxytocin affects a variety of cognitive, grooming, affiliative, sexual, and reproductive behaviors that bear a relationship to symptoms of OCD; these investigators have hypothesized that some forms of OCD are at the extreme end of a range of normal behaviors mediated by oxytocin [36]. The relationship of these findings to parenting behaviors is currently under study by Leckman and his associates at the Yale Child Studies Center. The question of the role of oxytocin—which is released during lactation—in various disorders is a topic of study [37-39]. However, the role of physical activity in regard to OCD and parenting behaviors remains to be examined.

The release of prolactin during the postpartum period significantly decreases anxiety in lactating women [40]. It is logical that the changing hormonal environment works to the benefit of the survival of the offspring. Taken as a whole, these changes may well represent nature's way of ensuring that the mother will behave repetitiously to meet the ongoing needs of the infant, while relieving anxiety and thereby stripping her of a pressing sense of the need to focus on herself. Certainly, there is evidence that the postpartum experience intensifies the perception of time and energy barriers to exercise by placing such a strong focus on meeting the needs of the infant [41].

The Social Challenge of the Postpartum Period

For women in the childbearing years, the postpartum period represents a strange mix of potentials. On the one hand, positive cardiovascular changes associated with pregnancy continue for some time following birth, providing the new mother with survival enhancements during this stressful period. On the other hand, compared to any of a woman's other roles in life, motherhood produces the greatest barriers to participation in exercise [42]. Modern influences can lead to a mothering lifestyle that is detrimental to physical and psychological well-being. Without appropriate informal social support, institutional supports for child care, appropriate programs, education on healthy behaviors, and safe environments or transportation, women in a variety of settings undergo lifestyle and psychosocial changes that lead to postpartum weight gain, inactivity, isolation, and depression. One British study has demonstrated that women with postpartum weight gain are at increased risked of long-term weight gains [43], raising their long-term disease risk.

For women of color these problems are exacerbated by an even greater lack of exercise settings that encourage them to participate [44]. Poor women and adolescent mothers are other groups disenfranchised by a lack of suitable, accessible programming and education. Yet bringing recreational exercise or an active lifestyle to these populations is possible and can provide benefits in both short- and long-term well-being.

After bringing forth a new human being through the auspices of her body, a woman faces extreme adaptations. In the United States she often does this in isolation. As her hormones shift following birth, she is "blue." She may even become depressed. A psychiatrist may offer drugs. After six weeks, her obstetrician pronounces her no longer postpartum since her uterus is now a non-pregnant size. At this time of life—perhaps more than at any other time—support is a critical component con-tributing to self-efficacy. Without adequate support a woman may lose belief in her ability to care for herself and her infant.

If she is in a setting where she receives social support, she still may not be encouraged to pursue physical activity, but rather to take it easy. Yet we know that one of the topics women want information about following birth is exercise and nutrition, and that women who are physically active before their six-week postpartum medical checkup may adapt more easily to motherhood and the recovery process. How well does their environment—including the health care providers with whom they come in contact—supply these women with the information, support, or prompting necessary to ensure they will participate in physical activity? How often do persons or circumstances around a postpartum woman enable her to make beneficial lifestyle choices?

PROVIDING PROGRAMS THAT MEET POSTPARTUM NEEDS

The childbearing years constitute a critical window for introducing women to or retaining them in meaningful physical activity. But, as with adolescence, the postpartum period is a time when women become alienated from recreational physical activity or an active lifestyle. Programs that provide a place for women to grow and develop as mothers, that attract them as social beings (with situational limitations, cultural perspectives, and personal needs and motivations), and that address specific physical needs following birth are at a premium. And for many women, such programs are simply unavailable or unattainable. So the job of those who provide programs and study postpartum women's fitness includes not only determining what kind of programs or interventions are effective for women, but also learning what can be done to make programs or interventions meaningful and accessible.

A woman with major body changes, a new infant to care for, and a new identity as mother of a new baby has health and fitness needs that are far different from those of the average denizen of the gym. As a group, these women need programs that will specifically benefit their situation by providing a high degree of social support and learning, focusing on the recovery of the postpartum body and mind, and facilitating mother-baby interaction. Before the discussion of postpartum program design in chapter 11, the next chapter examines the goals and priorities of postpartum fitness, so that the programs themselves can be designed to meet the needs of this population.

REFERENCES

1. Crittenden, A. 2001. *The price of motherhood*. New York: Henry Holt.

2. Thomas, D. 1990. Intra-household resource allocation. *Journal of Human Resources* 25(4):635.

3. Waldenstrom, U., Bergman, V., and Vasell, G. 1996. The complexity of labor pain: Experiences of 278 women. *Journal of Psychosomatic Obstetrics and Gynecology* 17(4):215-228.

4. Nesse, R.M., and Williams, G.C. 1995. *Why we get sick*. NY: Times Books.

5. Morse, J.M., and Morse, R.M. 1988. Cultural variation in the inference of pain. *Journal of Cross-Cultural Psychology* 19:232-242.

6. Vettrmann, J., Thomas, H., Lischke, V., and Asskali, F. 1996. Repeated addition of fentanyl to bupivacaine peridural analgesia in labor. Clinical action and fentanyl plasma level (German). *Anaesthesist* 45(5):428-436.

7. Clapp, J.F. 3rd, Kett, A., Olariu, N., Omoniyi, A.T., Wu, D., Kim, H., and Szeto, H.H. 1998. Cardiovascular and metabolic responses to two receptor-selective opioid agonists in pregnant sheep. *American Journal of Obstetrics and Gynecology* 178(2):397-401.

8. Chung, J.H., Sinatra, R.S., Sevarino, F.B., and Fermo, L. 1997. Subarachnoid meperidine-morphine combination. An effective perioperative analgesic adjunct for cesarean delivery. *Regional Anesthesia* 22(2):119-124.

9. Simkin, P. 1995. *Comfort measures for childbirth with Penny Simkin, PT*. VHS video tape. Seattle: Penny Simkin, Inc.

10. Morse, J.M., and Park, C. 1988. Home birth and hospital deliveries: A comparison of the perceived painfulness of parturition. *Research in Nursing & Health* 11:175-181.

11. Kusman, L.E. 1975. Reduction of pain in childbirth by the alleviation of anxiety in pregnancy. *Journal of Consulting and Clinical Psychology* 43(2):162-165.

12. Morgan, W.P. 1994. Psychological components of effort sense. *Medicine and Science in Sports and Exercise* 26(9):1071-1077.

13. Morgan, W.P. 1985. Affective beneficence of vigorous physical activity. *Medicine and Science in Sports and Exercise* 17(1):94-100.

14. Morgan, W.P., Horstman, D.H., Cymerman, A., and Stokes, J. 1983. Facilitation of physical performance by means of a cognitive strategy. *Cognitive Therapy and Research* 7(3):251-264.

15. Morgan, W.P., and Horstman, D.H. 1978. Psychometric correlates of pain perception. *Perceptual and Motor Skills* 47(1):27-39.

16. Morgan, W.P. 1978. The mind of the marathoner. *Psychology Today* 11(11):38-40.

17. Morgan, W.P., Raven, P.B., Drinkwater, B.L., and Horvath, S.M. 1973. Perceptual and metabolic responsivity to standard bicycle ergometry following various hypnotic suggestions. *The International Journal of Clinical and Experimental Hypnosis* 21(2):86-101.

18. McCaul, J.F. 4th, Rogers, L.W., Perry, K.G., Jr, Martin, R.W., Allbert, J.R., and Morrison, J.C. 1997. Premature rupture of membranes at term with an unfavorable cervix: Comparison of expectant management, vaginal prostaglandin, and oxytocin induction. *Southern Medical Journal* 90(12):1229-1233.

19. Keirse, M.J., Ottervanger, H.P., and Smit, W. 1996. Controversies: Prelabor rupture of membranes at term: The case for expectant management. *Journal of Perinatal Medicine* 24(6):562-572.

20. Duff, P. 1996. Premature rupture of the membranes in term patients. *Seminars in Perinatology* 20(5):401-408.

21. Shaley, E., Peleg, D., Eliyahu, S., and Nahum, Z. 1995. Comparison of 12- and 72-hour expectant management of premature rupture of membranes in term pregnancies. *Obstetrics and Gynecology* 85(5 Pt. 1):766-768.

22. Saropala, N., and Chaturachinda, K. 1993. Outcome of premature rupture of membranes (PROM) at term: Ramathibodi Hospital, 1988. *Journal of the Medical Association of Thailand* 76(Suppl 1):56-59.

23. Morales, W.J., and Lazar, A.J. 1986. Expectant management of rupture of membranes at term. *Southern Medical Journal* 79(8):955-958.

24. Capeless, E.L., and Clapp, J.F. 1991. When do cardiovascular parameters return to their preconception values? *American Journal of Obstetrics and Gynecology* 165(4):883-886.

25. Clapp, J.F. 2000. Report on Postpartum Exercise, 2nd Yale Conference on Women's Health and Fitness, Yale University, New Haven, CT.

26. Varney, H. 1996. *Varney's midwifery*, 3rd ed. Boston: Jones & Bartlett, p. 627.

27. McIntosh, E.N. 1999. Personal conversations with the president of The Johns Hopkins Program for International Education in Reproductive Health, Inc.

28. Beck, C.T. 1995. Screening methods for postpartum depression. *Journal of Obstetric, Gynecologic, and Neonatal Nursing* 24(4):309.

29. Weinberg, M.K., Tronick, E.Z., Beeghly, M., Olson, K.L., Kernan, H., and Riley, J.M. 2001. Subsyndromal depressive symptoms and major depression in postpartum women. *American Journal of Orthopsychiatry* 71(1):87-97.

30. Eyer, D.E. 1992. *Mother-infant bonding: A scientific fiction*. New Haven, CT: Yale University Press.

31. In the author's practice, the most common client comment on evaluation forms and personal communications from clients is that exercising in the group was the most critical factor for maintaining a sense of well-being in the postpartum period.

32. Koltyn, K.E., and Schultes, S.S. 1997. Psychological effects of an aerobic exercise session and a rest session following pregnancy. *Journal of Sports Medicine and Physical Fitness* 37(4):287-291.

33. Sampselle, C.M., Seng, J., Yeo, S.A., Killion, C., and Oakley, D. 1999. Physical activity and postpartum well-being. *Journal of Obstetric, Gynecologic, and Neonatal Nursing* 28(1):41-49.

34. Lederman, R.P., Weingarten, C.T., and Lederman, E. 1981. Postpartum self-evaluation questionnaire: Measures of maternal adaptation. In R.P. Lederman, B.S. Raff, and P. Carrol (eds.), *Perinatal parental behavior: nursing research and implications for newborn health*. NY: Alan R. Liss, Inc.

35. Altshuler, L.L., Hendrick, V., and Cohen, L.S. 1998. Course of mood and anxiety disorders during pregnancy and the postpartum period. *Journal of Clinical Psychiatry* 59(Suppl. 2):29-33.

36. Leckman, J.F., Goodman, W.K., North, W.G., Chappell, P.B., Price, L.H., Pauls, D.L., et al. 1994. The role of central oxytocin in obsessive compulsive disorder and related normal behavior. *Psychoneuroendocrinology* 19(8):723-749.

37. Epperson, C.N., McDougle, C.G., and Price, L.H. 1996. Intranasal oxytocin in obsessive-compulsive disorder. *Biological Psychiatry* 40(6):547-549.

38. Leckman, J.F., Goodman, W.K., North, W.G., Chappell, P.B., Price, L.H., Pauls, D.L., et al. 1994. Elevated cerebrospinal fluid levels of oxytocin in obsessive-compulsive disorder. Comparison with Tourette's syndrome and healthy controls. *Archives of General Psychiatry* 51(10):782-792.

39. Swedo, S.E., Leonard, L.H., Kruesi, M.J., Rettew, D.C., Listwak, S.J., Berrettini, W., et al. 1992. Cerebrospinal fluid neurochemistry in children and adolescents with obsessive-compulsive disorder. *Archives of General Psychiatry* 49(1):29-36.

40. Asher, I., Kaplan, B., Modai, I., Neri, A., Valevski, A., and Weizman, A. 1995. Mood and hormonal changes during late pregnancy and puerperium. *Clinical and Experimental Obstetrics and Gynecology* 22(4):321-325.

41. Godin, G., Vezina, L., and Leclerc, O. 1989. Factors influencing intentions of pregnant women to exercise after giving birth. *Public Health Reports* 104(2):188-195.

42. Verhoef, M.J., and Love, E.J. 1994. Women and exercise participation: The mixed blessings of motherhood. *Health Care for Women International* 15:297-306.

43. Harris, H.E., Ellison, G.T., and Clement, S. 1999. Do the psychosocial and behavioral changes that accompany motherhood influence the impact of pregnancy on long-term weight gain? *Journal of Psychosomatic Obstetrics and Gynecology* 20(2):65-79.

44. Carter-Nolan, P.L., Adams-Campbell, L.L., and Williams, J. 1996. Recruitment strategies for black women at risk for noninsulin-dependent diabetes mellitus into exercise protocols: A qualitative assessment. *Journal of the National Medical Association* 88(9):558-562.

CHAPTER 10

GOALS AND PRIORITIES OF POSTPARTUM FITNESS PROGRAMS

This chapter sets forth goals and priorities for effective postpartum fitness programs. It distinguishes between goals for the first six weeks postpartum, the medical period referred to as the *puerperium,* and goals for the extended postpartum period—the period following the first six weeks that often lasts six months to a year. Many women think this extended period truly reflects the time required to recover from pregnancy and birth. The chapter also distinguishes between goals for mom and goals for baby. Those for mom include assisting the immediate recovery, restoration of bony alignment and muscle balance, and mental and physical well-being. And goals for baby include interactions with mom, interactions with others, and a stimulating environment for development. Once again, the priorities for this population—both mom and baby—are safety, effectiveness, and community.

From the discussion in the previous chapter, it should be clear that two factors generate differences between postpartum programs and other programs. One factor is the unique nature of the recovery from pregnancy and birth, and the other factor is the baby. Because birth is usually a long-duration event and because it involves the expulsion of the baby from her body, a woman immediately postpartum is tired and bruised. Her body needs time to recover from birth itself, and then—over a longer duration—to return to a nonpregnant upright and restored muscle balance; and she needs time to adapt to her new identity. She has to get used to caring for the new person

who has come into the world, which can require many adjustments in her life. The baby needs care for survival, including stimulation for growth and development. Even if the woman has a partner who shares the caregiving, much of the physical labor falls to her in the first few weeks, months, or years.

Although there is less scientific research on the interaction of exercise with the postpartum period than with pregnancy, we have sufficient evidence to conclude that appropriate exercise has both physical and psychosocial benefits for mothers and infants. Many women find it reassuring that they will be able to exercise and interact in a meaningful way with their babies during an activity session. Postpartum women and young mothers represent a largely underserved population, but one that is motivated. The appearance and rapid proliferation of stroller exercise programs in the early 1990s demonstrate the importance of a format that involves activity inclusive of both mother and offspring.

In preparing programs for this population, it is important to distinguish between goals that primarily benefit the mother and those that primarily benefit the baby. None of the goals exclusively benefit only one or the other. After all, a healthy and fit mom has more stamina, strength, and patience for dealing with an infant. A baby who is stimulated to develop motor skills, mental capacities, and emotional security contributes to her mother's well-being. But programming and individual exercise design are simpler if we place goals in one category or the other. And because some mothers—those who give up their babies, those who are professional athletes returning to their sport, those who wish to work out on their own, or those whose infants are hospitalized or die—may exercise without infants, it is good to have some clear goals that are exclusively for the woman.

SETTING GOALS FOR MOM

Although women who exercise through their pregnancies are more likely to engage in exercise afterward than those who do not [1], significant numbers of women who were not active during pregnancy do join postpartum fitness programs, and very likely more would join a program if it were accessible. In a survey about self-care and baby care topics of interest among women at seven weeks postpartum, Moran et al. found that over three-fourths of the 1161 women responding wanted more information on at least one topic and that the highest percentage wanted more information on exercise, diet, and nutrition [2].

Immediate Needs

As in the prenatal period, women come to postpartum exercise with a variety of fitness histories. However, they bring a common motivation: *the third body*—that strange venue in which they find themselves housed after birth. They need information on how to operate this body, and they know they need information. While exercise during pregnancy improves birth outcomes, relieves discomforts, promotes the sense of well-being, and helps prevent unwanted weight gain as well as a number of disorders, it is the course of activity in the six-week recovery period that helps establish the long-term weight gain or loss and that affects energy level and vitality.

In practice, we have found it effective to bring women through an immediate recovery program at their point of entry into postpartum exercise. Ideally, this occurs in the six weeks following birth; but at any point when a woman starts exercise after giving birth, it is useful to ensure that she meets the goal of immediate recovery before engaging in a regular exercise regimen. A woman who joined the author's postpartum program at four years following the birth of her daughter provides a case in point. At the outset, she was unable to contract her transverse abdominal muscle and maintain the compression or hollowing of the abdomen during a curl-up. She had a diastasis of three fingers, both lower and upper back pain, and stress incontinence. After she went through the recovery phase, all of these problems lessened and she was able to participate in vigorous exercise.

Continuing Needs

Once the immediate recovery period is over and a woman is ready to begin more vigorous and sustained activity of longer duration, is she ready to pick up where she left off prior to pregnancy? Some women may be, but experience tells us most women are not. For one thing, there is the matter of what to do with the baby. And, for another, the body still needs to make adaptations to the change in the center of gravity. The alteration in identity—especially for a first-time mother—may also affect her comfort with former exercise associates if they are primarily young single people. The support of other mothers and babies in a postpartum group program is often a lifeline for the group fitness fan. For the new mother who is older, a trainer who works regularly with the postpartum population and who will travel to her may be the answer. In both cases, six months or a year is not an unusual period of time to consider oneself as being in a transitional mode.

FIRST GOAL FOR MOM: ASSIST THE IMMEDIATE RECOVERY

Whether from a spontaneous vaginal delivery or an emergency cesarean at the end of a prolonged labor, there are physical effects of birth. The six-week period following this event ideally includes living and moving in a way that promotes the healing of tissues, begins the process of realigning the body toward a normal posture, and includes stress management techniques to help adjust to the demands of meeting the baby's needs. And the blocks of time dedicated to these goals should be short, as the call of a newborn takes the number-one spot in a new mother's life. But even if the mother is not caring for a newborn—she has given the baby up for adoption, has live-in help, or has lost a baby—she needs to care for her own body so it will recover and function normally.

Although research is limited, it is clear that exercise during the six-week puerperium produces both physical and psychosocial benefits for the mother (see chapter 9). There is also extensive anecdotal evidence that appropriate recovery activities—such as Kegels, abdominal compressions or hollowing exercises, relaxation, and walking—assist new mothers in the transition. Keeping track of one's own nutrition and fluid intake can easily take a back seat to the role of caregiver, but sometimes a glass of milk or fruit juice and a few deep abdominal breaths can do wonders. It is beneficial to set aside a few minutes here and there during the day to focus on these recovery activities while the baby is napping or playing with the grandparents.

SECOND GOAL FOR MOM: RESTORE BONY ALIGNMENT AND MUSCLE BALANCE

The postural dynamics discussed in chapter 5 serve as a starting point for evaluating particular biomechanical issues that may confront a given woman. Specific changes in bony alignment—resulting from the prenatal shift in the center of gravity—may be present for some time, including increased lumbar lordosis, anterior pelvic tilt, increased flexion in the iliofemoral joint, increased kyphosis (thoracic spine curve) and cervical curve, coccyx pushed back during delivery, and alterations in the angles of peripheral joints to keep the head and body upright against gravity.

Effects of Misalignment

Neurological problems that may have occurred as a result of changes in bony alignment derive from erosion of joint surfaces, abnormal compression forces on discs and facets, and decreased joint spaces leading to nerve or blood vessel entrapment. In addition, postpartum inflammatory responses generated by the changing hormone status may be aggravated by these effects of bone misalignment (discussed in more detail later).

Because of bony shifts, muscles can be improperly aligned, causing the following alterations in muscle action:

- Shortening and tightening of low back and iliopsoas (hip flexors)
- Shortening of thoracic spinal flexors and pectoral muscles
- Overstretching and weakening of gluteals and hamstrings
- Overstretching and weakening of abdominals and pelvic floor
- Overstretching and weakening of upper back muscles

Each of these areas should be addressed to the extent necessary so that each woman develops a healthy postpartum alignment, permitting her to deal with the demands on her body without undue discomfort or stress. It is reasonable to expect that through proper exercise programming and attention to compliance, postural dynamics will move toward a healthy postpartum resolution. In a group setting, it is feasible to deal in a balanced way with all these areas of the body and then devote a period of time to work on specific individual challenges. Some persons and some conditions require very little

assistance, and others require a great deal of assistance. For example, a woman with a very tall, ectomorphic body type may find that the alignment problems of pregnancy were limited to the last month or two and that her body returns to a healthy posture and normal elasticity a few weeks following birth. Such a woman may need less compensatory muscle strengthening and stretching than a woman with a shorter, endomorphic body type.

Dealing With Competitive Athletes

Athletes seeking to return to competition, especially professionals, form an interesting subgroup. If they fail to attend to the recovery of upright and the kinesthesia required to work in a centered way following birth, they can find themselves several months postpartum with nagging biomechanical problems. Despite having regained a competitive level in the performance of their event, they can have serious damage affecting their long-term output. Taking a small amount of time early in the postpartum period to focus strictly on the recovery process can minimize this situation.

THIRD GOAL FOR MOM: PROMOTE PHYSICAL AND MENTAL WELL-BEING

Perhaps at no time in the life cycle does gender affect the health of a woman as much as in the extended postpartum period. The complexity of hormones and other factors related to pregnancy may be responsible for biochemical disorders that manifest themselves in a woman's physical and mental health.

Effects of a Changing Biochemistry

High levels of placental corticotropin-releasing hormone in late pregnancy are associated with the timing of labor and lead to hypercortisolism, which causes a transient postpartum adrenal suppression. Together with estrogen withdrawal, this helps explain the mental depression and autoimmune/inflammatory phenomena associated with the postpartum period [3]. While social factors and personal history undoubtedly contribute to depressive conditions, it is important to understand that the changing neuroendocrine status of postpartum women can predispose them to depressive states.

Changes in endocrine function during pregnancy and the postpartum period, and their effect on autoimmune disorders, are currently under scrutiny. Both prolactin [4] and fetal cells that persist in the mother's blood after delivery [5] have been implicated in the development of such disorders in women, who constitute 80% of the individuals afflicted with Graves disease and Hashimoto's disease (both of which affect the thyroid), lupus, rheumatoid arthritis, Sjogren's syndrome (inability to make saliva or tears), multiple sclerosis, and other related disorders. Some conditions—such as tendinitis in the shoulders or wrists, or joint pain or swelling in the knees—might at first appear to be biomechanical in origin, but it may be that poor movement is only exacerbating an underlying autoimmune or inflammatory response. Consequently, when postpartum clients develop such problems, it is important to have a medical opinion about the possible origin. Because these problems often show up several months to years postpartum, it is not just postpartum instructors who need to be aware of this scenario.

The positive effect of physical activity on the biochemistry of immune function, mood, and vigor may well help to counter these problems. While we can assume that some of the mechanisms involved are similar to those evident in a non-childbearing population, there is much yet to be uncovered regarding the mechanisms by which exercise interacts with the changing neuroendocrine status that characterizes the postpartum period.

The Role of Physical Activity in Postpartum Mental Health

The mental and emotional states of postpartum women may be affected by factors we have observed previously in pregnant women. Such elements as neurological reprogramming of the sense of upright or development of greater kinesthestic awareness of the center of one's body contribute to self-image. And, if the infant is present and participating, the mother experiences herself as accomplishing physical work while simultaneously relating to her infant. The myth that a woman cannot be a good mother and care for herself at the same time can be dispelled.

Being healthy and fit also permits an individual to see herself as capable. When it's time to get up in the middle of the night, the woman who has eaten well, has cared for herself through exercise and relaxation sessions, and feels confidence in her body's ability to achieve motor tasks has clear advantages over the woman who is unhealthy and unfit. If the mother intends to return to work, it is also to her advantage to be healthy and fit. If she plans to stay home with her children, she will benefit from being strong, having endurance, and being experienced in facilitating her child's development. The same positive effects of fitness that any individual derives in terms of healthy cells, organs, and systems (including the mind) also accrue to the new mother.

One area in which a postpartum woman obtains a unique mental benefit from exercise is the positive reinforcement she receives from her instructor or trainer, or from other women if she is in a group. When a new mother responds to her crying infant, picking her up, holding her, or checking for problems, she receives encouragement. If she is with a group and is a brand-new mom, the more advanced mothers often help her. The mother network helps women figure out how to interact appropriately when their infants exhibit a variety of behaviors. And there is always a patient adult around to lend a hand when a mother is fatigued or exasperated.

Taking a Practical Tack Toward Weight

If women have eaten a healthy diet during pregnancy and continue to do so postpartum, body mass index should become healthy, provided that there is not an underlying medical condition. How long this takes depends on factors that include genetics, diet, level of activity, and breastfeeding. Before setting individual goals, women should take stock of all of these factors. Instructors can help women develop realistic expectations. Objectives need to be practical as well as realistic, such as fitting into an outfit for a special occasion two months in the future when there are 10 or 12 pounds to lose and the abdominals to be tightened. If there are 40 pounds to lose, an instructor or trainer might help the new mom consider another objective.

SETTING GOALS FOR BABY

What can a baby gain by being in a room full of exercising postpartum women and other babies? Why take a baby out of her warm, cozy home at six or eight weeks and expose her to all that sweat? How can a mother pay adequate attention to her baby if she is trying to figure out which foot to step onto? What if a baby needs to nurse in the middle of the cardiovascular workout? These and other questions plague the minds of the uninitiated! Working with mothers, babies, and exercise has its own set of rules—it is a complex task—but when done well, it is very effective.

It is helpful to keep in mind that people can accomplish more than one thing at the same time in a well-run class or workout session. Figure 10.1 shows a group of women doing abdominal exercises. While one mother does her curl-ups, she is also playing peek-a-boo with her baby. Others' infants are sleeping nearby, and those mothers have a chance to work on their technique.

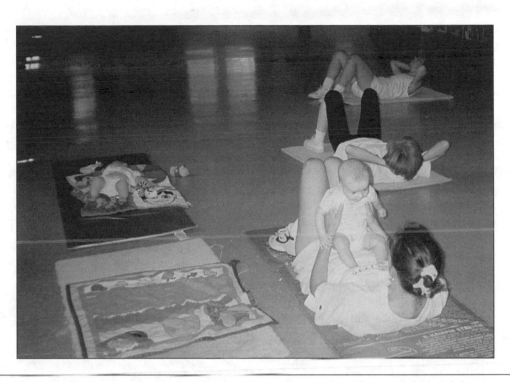

Figure 10.1   Meeting babies' needs can mean more than one thing at the same time. Here one baby is helping mom with her curl-ups while other babies sleep. Not everyone has to be doing the same thing in a postpartum group exercise class.

When babies are present in the exercise setting, it is important to ensure that some portion of most sessions includes time for mother-infant interaction. And because babies learn from each other, there can also be opportunities for babies to interact. This can be accomplished informally, by arranging the babies on mats in the center of the room and having moms jog or dance around them in a circle. One or two moms can be assigned the job of being the "eyes on the babies." Another element of a mother-baby class is working on the baby's developmental tasks; for example, the baby can learn to hold her head up while lying on her stomach. It is easy to combine this with interaction with mom. A critical strength element for mom is upper back extensions, which she can work on while lying on her stomach, *en face* with baby, and raising her head and chest off the ground while the baby does the same. The activity is generated by the baby's attempt to develop this skill and the mother's or instructor's perception that this is what is occurring.

FIRST GOAL FOR BABY: ENCOURAGE INTERACTION WITH MOM

One of the most important opportunities a mother-baby program provides is that of accomplishing things together. Just getting out of the house and arriving at a first class is an activity worthy of positive reinforcement. Mom and baby are two beings obliged to find workable systems for together achieving a variety of objectives (preparing food and eating, cleaning up, doing stimulating activity, getting rest, etc.). Exercise class is a place where this goal can be worked on. Bringing in all the equipment and supplies from the car without losing track of the baby might sound easy. But, as with any new psychomotor skill, people need practice in order to do such tasks efficiently and to feel comfortable while doing them.

Mom is a major being in the life of an infant. At first, babies recognize little more than the smell of the energy vortexes (we call them people) who approach them. The smell of mom is important. Also important are mom's heartbeat and breathing rhythm, things that are familiar from the womb. As an infant progresses and becomes aware of things outside its one-dimensional environment, mom (or primary caregiver) is the safest avenue into the two- and three-dimensional world. During a newborn's alert periods, a new mom can gently stimulate her baby by responding to reflex actions and through massage and gentle stretching.

The first time an infant comes to a class, it may not be possible for the mother to accomplish a lot of exercise; but if she is patient and comforting, she is teaching her infant that this is a safe place. We find that infants who are given comfort and attention for the first one or two sessions quickly settle into a routine in which they relax, enjoy the stimulation of the environment, and let us know when they are truly hungry, wet, tired, or having a little existential angst.

Mom is not the only one who benefits from the assistance she receives from other mothers. The interaction of mother and child bears on early development, and modeling by other mother-baby dyads also benefits a new baby's development. For example, one study uncovered evidence that babies traditionally labeled as having *infantile colic* are perceived by their mothers as more bothersome, withdrawn, intense, and negative than noncolicky babies and that they receive less stimulation from their mothers than noncolicky controls [6]. This difference in treatment, the study authors concluded, may contribute to a temporary developmental delay. At six months, these infants scored significantly lower on Bayley Mental and Psychomotor Development scales, while there was no significant effect at 12, 18, or 24 months [6]. An infant with colic can be difficult to deal with. Having a place to go where a mom can get recharged and receive advice and assistance, and where her infant can get some extra stimulation, benefits that infant.

SECOND GOAL FOR BABY: ENCOURAGE INTERACTION WITH OTHERS

Watching babies interact with each other can be a revelation. Having so long been verbal, many adults forget that humans also communicate with body language and simple sounds. And we learn by watching as much as by listening. When babies are busy participants in this primitive interactive process, they are learning from each other.

One baby's ability can serve as the impetus for other babies' learning. On one occasion, the author observed that her class included several infants ranging in age from 12 to 18 weeks, none of whom had shown interest in sitting. Another baby, 20 weeks old, joined the class. This baby could sit without assistance. Within a week, all of the other babies in the 12- to 18-week age range were sitting alone for brief periods or were working on it. The interaction was more complex than just the observation by the babies that the new baby could sit. After all, their mothers had to assist them initially. But the new baby served as a catalyst for developmental behavior on the part of the other babies through their observation of the newcomer.

We know that although babies have their own rhythm of development, they are also stimulated to develop by environmental pressures. The example of sitting serves to demonstrate the role of peer leaders, even at this young age, as one significant form of environmental stimulation. Over the years, we have watched the interaction of infants and toddlers in postpartum and stroller exercise programs and have come to realize the importance of this facet of the program. In the past, extended families provided such play groups, but now more commonly we must provide a setting in which babies can flourish through interactions with others of a similar age.

Babies also flourish through interaction with other mothers or the instructor/trainer. A regular group of experienced adults forms a basis of comparison for the infant. Recognizing mother (and hopefully, safety) becomes a reliable event. In addition, the baby comes to trust other adults. Different styles of interaction help the baby expand its repertoire of behavior.

THIRD GOAL FOR BABY: PROVIDE STIMULUS FOR DEVELOPMENTAL TASKS

Infants and toddlers have many motor skills to learn: holding their own heads erect, reaching, grabbing, sitting, rolling over, crawling, standing, walking, and so on. Some actions, such as sucking, are reflex responses to a stimulus, in this case touching the face near the lips. Beginning with primitive reflexes, postural reactions, and locomotor reflexes, patterns of movement are acquired, accreted, and refined.

Haywood [7] reminds us that the technique employed in motor skills (*movement process*) affects the outcome of the movement (*movement product*) and that technique is affected, in turn, by outcome. The phenomenon is characterized at each stage of motor development for a given skill. The life of an infant is a symphony of acquiring new skills—elements of these skills appear and are refined, hopefully achieving better results, and develop into more and more complex behaviors by stages. How does the infant acquire effective technique? By being successful—grabbing that toy or pushing on the mat with its hands to help raise its head. The adult watching has the option of encouraging every element of skill development. For our children to develop self-efficacy, it is our support of their efforts, not our efforts to control their behavior, that allows this symphony to be written.

How much does an instructor or trainer need to know about infant development to design a truly effective mother-baby program? Learning as much as possible through reading and experience, of course, leads to improvements in program design and facilitation. However, no matter how much one knows, there remain a few simple principles that should guide an exercise leader when working with mothers and infants. First, the leader must not undermine the mother's authority. Second, observation is the best way to figure out what the baby wants to be able to do (babies are self-organizing organisms). Third, it is important to motivate the baby to figure out how to accomplish what it wants (as long as it's safe) through encouraging sounds and expressions. And, fourth, both baby and mother should be congratulated when the baby accomplishes what it wants.

By supporting mothers in their struggle to see the baby for itself, an instructor or trainer can have a profoundly positive effect on the lives of both mother and child. One needs to play this hand with a light touch and to treat with enormous respect the mother-infant bond. No matter how experienced an instructor or trainer may be as a parent, every baby and every mother is an individual. To see these individuals afresh each time one encounters them is a skill to be practiced.

PRIORITIES

The priorities for postpartum exercise remain the same as for the prenatal period, although the particulars change. Obviously, safety is paramount. In the postpartum period, this means three things: first, ensuring that the mother's activities will help her recover from the stresses of pregnancy and birth; second, ensuring that the baby's needs are met; and third, ensuring that all equipment (such as strollers or toys) is safe.

Another important priority is effectiveness. Is the mother achieving postural realignment and muscle balance? Is she strong enough to minimize the biomechanical problems of lifting, carrying, and transferring an infant, as well as the accoutrements of infancy such as car carriers, diaper and bottle bags, and so on? Is she developing techniques that allow her to function in a healthy, fit manner?

The development of a supportive community for this population is also a high priority. The factors already discussed in this and the previous chapter make it clear that during the postpartum period, women and their infants benefit from group support. In practice, we periodically see groups of women who, having bonded through their pre/postnatal exercise program, begin play groups when their infants develop into toddlers. Their comments about this experience always include a note that they do this as much for themselves as for their children [8].

FIRST PRIORITY: SAFETY

The three areas in which safety must be accounted for— the mother's recovery, the baby's needs, and equipment safety—must each be assessed. The one overriding skill that helps the instructor or trainer succeed in all three areas is an ability to use common sense in making judg-

Safety Issues for Postpartum Recovery

1. Monitor screening factors (especially the lochia) and complications.
2. The mother should begin with basic core body exercises (Kegels and hiss/compress) and walking.
3. She should avoid quick abduction of the legs for about 8 or 10 weeks.
4. She should avoid percussive, ballistic, or high-impact movements until core body strength is restored and joint laxity or soreness has disappeared.
5. She should maintain a healthy diet and adequate fluid intake, especially if nursing.

ments about whether or not to allow an activity to take place. For example, if a mother who is two weeks postpartum has a serious diastasis (abdominal separation) and has stitches in her perineum from an episiotomy says she wants to do martial art kicks, the instructor might advise her to wait a few more weeks until she has recovered sufficiently. Or, if a mother brings a piece of equipment (e.g., carriage, stroller) that the instructor, on first glance, knows she would not put her own child into, this is a clue that the instructor should examine the item carefully.

Mother's Recovery

Detailed procedures for the safe return to a full exercise regimen are given in chapter 11, including what to do from the first few days through the return to a class or regular workout.

The sidebar above lists issues discovered through practice that dramatically affect the safe recovery for a new mother.

Meeting the Baby's Needs

Babies let us know when something needs attention by crying or fussing. If the catalogue of obvious problems has been attended to (hungry, wet, sleepy, cold, hot, stuck, wants to play, etc.) and a baby continues to be fussy, it may be experiencing a moment of angst. The baby could be preparing to grow physically or neurologically, having absorbed and organized some food energy or movement pattern. Holding the baby, talking, and fussing over the baby are often all that's required. One of the most effective ways to meet baby's needs within the class or workout session is to integrate infants into activities such as curl-ups. Older babies and toddlers enjoy stroller work-outs, with mom pushing the stroller while doing a variety of locomotor patterns.

How does one reconcile the baby's needs with the demands of a workout session? The first rule is always that babies come first. For the situation to be one in which this does not produce upset or frustration when a baby "interrupts" a mother's workout, this rule must be clearly understood by participants. What does this mean? All incoming mothers in a group setting need to agree not only that they will not judge other people's babies if they need a lot of attention, but also that they will not feel they are imposing on people if their own babies require attention. Handling this in a light and humorous way—such as saying "we run on baby standard time!"—allows the mother to relax. This, in turn, helps all the participants relax, thus reducing the possibility that tension will keep women from accomplishing their workout.

In a group setting, being able to keep an eye on women's biomechanics and babies' safety requires attention to detail. This is an important skill, as is the ability to prioritize based on how the babies are behaving on a given day. In a postpartum program there are some days when the babies are very quiet and it is hard to distinguish between this class and a general-population fitness class, but on other days the class becomes a stroller exercise class because motion is the only way to pacify many of the babies.

Safe Equipment

Car seat carriers and strollers (or carriages) are the two most commonly used baby transport devices that we see in mother-infant classes. Carriers need to be stable, constructed of sturdy materials, and placed out of the path of locomotor activities. One must never place a car seat carrier with a baby in it on a table or other elevated surface.

Strollers and carriages need to be well constructed, with sturdy wheels that are securely attached. The center of gravity of a stroller or carriage should be low. Some carriages have an area at the top that a car seat carrier fits

---

Safety Features of Carriages and Strollers for Mother-Infant Exercise Programs

1. Solid construction with wheels securely attached
2. Low center of gravity
3. Proper handle height for mom
4. Good brakes
5. Seat belt

---

into. In this case, to lower the center of gravity, one must be sure that something heavy is placed in the compartment usually found near the bottom of the carriage. This minimizes the risk of the carriage's tipping over. The prevalence of stroller-related injuries is not known, although it is known that mild head injuries are the most common type [9].

Another important characteristic of a stroller or carriage to be used for physical activity is the height and arrangement of the handles. The handles should be located so that there is no strain on the mother's arms or shoulders due to poor positioning. Also, a dependable braking mechanism for the wheels must be present. A seat belt that will prevent an infant or toddler from falling out of the stroller or carriage is important. Parents should examine the clasp and strap arrangement carefully, as some seat belts are more easily manipulated by toddlers than others [10]. The sidebar at the bottom of this page reviews safety features for carriages and strollers.

People using baby joggers and front-facing strollers need to pay attention to the environment also. When moving fast enough, the equipment may stop suddenly if it encounters an obstacle and an infant may be propelled forward with no protection, so a sturdy restraining system is mandatory. Car exhaust or other contaminants can irritate the baby's eyes or breathing. Joggers usually require that the baby weigh enough to help ground the equipment. Large, sturdy wheels are a must on joggers.

Another device that occasionally turns up in a mother-infant class is an infant walker. This is a controversial device in which a seated baby can move about on wheels by kicking and pushing off the floor with its feet. Walkers frequently also have a circular shelf or tray, with a hole in the center for the suspended cloth seat. The safety of such devices has been questioned, particularly the braking mechanisms, which have not been found to be effective in preventing falls down stairs [11]. In an attempt to prevent the problems of walkers, some manufacturers have placed a curved pan that serves as a rocker under the feet to prevent locomotion. However, also of significance regarding infant walkers and rockers, two studies have concluded that such devices delay the infant's motor development [12, 13]. This equipment prohibits the baby from seeing what its lower body is doing. Although mothers may find these devices convenient for occupying an infant while they exercise, their use should be discouraged. Providing literature about the safety and developmental issues can be helpful in dissuading a well-meaning parent interested in a device of questionable safety.

Sometimes mothers want to participate in exercise with their infants in a wrap or sling device. Unfortunately, this is the equivalent of working out with a 10- or 15-pound bowling ball hanging off the mother's body. The biomechanical stress is unacceptable. The mother's body should not be subjected to the momentum that is created, and the child is at risk for shaken baby syndrome. Consequently, it is best to make clear to mothers that their infants can be in a stroller or car seat or on a blanket or mat while mom exercises, with the mom during mother-baby exercises, or—if the baby needs more attention—with the mother while she directs her attention to the baby's needs. When mothers and babies want to be together during locomotor or standing movement, small babies can be held at the shoulder, and all babies can be carried in a colic hold (see figure 11.8a) for brief periods. However, care must be taken to avoid impact or shaking.

SECOND PRIORITY: EFFECTIVE ACTIVITY

If a woman is strong, flexible, and aerobically fit, if she is having little or no discomfort, if she is well nourished and able to manage most of her daily activities with equanimity, and if her child is thriving, these are all good signs that her regimen is working. To be effective, a postpartum program can be expected to enable women to make gains in their recovery and adapt to the new demands on their bodies; to allow women to maintain or increase strength, endurance, and flexibility; to provide women with a safe place in which to commit themselves to their own and their infants' wellness; and to be a place where women can find valid information and referrals for common postpartum problems.

Effective Exercise Components

The exercise components involved in accomplishing the physical elements of recovery include cardiovascular or aerobic conditioning, strength training, flexibility exercises, and mind/body activities such as centering and relaxation. It is also helpful for women, during rest in the constructive rest position, to use imagery or mental rehearsal of the body's return to a healthy alignment.

The catalogue of potential postural problems outlined at the beginning of this chapter can be alleviated through a combination of passive and active approaches to movement. In an effective program for postpartum women, difficulties associated with prenatal postural shifts should be minimized as much as possible. Women should be learning new skills for lifting and carrying infants. They should be able to maximize their workout time through efficient program design, incorporating the baby as needed.

Effective Programming for a Split Demographic

Although exercise, especially in groups, can obviate many of the physical and mental health concerns in the postpartum period, it is important not to confuse this benefit with long-term solutions to the social context in which these concerns arise. The economic disadvantages and lack of large-scale cultural support for mothers have produced a remarkable phenomenon: the bifurcation of the childbearing population into adolescent mothers and women who delay childbearing until the third and fourth decade of their lives [14]. Women of the middle and upper-middle economic classes now frequently wait until a career path is well established and they can afford motherhood. But they often lack the extended family of the past that provided a major measure of support and relief. As the form of the American family continues to shift, more social policy supportive of mothers is greatly needed. In the design of postpartum fitness programs, the importance of community building cannot be overemphasized, for association among new mothers is a powerful force in prompting the changes that are needed.

Adolescent childbearing—which was a normal part of life until industrialization and the eventual absorption of women into the workforce—is now considered by many politicians and policy makers to be the unplanned cause of a downward economic slope for the young parent that runs counter to society's interests [15]. However, a closer look reveals that the assumptions underlying this notion are not substantiated in the research; rather, teenage parenthood does not change long-range financial outcome and may be a smart move for some socially and economically disadvantaged girls who can take advantage of an extended family [16]. While the older mother forms a lucrative income source for the properly trained postpartum fitness expert, a second maternal population of adolescent mothers could benefit from the establishment of school-based postpartum fitness and parenting programs. Programming for both populations is covered in chapter 11.

THIRD PRIORITY: COMMUNITY

The fact that groups contribute to positive outcomes for women is well established. Clearly, women learn from each other. In the postpartum period, the opportunity to see other moms and other babies not only satisfies a social need many women feel, but also provides a source of information and enables women to receive the support, encouragement, and respect they are due.

But what do we really know about the outcomes of women in postpartum exercise groups? Anecdotal evidence tells us women feel good about the experience. Certainly, we see women getting fit. They tell us they thrive on the companionship. In the author's practice, women who became associated during childbearing, organized play groups together, and sent their children to the same schools are now watching them go off to college. The women remain close to each other, and some of the children have established their own bonds. It is thrilling and a little frightening to see how profoundly these women's life experience has been affected by the decision to join a pre/postnatal exercise program.

As the numbers of these women grow, there will be much information to be gathered concerning how their lives have been affected. Whether their health and fitness are better or worse than for their nonparticipatory counterparts is but one question. Has a postpartum exercise group affected their career choices? Their socioeconomic status? Is this phenomenon different depending on race? And, what happens to their offspring? All of these are fascinating questions that researchers need to ask. In the meantime, the preliminary evidence seems overwhelming that the development of meaningful postpartum exercise programs has at least short-term benefits for both mother and baby. Designing meaningful programs for this population is the topic of the next chapter.

REFERENCES

1. Devine, C.M., Bove, C.F., and Olson, C.M. 2000. Continuity and change in women's weight orientations and lifestyle through pregnancy and the postpartum period: The influence of life trajectories and transitional events. *Social Science and Medicine* 50(4):567-582.
2. Moran, C.F., Holt, V.L., and Martin, D.P. 1997. What do women want to know after childbirth? *Birth* 24(1):27-34.
3. Chrousos, G.P., Torpy, D.J., and Gold, P.W. 1998. Interactions between the hypothalamic-pituitary-adrenal axis and the female reproductive system: Clinical implications. *Annals of Internal Medicine* 129(3):229-240.
4. Walker, S.E., and Jacobson, J.D. 2000. Roles of prolactin and gonadotropin (Review). *Rheumatic Diseases Clinics of North America* 26(4):713-736.
5. Evans, P.C., Lambert, N., Maloney, S., Furst, D.E., Moore, J.M., and Nelson, J.L. 1999. Long-term fetal microchimerism in peripheral blood mononuclear cell subsets in healthy women and women with scleroderma. *Blood* 93(6):2033-2037.
6. Sloman, J., Bellinger, D.C., and Krentzel, C.P. 1990. Infantile colic and transient developmental lag in the first year of life. *Child Psychiatry and Human Development* 21(1):25-36.
7. Haywood, K.M. 1993. *Life span motor development*, 2nd ed. Champaign, IL: Human Kinetics, p. 89.
8. Personal communications with two groups of the author's clients. Also communications with four instructors in the author's programs about their clients.
9. Lee, A.C., and Fong, D. 1997. Epidural haematoma and stroller-associated injury. *Journal of Paediatrics and Child Health* 33(5):446-447.
10. Ridenour, M.V. 1997. How child-resistant are stroller belt buckles? *Perceptual and Motor Skills* 84(2):611-616.
11. Ridenour, M.V. 1997. How effective are brakes on infant walkers? *Perceptual and Motor Skills* 84(3 Pt. 1):1051-1057.
12. Thien, M.M., Lee, J., Tay, V., and Ling, S.L. 1997. Infant walker use, injuries and motor development. *Injury Prevention* 3(1):63-66.
13. Siegel, A.C., and Burton, R.V. 1997. Unpublished study reported in J.E. Brody, Baby walkers may slow infants' development. *NY Times* October 14, 1997, p. F9.
14. Luker, K. 1996. *Dubious conceptions*. Cambridge, MA: Harvard University Press.
15. Geronimus, A.T. 1997. Teenage childbearing and personal responsibility: An alternative view. *Political Science Quarterly* 112:405-430.
16. SmithBattle, L. 2000. The vulnerabilities of teenage mothers: Challenging prevailing assumptions. *ANS Advances in Nursing Science* 23(1):29-40.

CHAPTER 11

POSTPARTUM PROGRAM DESIGN

This chapter presents procedures for designing, monitoring, and evaluating postpartum fitness programs. It begins with intake procedures, including provisions for those who are coming directly from a prenatal program into a postpartum program, those who are entering from the outside who have been active, and those who have had a sedentary pregnancy. Next, the chapter outlines a sample six-week immediate recovery program that women can accomplish at home during the *puerperium* (the six weeks immediately following birth) and includes procedures for monitoring safety. We then consider selecting exercise components for the extended postpartum period, as well as formatting and evaluating programs. The chapter concludes with a discussion of postpartum adolescents in a school- or community-based program. As with prenatal exercise, adaptations of other health care and fitness protocols, clinical observations, and experimentation have resulted in some procedural norms. However, there is much research to be done in this area.

INTAKE PROCEDURES FOR POSTPARTUM EXERCISE

The intake process for the puerperium and extended postpartum period involves ongoing needs assessment for several months. It includes listening to the birth story, facilitating the immediate recovery period, assessing factors that affect commencing the extended postpartum exercise regimen, medical screening, and assessing the

impact of conditions that may have resulted from pregnancy or birth.

Listening to the Birth Story

Telling one's birth story serves as a base for a meaningful postpartum experience. Whereas birth education and prenatal fitness help a woman recognize the stages and nuances of her labor while it is happening, telling the story afterward serves as a debriefing that helps her comprehend what she has been through. Just as each pregnancy follows its own course, so does each birth. Consequently, there are as many stories as there are births.

Listening to each woman's story also provides the instructor or trainer with an opportunity to do two things. The first is to be *sympatico*—to listen and to validate the woman's experience by adding "ooh's" and "aah's" at the right moments so the woman knows she is supported in her feelings about this amazing event. Second, this listening process allows one to collect data—to find out whether it was a long or short labor, whether the woman had a spontaneous vaginal or a surgical delivery, whether the baby was large or small, whether the mother did or didn't have an episiotomy or tear, whether she did or didn't have drugs, and other details that may influence her needs for both immediate recovery and long-term well-being.

A birth story full of joy, awe, and empowerment reflects more than just a woman's disposition or physical prowess in birthing. It also indicates a labor and delivery that allowed her to attain these feelings. A story full of anger and disappointment might indicate a birth in which things did not go well, for which she was poorly prepared, or during which she may have been badly treated. In such cases, some repair to the self-esteem, self-schema, or self-efficacy may be in order. Various scenarios can have vastly different effects on physical activity following birth.

If a prenatal instructor or trainer is consistently seeing her clients upset about their births, she might inquire into their preparation for birth. It is reasonable to expect a well-run pre/postnatal fitness program to provide activities and support that are effective for labor, but there are other factors as well. The instructor may want to look at whether some obstetrical practices or childbirth educators in her community are associated with unhappy postpartum women while others are associated with well-adjusted clients. The initial collection of information following birth is one key element in devising strategies to help other women cope with the rigors of birth.

One of the great joys of working with this population is hearing from a new mother soon after birth. On occasion, women who are continuing on from a prenatal program call their instructor from the delivery or recovery room because they are so excited to talk about their experience. If a woman is not present for group classes and does not check in around her due date, a call to find out if she has given birth, to make sure everything is all right, to be reassuring, or to check that she is receiving support if needed, is entirely appropriate.

In extremely rare cases, a fetal death, stillbirth, neonatal death, or elective abortion due to multiple congenital anomalies may occur. In the author's practice, of the first 5000 women through the program, there were 5 such cases. This is a low number, one in a thousand; and none of these cases were related to maternal exercise. Women differ in whether or not they want contact following such an event, and the instructor should determine the woman's preferences. Having an advisory board member who is a psychologist specializing in maternal grief is a great asset in such a case.

Facilitating the Immediate Recovery

Because the birth itself affects physical activity, it is a good idea to hear about the birth as soon as possible. Continuing to be in contact with the new mother through her recovery period is part of the postpartum intake process with clients who are carrying over from prenatal to postpartum classes. How a woman progresses through activities during the puerperium influences how fast she can return to regular, vigorous exercise.

Preparation for exercise in the postpartum period can begin prior to birth if a woman is planning to transfer from a prenatal group class to a postpartum group class within a coordinated program. During the final weeks of her pregnancy, a woman can review an immediate recovery program with her instructor, be reminded to contact her instructor shortly after birth, and be assigned a postpartum buddy who will follow up with the new mom to help smooth her transition into the postpartum class.

If the postpartum woman is unfamiliar and presents herself several weeks after birth, it is important to inquire into her prenatal fitness and her birth and recovery process, including what activities she may have been doing on her own since the birth. If she was sedentary during her entire pregnancy, stopped exercising, or was on bed rest at the end of her pregnancy, it is still important to ask about the birth and recovery process and to ascertain whether or not the woman is still sedentary. However, with women the instructor or trainer does not know, or with sedentary women, it is necessary to wait for medical clearance before commencing a discussion of recommended activities.

Factors That Affect Commencing the Extended Postpartum Exercise Routine

Once the birth story, its consequences, and the immediate recovery program have been reviewed, it is time to assess the factors that affect the physical process of returning to an extended postpartum program and regular exercise activities. A mother may feel she is or is not having a good adjustment period, but observing in person provides additional clues to how she is doing and what she needs in the way of physical activities. Some new mothers need to exert themselves more and others need relaxation.

Three factors influence the process of returning to regular exercise in the extended postpartum period: prenatal fitness; the course of labor, birth, and immediate recovery; and the maternal/infant adjustment. It is important to keep in mind that this is a fluid situation. The three factors weigh differently in different situations. And things may change. Mom, baby, or both may develop a complication.

Prenatal Fitness

A woman's level of fitness going into birth plays a large role in her recovery. The same physiological augmentations that enhanced oxygen and nutrient delivery in the prenatal period enhance tissue recovery in the period immediately following birth. The general rule is the more fit someone is going into the birth, the more fit the person is coming out and the faster the return to activity.

If the woman is familiar to the instructor or trainer, it may not be necessary for her to fill out an exercise history before she returns to a workout regimen or class, provided the instructor or trainer is aware of her progress through the first few weeks postpartum. However, with a new client, such a history is essential. The form "Exercise History (Postpartum)" is an appropriate exercise history form. Exercise testing is a reliable method of determining functional capacity when this information is required, although it should be deferred until the health care provider approves.

Course of Labor, Birth, and the Immediate Recovery

A fit woman with a relatively easy labor and no complications may be walking or even jogging a mile or two every other day by the end of the second week postpartum. At the other end of the spectrum, an inactive woman with a difficult labor may not be able to execute all of her activities of daily living by the end of the second month. The range of variations is so great that it is helpful to review the information on an individual woman's labor and birth and to ask about what activities the woman was able to execute at the two-week point. The new mother can complete the form "Exercise Assessment at Two Weeks Postpartum" at home for the purpose of recording her activities at this point.

At two weeks, it is helpful if the new mom assesses her abdominal muscles for separation, or *diastasis*. The procedure for this assessment is shown in figure 11.1. The instructor or trainer should also review her two-week assessment form with her to find out whether or not she has begun abdominal strengthening exercises and pelvic floor exercises and whether she has been able to take some brief walks. If not, and if there is no medical problem, she can be encouraged to try these. If she has had a cesarean, and feeling is returning to her lower abdomen, she may be ready to begin gentle abdominal compression. In practice we are well aware that women who manage to do these activities right away spare themselves much of the discomfort, posture problems, and stress incontinence that can occur following birth. If a woman complains of difficulties in these areas, she should be encouraged to seek medical assistance. She needs support; if she feels her problems are serious, do not let her be dissuaded from seeking further help if her concerns are initially dismissed.

Unless there are medical problems, women whom the instructor or trainer knows can be encouraged to progress through the immediate recovery program at their own pace. They must be reminded to be cautious and to pay attention to warning signs such as discomfort, pain, bleeding, swelling in the leg, and fever. If the instructor or trainer is not familiar with a woman who is inquiring about postpartum exercise, it is appropriate to wait until she has approval from her health care provider before proceeding with intake procedures and recovery exercises.

Maternal/Infant Adjustment

The baby's disposition and the adjustment of the new mother-baby dyad play a significant role in the commencement of a regular exercise program. If it is easy for the mother to deal with the baby and the mother is getting some regular periods of sleep, it is likely she will be able to do some fitness activities in the first few weeks. On the other hand, a difficult adjustment may prolong the start of activities other than essentials.

For a first-time mother today, bringing a baby home can be a shocking experience. For women who find it difficult to adjust but who are connected with an ongoing exercise group, it can be very beneficial to return to the group for support even if the actual exercising has to wait. Exercise also helps alleviate depression and, once resumed or even taken up for the first time, is a great asset to the new mother.

Medical Screening

Most women who are fit and able to work on abdominals, pelvic floor, and walking in the first few weeks are ready to begin a structured exercise regimen by six weeks. At first, they need to monitor themselves carefully for fatigue or discomfort. The most desirable settings for them at this point are group postpartum classes, personal training, or small, familiar personal training groups.

Before a woman begins a regular exercise program at about six weeks that involves sustained activity, a number of conditions should be medically screened or assessed. The lochia should have ceased or nearly ceased, and walking a mile should not cause an increase in flow the next day. In any case, there should be no bright red blood. An episiotomy should be healed sufficiently and should present little or no discomfort and no infection. A cesarean closing should be healed sufficiently, and no infection should be present. Any pelvic relaxation should have lessened. There should be no stress incontinence due to muscle laxity. Abdominal tone should be sufficient to enable the woman to tighten the transverse by hissing/compressing; diastasis should be reevaluated. Conditions resulting from birth (see next section) should be evaluated. If the woman is nursing, milk production should be satisfactory. One should also make note of physical activities at six weeks, and may refer to the woman's two-week assessment. The form "Six-Week Postpartum Medical Screening and Exercise Assessment" is appropriate for medical screening and exercise assessment at six weeks.

Exercise History (Postpartum)

Name: _____ Age: _____ Today's date: _____

Baby's birth date: _____ Baby's name: _____

1. During your pregnancy, which of these things did you do regularly?

   ☐ *Aerobic exercise*: # of sessions/week _____; approx. length of each session: _____.

   What was your target heart rate range? _____ bpm.

   What was your RPE (rate of perceived exertion) range? (Circle lowest intensity and highest intensity.)

   Very light   Light   Fairly light   Somewhat hard   Hard   Very hard   Very, very hard

2. List your activities (running, aerobic dancing, etc.):

   _____

   ☐ *Strength activities (weightlifting, calisthenics, etc.):*

   # of sessions/week _____ Hip and knee flexors/extensors and ab/adductors

   _____ Chest and back; shoulders and arms

   _____ Abdominals; spine (core strength)

   _____ Pelvic floor

   ☐ *Flexibility activities (yoga, stretching, dance, etc.):* # of sessions/week _____

   ☐ *Combination activities (advanced dance, martial arts, basketball, etc.):* # of sessions/week _____.

   List your activities: _____

   _____

   ☐ *Relaxation (progressive relaxation, autogenic training, hypnosis, etc.):* # of sessions/week _____

   ☐ *Centering (meditation, dance, tai chi, etc.):* # of sessions/week _____

3. Did you remain active until delivery? ☐ Yes ☐ No   If No, when did you stop (how long before birth)? _____

4. Do you have one or more children in the 1- to 5-year-old range who are very active? ☐ Yes ☐ No
   If yes, how much time do you spend with her/him/them?

5. If you work, have you returned to your job? ☐ Yes ☐ No   Is it a physically demanding job? ☐ Yes ☐ No
   Is it stressful? ☐ Yes ☐ No   Are you on your feet a lot? ☐ Yes ☐ No

   Describe your work activities: _____

   _____

   _____

6. Describe your exercise and/or other physical activities since the birth of this child, including housework, cooking, etc: _____

   _____

A.F. Cowlin, 2002, *Women's fitness program development* (Champaign, IL: Human Kinetics).

Exercise Assessment at Two Weeks Postpartum

Name: _____ Today's date: _____

Baby's birth date: _____ Days postpartum: _____

Lochia (bleeding/flow due to the separation of the placenta) ☐ has ceased ☐ has not ceased.

Have you walked (or jogged) continuously for at least 1 mile or 15-20 minutes? ☐ Yes ☐ No

If yes, did you have any problems or increased bleeding as a result? ☐ Yes ☐ No

If yes, how many days postpartum were you at the time? _____

What is the most vigorous activity you have done? _____

How many days postpartum? _____ Any problems? _____

Increased flow or bleeding? ☐ Yes ☐ No

Episiotomy: Stitches have dissolved? ☐ Yes ☐ No   Discomfort? _____

Numbness? ☐ Yes ☐ No   Infection? _____

Cesarean closure: Stitches have dissolved? ☐ Yes ☐ No   Discomfort? _____

Numbness? ☐ Yes ☐ No   Infection? _____

Pelvic relaxation: Do you feel that your pelvic bones are stable? ☐ Yes ☐ No If no, describe
_____

Pelvic floor: Can you stop the flow of urine during a Kegel? ☐ Yes ☐ No ☐ Don't Know

Abdominal tone: Do this test. Lie on your back, knees bent, feet on floor. Inhale, relax abdomen. Exhale, hiss and compress abdomen. Can you suck in your abdomen? ☐ Yes ☐ Somewhat ☐ No

Conditions resulting from birth (& notes): Diastasis—Repeat the hiss/compress, then hold your breath and curl up. How many fingertips fit between the sides of your abdominal muscles 1 inch above your belly button?
☐ 1 fingertip ☐ 2 fingertips ☐ 3 fingertips ☐ more than 3

☐ Symphysis separation?

☐ SI joint?

☐ Broken coccyx?

☐ Back pain?

☐ Lower body?

Milk production, if nursing: Properly established? ☐ Yes ☐ No

Notes: _____

_____

_____

_____

_____

_____

_____

_____

_____

A.F. Cowlin, 2002, *Women's fitness program development* (Champaign, IL: Human Kinetics).

Six-Week Postpartum Medical Screening and Exercise Assessment

Note: Fill this out with your care provider and bring it to your instructor or trainer.

Name:_____ *Today's date: _____

Weeks postpartum:_____ Care provider's signature: _____

Lochia (bleeding/flow due to the separation of the placenta) ☐ has ceased ☐ has not ceased.

What is the most vigorous activity you have done? _____

Any problems? _____

Episiotomy: Discomfort? _____

Cesarean closure: Discomfort? _____ Numbness? ☐ Yes ☐ No

Pelvic relaxation: Are the pelvic bones stable? ☐ Yes ☐ No

If not, describe _____

Pelvic floor: Can you stop the flow of urine during a Kegel? ☐ Yes ☐ No ☐ Don't Know

Abdominal tone: Do this test: Inhale, relax abdomen. Exhale, hiss and compress abdomen. Do a curl-up. Does your abdomen stay compressed? ☐ Yes ☐ No, It Bulges

Conditions resulting from birth (& notes): _____

   ☐ Diastasis recti   ☐ Broken coccyx

   ☐ Symphysis separation ☐ Back pain

   ☐ SI joint   ☐ Lower body

Other: _____

Milk production, if nursing: Any problems? _____

What do you do weekly in each of the following components?

  1. Centering: _____

  2. Cardiovascular or aerobic conditioning: _____

  3. Core strength: ☐ Hiss/compress ☐ Curl-ups

  4. Upper-body strength: ☐ Upper back ☐ Push-ups

  5. Relaxation: _____

  6. Realignment: _____

  7. Mother-baby activities: _____

  8. Support: _____

*Notes: _____

_____

_____

_____

*These items should be filled out by your care provider.

© 1998 Ann Cowlin. Used by permission.

A.F. Cowlin, 2002, *Women's fitness program development* (Champaign, IL: Human Kinetics).

In addition to special postpartum screening, one or more of the standard health and/or fitness questionnaires or screening forms may be in order. The SF-36 health survey [1], PAR-Q [2], or American College of Sports Medicine (ACSM)/American Heart Association cardiovascular screening [3] may be useful. A comprehensive questionnaire can be devised following ACSM's guidelines [4], or an existing form already in use at a facility may be available. In addition, the Childbirth Impact Profile—Form MQ measures functional ability and status of mothers after childbirth [5].

Conditions That May Result From Pregnancy or Birth

The conditions discussed in this section result from the structural stresses of pregnancy and birth. The first—diastasis recti—is common, although often negligible in many fit women. All these conditions need to be evaluated, and if found, need to be assessed for their impact on movement range and possible exercise restrictions. The primary health care provider needs to be made aware of these conditions if they are discovered by the instructor or trainer.

Diastasis recti is the separation or tearing of abdominal muscles away from the linea alba or a plastic stretching of the linea alba that results in a widening and/or deepening of the trough between the recti abdominal muscles. Figure 11.1 illustrates the process of assessing the trough, or space along the linea alba that separates the right and left sides of muscles of the abdomen. To check for diastasis recti following birth, have the client, from a supine position with knees bent, exhale, execute a curl-up, and hold the position. Palpate the linea alba about an inch above the belly button; then run the finger(s) along the trough. The width and depth of the space between the two recti abdominal muscles indicates whether there has been tearing of the muscles away from the linea alba. If there are two or more finger-widths between the

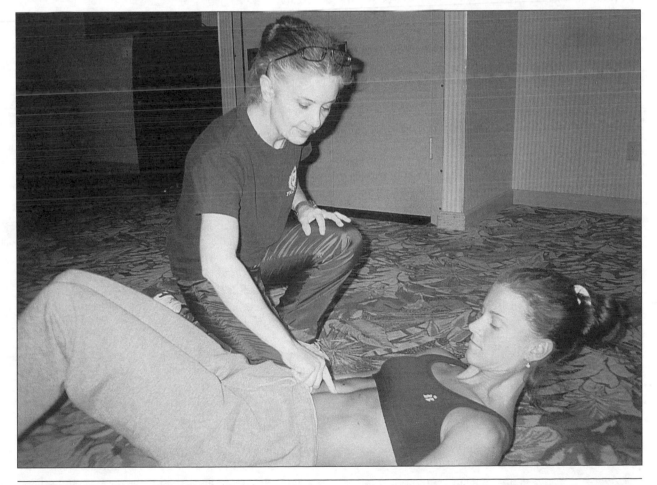

Figure 11.1   Checking for diastasis recti. The width and depth of the space between the two recti abdominal muscles indicates whether there has been tearing of the muscles away from the linea alba. Here, the author palpates an intact abdomen. Only one finger can be placed between the sides of the recti abdominal muscles, and the trough is not deep.

sides of the recti muscles, the client is asked to splint her abdomen while doing head lifts or curl-ups until the situation improves. If the trough is deep, she should be asked to focus on the hiss/compress exercise and not begin head lifts or curl-ups for a few more weeks until the transverse muscles have strengthened.

In time, an instructor or trainer learns to see various types of damage, unbalanced development, and strengths and weaknesses resulting from diastasis recti. It is the author's experience that deep separations are far more serious than wide separations—providing that the wide separation is not deep. A deep separation indicates that the transverse muscle is weak or torn. In the case of serious deep separations that do not improve, evaluation by a physical therapist or orthopedist is necessary.

A wide separation requires splinting of the abdomen during curl-ups: the woman places her hands on either side of the abdomen and pulls toward the center when curling up. She can continue this for a few weeks until the situation improves. A deep separation requires delaying curl-ups until the transverse abdominal muscles can be strengthened, perhaps two to four weeks. Attention to the abdomen in the first few weeks postpartum is critical to a woman's recovery process. If the mother is diligent and the condition does not begin improving by six weeks, referral to a physical therapist is appropriate.

Separation of the symphysis pubis occurs occasionally. The connective tissue located in the symphysis pubis breaks or becomes plastic to the extent that the two pubic rami move independently. This usually happens in the third trimester and is accompanied by sharp pain and sometimes difficulty walking. Postpartum, the woman must avoid a wide lateral stance for two or three months. If the condition does not gradually abate, medical attention is imperative.

Sacroiliac dysfunction and/or *sciatica* are not uncommon. Check for sacroiliac slippage, spasm in the medial gluteal, or, if sciatica is suspected, spasm in the piriformis muscle. In the latter case, the special exercise for the piriformis given to pregnant women (see pp. 166-167) may also be useful. Constructive rest may be helpful in the case of slippage or muscle spasms in the low back by allowing relaxation so that bones are not pulled out of normal alignment. If simple measures are not helpful, a physical therapist is the appropriate next step.

A *broken coccyx* can occur during delivery. The coccyx bones may be pushed back severely enough to cause a break. This may restrict exercise for six to eight weeks. The woman should sit on her ischial tuberosities (sitsbones) and should not sit on a rubber donut, as this puts weight directly on the broken coccyx.

Upper back pain is also not uncommon. Check for positioning of the baby during nursing. Sometimes mothers hold their infants in such a way that they must bend over them to nurse. This is neither satisfactory for the mother nor particularly helpful to the infant. Assistance with positioning from a lactation consultant or La Leche League leader is useful. In the early postpartum period, muscle spasms resulting from extreme shoulder tension in labor, or from a difficult position held for a long time during the second stage of labor (pushing), sometimes cause pain. Designing relaxation positions to relieve this area can prove beneficial. Again, check the nursing position for ergonomics.

In cases of *low back pain* and/or *midback pain,* check biomechanics and abdominal strength. This type of pain can also arise from postepidural discomfort. Ascertain whether there is actually pain, numbness, or lack of motion associated with the midspine area, or whether there is a more generalized discomfort that may be part of the mental association of having a needle inserted into one's spine. In the latter case, reassurance that the area is intact may be all that is required. If not, referral to a qualified professional is necessary. Back discomfort stemming from fatigue abates in the deeply folded position (see figure 8.14, in chapter 8).

Slow-healing surgical closures are sometimes a problem and may be a result of infection. Delay the start of strength work, stretching, or strenuous aerobic exercise. Be sure that the primary health care provider is satisfied that it is safe to commence physical activity. In addition to the physical healing process, it may be that a real mental or emotional healing process needs to take place. In the case of cesarean delivery, for example, a woman may have feelings of anger about the way she was treated. With each postcesarean client, it is important to determine not only the state of her physical being, but also how she conceives of what happened and where she is in the healing process. While some clients have no difficulties with the need for surgery or the treatment they received, others have issues with the procedure. After asking permission, try gently placing hands on the woman's abdomen and reminding her that all is whole again. Sometimes she is able to feel that she controls her body again. If not, referral to a mental health professional may be necessary.

Cystocele is the term referring to a bulging of the bladder into the vaginal wall. A first-degree cystocele is common in women who have borne a child [6]. Second- or third-degree cystocele is more pronounced. First- or second-degree cystocele without symptoms (no incontinence or sexual dysfunction) is not treated. However, a symptomatic second-degree or a third-degree cystocele requires referral for treatment. This affects exercise prescription in obvious ways. Impact activities are contraindicated, as are activities that may encourage bearing down, such as heavy lifting. Other modifications should take place in consultation with the care provider.

Lower limb problems include circulation disorders, such as those mentioned in chapter 9, and biomechanical problems of the lower leg resulting from physiological changes in pregnancy, discussed in chapters 5 and 6. Women with circulation problems must be under medical supervision. When joint laxity occurs, researchers believe that discomfort and instability problems associated with late pregnancy and the postpartum period are largely due to biomechanics [7, 8]. One study on elite female athletes indicated that weakness in the hamstrings (vs. quadriceps), and the pattern of fiber recruitment, made women vulnerable to anterior cruciate ligament injury [9]. In practice, one can help limit lower leg problems by using centering techniques; strengthening the abdominals, gluteals, and hamstrings; limiting leg abduction in the first two or three months postpartum; and focusing on the development of leg strength through a large range of motion.

Special needs of postpartum women relate to both physical and psychological problems. Following birth there can be structural damage to the pelvic region. Common results—such as a broken coccyx or sacroiliac joint dysfunction—can cause discomfort, but generally resolve in time and with careful mobilization. Less common problems—nerve or muscle damage in the pelvic floor due to surgery or tearing, infection, or psychological trauma—can be devastating. Encouraging clients in these situations to get proper medical or psychiatric attention, as well as the support of their peers, is an act of compassion that the postpartum health and fitness professional can undertake. Depression and difficulty adapting to a changing identity can also be traumatic, and in these cases it is equally important that the instructor or trainer maintain compassion. The information on group cohesion from chapter 8 also applies in this setting. Psychology professionals are good resources.

Scope of Practice and Liability Issues

Perinatal fitness specialists are often called on to explain pregnancy- and birth-related conditions to their clients and help them with bodywork to improve some situations. As healing continues, most of these conditions improve with appropriate exercise. Because of the variations in recovery factors, women are ready to join an extended postpartum class or return to regular exercise activities anywhere from three to eight weeks. However, the medical postpartum period is considered six weeks, and many programs require that women wait to see their health care provider and receive medical clearance at their six-week checkup before participating in vigorous activity. As with any physical activity program for a special population, medical screening and a waiver of liability are standards of practice.

Developing Research Questions

Readers interested in developing research questions may wish to look at additional instruments for gathering information about this population. Topics addressed by such instruments include demographics [10-12], maternal adaptation [13-16], postpartum function [17-23], psychosocial factors [24-37], abuse [38-43], the effects of preparation and experience on outcome [44-49], issues related to infants and children including breastfeeding [12, 50-58], and factors related to adolescent mothers [59-64].

SIX-WEEK IMMEDIATE RECOVERY PROGRAM

Postpartum fitness begins when the new mother takes stock of her body. This may happen as soon as the baby has its first quiet moments an hour or two after birth, or years later, depending on a woman's habits and orientation. In practice, we encourage women to take stock at some point on the first day by making a mental scan of the body from head to toe. Women without medical complications can begin exercising at home within a few days of giving birth. The program consists of these six elements:

- Constructive rest and relaxation
- Kegels or pelvic floor exercises
- Abdominal exercises
- Essential strength exercises
- Essential stretches
- Walking or other nonimpact cardiovascular activity

The form "Schedule for Sample Six-Week Immediate Recovery Program" summarizes a sample recovery program, which is detailed in the following sections.

Week One

If there have been no complications with a vaginal birth, women may try to do Kegels—or tighten and relax the pelvic floor muscles—within a few hours after delivery. Women should be able to stop the midstream flow of urine by their six-week postpartum checkup. If unable to do this, they must tell their health care provider at that time. If a woman has had a cesarean section, she can start Kegeling as soon as this activity is comfortable. If a woman has difficulty getting to the floor in the first few days after delivery, she can do pelvic floor exercises in

Schedule for Sample Six-Week Immediate Recovery Program

Day	1	2	3	4	5	6	7
Week 1							
Constructive rest	x	x	x	x	x	x	
Kegels*	x	x	x		x	x	
Hiss/compress*†	x	x	x		x	x	
Walk 5-10 minutes	x	x	x	x	x	x	
Week 2							
Constructive rest	x	x	x	x	x	x	
Kegels*	x	x	x		x	x	
Hiss/compress*	x	x	x		x	x	
Diastasis check						x	
Head lifts* (splint, if needed)	x	x	x		x	x	
Gluteals, strength*	x		x		x		
Gluteals, stretch^	x		x		x		
Upper back, strength*	x		x		x		
Upper back, stretch^	x		x		x		
Chest, stretch^	x		x		x		
Walk 10-20 minutes	x	x	x		x	x	
Weeks 3-6							
Constructive rest	x	x	x	x	x	x	
Kegels*	x	x	x		x	x	
Hiss/compress*	x	x	x		x	x	
Curl-ups* (splint, if needed)	x	x	x		x	x	
Strength*#	x		x		x		
Stretch^#	x		x		x		
Whole-body stretches^	x		x		x		
Deeply folded stretch+	x		x		x		
Squats*	x		x		x		
Walk/jog 20-30 minutes‡	x	(x)	x		x	(x)	

* = Start with 5 reps, progress to 3 sets of 5, then 3 sets of 10.

† = As muscles get stronger, you can exhale without hissing to help prevent hyperventilation; resting between sets also helps prevent hyperventilation.

^ = 3 reps.

+ = 1 rep.

= Strength and stretch exercises include gluteals, hamstrings, upper back, chest/push-ups.

‡ = Some women are able to progress to more vigorous activities than others; confer with health care provider.

(x) = An optional activity on the given day.

A.F. Cowlin, 2002, *Women's fitness program development* (Champaign, IL: Human Kinetics).

bed. If she is able to do exercises on the floor, she must be sure to rise from the position slowly and carefully, rolling onto her side, then onto hands and knees, and then slowly standing up.

Constructive Rest and Relaxation

The constructive rest position uses gravity to help the body correct posture changes that occurred during pregnancy. Readers interested in more information on the development of this position may refer to Sweigard's text [23]. This position also allows muscles to relax before the woman begins abdominal or other strengthening ex-ercises, so that they are not used improperly. Some muscles assisted with posture during pregnancy and no longer need to work when one is not pregnant.

To get into the position, lie on the back with knees bent and feet flat, a comfortable distance from the but-tocks. Rest the hands on the abdomen, breathing deeply and slowly. Figure 11.2 shows this position with varia-tions. To help the body make postural changes, lie in this position for 20 minutes and rest. While resting, visualize the front of the abdomen narrowing and the spine length-ening. To relax muscles before exercising, stay in this position for 2 to 3 minutes; then begin with Kegels, fol-lowed by abdominal exercises.

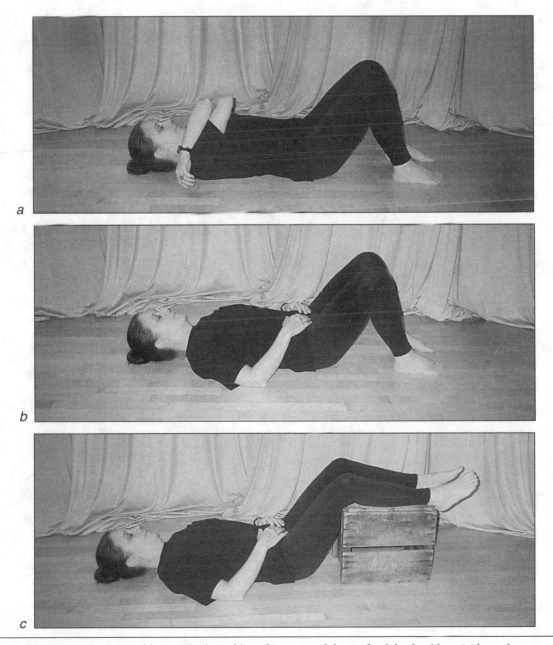

Figure 11.2 Constructive rest position: *(a)* basic position, *(b)* arms on abdomen for tight shoulders, *(c)* lower legs on stool or chair for tight lower back.

Kegels

To do the Kegel exercise postpartum, start in the constructive rest position. Draw the sitsbones together. Then squeeze the anus, vagina, and urethra. Then lift the pelvic floor. Hold for a count of 10 and relax. Breathe in and out. Do this five times to start; increase to three sets of 5; then increase the number of repetitions daily until reaching a goal of three sets of 10, for a total of 30 almost every day. As always, it is as important to relax the pelvic floor muscles as it is to contract and hold them.

Abdominal Exercise: Hiss/Compress

From the constructive rest position, begin work on the hiss/compress abdominal exercise for the transverse abdominal muscle. Inhale, relaxing the abdomen and expanding the lungs and lower abdomen. Then exhale, letting the air out with a hiss. Compress or hollow the abdomen by pulling the belly button toward the back of the waist. Repeat three times, then rest. Repeat the hiss/compress cycle two more times for a total of nine repetitions the first time. This action is shown in figure 11.3.

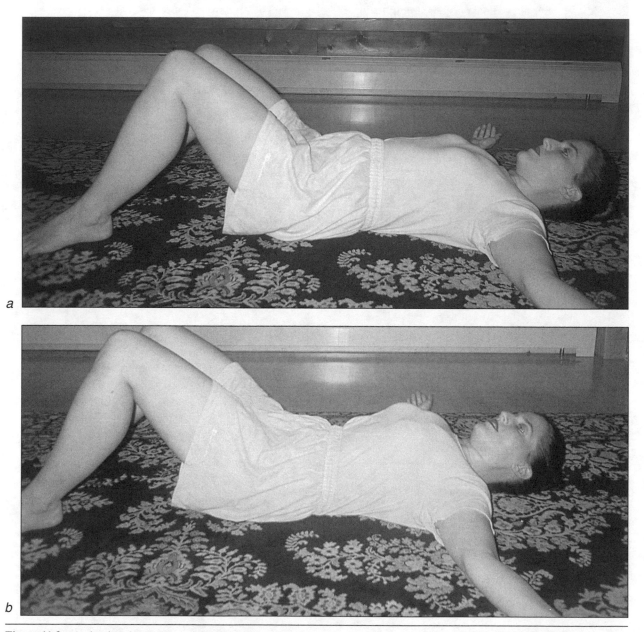

Figure 11.3   Activating the transverse abdominal muscle in the early postpartum period. *(a)* Inhale and relax the abdomen. *(b)* Exhale (hiss) and contract the transverse abdominal muscle, hollowing the abdominal contents and pulling the belly button toward the spine.

As the muscles get stronger, to help prevent hyperventilation one can exhale without hissing. Resting between sets also helps prevent hyperventilation. If a client has difficulty locating the transverse abdominal muscle, ask her to cough and to sense the deep muscles involved in this action. The back of the waist presses into the floor as a result; but it is best not to use this action as a motivating image. Pressing the back of the waist into the floor can also be accomplished by a pelvic tilt, which is not the purpose of the exercise. Using the image of pressing the back into the floor may confuse the woman as to what she should do.

Importance of Correct Abdominal Patterning. As the woman correctly activates the transverse abdominal muscle (the muscle of forced exhalation that supports the abdominal cavity and protects the low back), the core of the body begins to strengthen. This muscle lies beneath the abdominus recti, the internal obliques, and the external obliques—muscles responsible for motions of the abdomen such as the curl-up and twisting motions. During pregnancy, the transverse abdominal muscle and all the anterior and lateral abdominal muscles are stretched. When bearing down, or pushing the pelvic floor to open during delivery, the transverse abdominal can distend. It is not uncommon for postpartum women to begin a curl-up with this distending or bulging motion instead of compressing or hollowing the abdomen. It is imperative, therefore, to ensure that the new mother can activate (compress rather than distend) this deep muscle properly before beginning curl-ups or other motions that load the surface abdominal muscles. The transverse is distending if there is an upward bulging of the lower abdominal area as an individual begins a curl-up. Repatterning the transverse continues in week 2, as the new mother learns to integrate abdominal compression with three other abdominal actions.

Cesarean Variation. If the woman has had a c-section, she should wait a few days to two weeks to try the hiss/compress. When she does try it, she should feel only a gentle pulling where the stitches are as she exhales and tightens the muscle. If she feels pain or discomfort, she should stop the exercise and try again in a few days. By two weeks, she should be able to try the exercise. If she can't do it by three weeks, she should tell her health care provider.

Walking

The first week is also the time to begin walking. Women can start by walking at their own pace for 5 to 10 minutes every day. They should increase the pace as the week progresses. Some women are more comfortable walking on a treadmill or stair stepper. At the end of week 1, a woman should be able to do all the activities mentioned so far with little difficulty unless she has had a cesarean, in which case her recovery process may be delayed by two weeks.

Week 2

In week 2, women continue with constructive rest, Kegels, hiss/compress, and walking. At the start of the second week, they can do the head lift test to see if the transverse abdominal muscle is properly patterned and strong enough to stabilize the lower abdomen when the recti abdominal muscles are activated. If so, they can add head lifts. At the end of the week, a woman can fill out the two-week assessment form and perform a first check for diastasis. If necessary, she can use splinting when she does head lifts. She can also add strength and stretch exercises for the gluteals and upper back and can stretch the chest.

Abdominal Exercise: Head Lifts

To do the head lift test, start in the constructive rest position. Begin with a hiss/compress and hold the compressed or hollowed abdomen; then lift the head off the floor and look at the knees, chin tucked. Keep the abdomen compressed or hollowed. Lower the head and inhale, relaxing the abdomen. If the abdomen remains compressed or hollowed during the head lift, it is appropriate to begin doing sets of head lifts. Always start the head lift with the hiss/compress, and work slowly. However, if the abdomen bulges, do not do head lifts, but continue the hiss/compress exercises and check again in a few days. Be sure the abdomen stays compressed or hollowed during the head lifts.

Strengthening the Gluteals

For the gluteals, do pelvic tilt exercises from the constructive rest position. Exhale and squeeze the buttocks, lifting 2 to 3 inches off the floor, about the height of a fist. Lower to the floor, inhale, and relax.

Stretching the Gluteals

After each set of gluteal strengthening exercises, stretch the gluteal muscles while in the constructive rest position. Bring one knee toward the chest and keep the leg in that position by holding onto the back of the thigh. There should be a feeling of a pulling in the buttock; if not, rotate the thigh outward or inward slightly and pull the leg toward the chest, but do not pull on the foot, as this places torque stress on the knee. Hold for 15 to 30 seconds, breathing in and out slowly. Do two or three repetitions for each side.

Strengthening the Upper Back

Although a woman may be able to execute more strenuous upper back strengthening, it is worthwhile to begin with the following exercise, which requires core stabilizing and attention to alignment. To strengthen the upper back, start on hands and knees, squarely placed, with a flat back, supported by compressed transverse abdominals, and head in line with the spine. Exhale and lift one arm forward to shoulder height, maintaining the flat, supported back. Hold 5 seconds, inhale, and return to the starting position. Repeat on the other side.

Stretching the Upper Back

To stretch the upper back after completing the upper back strengthening exercises, sit cross-legged. Extend arms forward at chest height, hands clasped. Tuck the chin and curve the upper back until there is a feeling of a gentle pulling around the scapula. Hold 15 to 30 seconds, breathing in and out slowly. Do two or three repetitions.

Stretching the Chest

The following exercise to stretch the chest can be alternated with stretching the upper back. Remain seated and place hands on floor behind the back. Lift chest and face to the ceiling. Hold for 15 to 30 seconds, breathing in and out slowly. Do two or three repetitions.

Walking

For cardiovascular exercise, a woman can walk four or five days during week 2. If possible, she should increase the time to 20 minutes by the end of the week. The goal for week 2 should be to walk for 20 minutes without stopping. If able to do this before the end of the week, some women like to begin alternating walking and jogging. Many are more comfortable with a fast walk or a stair stepper at this point because impact is often uncomfortable. For those who want to jog, the recommendation is to alternate walking and jogging. Women should warm up with 2 to 3 minutes of walking, then jog for a minute, and walk for 2 or 3 minutes. They should repeat this walk/jog routine for up to 20 minutes. It is essential for a woman to monitor her lochia—an increase tells her she has done too much.

Check for Diastasis Recti at the End of Week 2

At the end of week 2, the woman can do a first check for abdominal separation, or diastasis, as described earlier and shown in figure 11.1. If the woman can fit two or more fingertips side by side into the space between the right and left recti abdominal muscles, there is a separation and she should splint her abdomen during head lifts. The separation should be checked once a week. If it does not begin to get smaller in six weeks, the woman should be reminded to tell her health care provider.

Weeks 3 to 6

Activities in weeks 3 through 6 continue with Kegels, constructive rest, hiss/compress, strength and stretch exercises, and walking. When able to do three sets of 10 repetitions of the head lifts while keeping the abdomen compressed or hollowed, the woman can try the curl-up test to see if she is ready to add curl-ups. In this period, she can also add whole-body stretches, other strength exercises if she is able to maintain abdominal compression during exertion, other stretches including the deeply folded stretch, and standing squats for leg strength.

Abdominal Exercise: Curl-Ups

When ready to try the curl-up test, start in constructive rest position with hands across the chest. Begin with a hiss/compress and hold the compressed or hollowed abdomen; lift head and shoulder blades off the floor, keeping the abdomen compressed or hollowed. Lower shoulder blades and head, and inhale. If a woman is able to keep the abdomen compressed during the curl-up, it is time to add curl-ups or replace head lifts with curl-ups. If the abdomen bulges, the woman is not ready to do curl-ups; instead she should continue with hiss/compress and head lifts and should test for curl-ups every few days until she is able do them while keeping the abdomen compressed. It's essential not to forget to splint the abdomen in case of a diastasis. When a woman can do three sets of 10 curl-ups with hands on her chest, she can do curl-ups with her hands behind her head, keeping the abdomen compressed. After she can do curl-ups and her diastasis is less than two finger-widths, she can begin oblique curl-ups.

Whole-Body Stretch

A way to perform a stretch for the whole body from the constructive rest position is to extend one leg at a time along the floor on the ground and extend the arms toward the ceiling. Then slowly lower the arms overhead onto the floor while maintaining the back of the waist on the floor and exhaling. Once fully extended, breathe in and out slowly, elongating from the hip sockets in both directions—up through the spine and down through the legs.

Other Strength and Stretch Exercises, Including Deeply Folded Position

In practice we have found that gluteal and hamstring exercises on the hands and knees, exercises from the prone position (on the stomach) to strengthen the upper back and thoracic spine, and push-ups on the wall or from the knees are also helpful in developing core strength. Following strength exercises on the hands and knees and from a prone position, the deeply folded position—shown in figure 8.14—is a particularly effective stretch. To alter the position for the nonpregnant body, the knees can be close together as one pulls the buttocks down over the heels to stretch the spine, low back, and gluteals. Following standing squats, standing stretches for the quadriceps, hamstrings, and calf muscles are also helpful.

Standing Squats for Leg Strength

The basic fitness squat for women—described in chapter 8—starts in standing with weight centered, parallel-leg position, feet 6 to 8 inches apart, no internal or external femoral rotation. Bending the legs, allowing slight internal femoral rotation and pitching the entire torso forward slightly, then pushing up by pressing against the floor recruits muscles from almost all leg groups. The depth of the squat depends on the strength and stability of the individual. The woman squeezes the gluteals and pelvic floor at the top of the action. Squats with legs open in second position are not suggested until 10 to 12 weeks postpartum.

Walking

Women can continue to walk, jog, or use a stair stepper for 20 to 30 minutes four to five times a week but should do so no less than three times a week. By the six-week postpartum checkup, many women can accomplish these activities and have no urinary incontinence and no more lochia. If a new mother has difficulty with any exercise or continues to have incontinence, lochia discharge, or any other symptom, she must tell her health care provider at her six-week checkup.

EXERCISE COMPONENTS FOR THE EXTENDED POSTPARTUM PERIOD

Once the new mom can perform these basic skills, and mom and baby have made their basic adjustment to each other, it is time to begin a more structured regimen. Chapter 10 outlined the exercise components that are safe and effective during the postpartum period: cardiovascular

or aerobic conditioning, strength training, flexibility exercises, and mind/body activities including centering and relaxation. Chapter 8 covered these exercise components in detail as they relate to pregnancy. Their application in the postpartum period requires moving clients slowly away from the special considerations and modifications described in that chapter toward nonpregnant norms. The following sections present information on this process. The frequency of exercise components depends on the preferences, experiences, and priorities of each woman. Two recommended weekly schedules are given in the form "Weekly Schedules for Exercise Components in the Extended Postpartum Period."

Cardiovascular or Aerobic Conditioning

For the first six months following birth, it may be helpful to consult the recommendations for first-trimester pregnancy in figure 8.12. The primary issue during this time is the potential for damage to the bones, muscles, connective tissue, and nerves from activities that produce biomechanical stresses. Although fitness is also an issue, the impacts of ground forces and ballistic motion are the greatest concerns in determining the suitability of an activity. As always, intensity is controlled mainly by modulating size and speed of movement.

Impact and Ballistics

During cardiovascular workouts, activities involving little or no impact are likely to be more comfortable than impact activities for many women for the first several months, although in practice, individual preferences vary greatly. In practice, we find that some women are very aggressive in their early return to vigorous exercise, especially if they have a treadmill or stair stepper at home. Those who wish to do moderate- or high-intensity cardiovascular work in the first few months postpartum must be monitored for biomechanical stresses; for although the heart and vasculature are willing, the structure is vulnerable. Choose movements that can have a small or a large range of motion, and reduce impact as much as possible. If a woman is moving without control, she must reduce the size of her movements until she can control her extremities.

Fit Women

The cardiovascular enhancements due to pregnancy continue for some time postpartum. In addition, women who begin vigorous physical activity within the first few weeks continue to see the beneficial effects associated with exercise, including increased blood volume, vasculature,

Weekly Schedules for Exercise Components in the Extended Postpartum Period

Less Active Women

Day	1	2	3	4	5	6	7
Centering	x	x		x		x	
Strength		x		x			
Flexibility		x		x			
Cardiovascular		x		x		x	
Relaxation	x	x		x		x	

More Active Women

Day	1	2	3	4	5	6	7
Centering	x	x	x		x	x	
Strength	x		x			x	
Flexibility	x		x			x	
Cardiovascular	x	(x)*	x			x	(x)*
Relaxation	x	x	x		x	x	x

*This exercise component is optional on the given day.

A.F. Cowlin, 2002, *Women's fitness program development* (Champaign, IL: Human Kinetics).

and heart strength. Waiting more than a few weeks to begin aerobic components of an activity regimen means that deconditioning becomes a factor. While we want a woman to take advantage of the aerobic benefit of pregnancy, it is critical for her to work at intensities and durations that do not produce discomfort or fatigue, because her primary obligation is the well-being of her infant. Women who are fit as they come into the extended-period program may need to be reminded that their preferred intensity level will vary from day to day depending on the baby—how the baby slept the night before, how much the baby is nursing—as well as other demands on the mom.

Women Who Are Unfit or Low in Fitness

Just as pregnancy can be a point of entry into fitness, the postpartum period can be a time when women decide to enter the fitness culture. It is not uncommon for a nonexercising woman who has had a baby in the last few months to turn up at a mother-baby program with a friend who is already enrolled. She may even have been active in the past but inactive for a year or more. Also, women who were regular exercisers prior to pregnancy and were

placed on bed rest or restricted to mild daily-living activities during pregnancy frequently wish to return to exercise following the birth.

Women who are unfit or low in fitness and who wish to begin regular exercise in the postpartum period must be medically screened and their fitness level assessed. Exactly how one proceeds depends on the point at which the woman makes contact with the program. If a woman makes contact early in the postpartum period, or even before she gives birth, she can be instructed in intake procedures and early postpartum activities, when appropriate. If she makes contact several weeks or months after the birth of her baby, then screening and exercise testing are used to determine a starting level.

Strength or Resistance Training

During the early postpartum period there is still an emphasis on strength training for the upper back, abdominals, pelvic floor, gluteals, and hamstrings as a way of helping the body realign. As time passes, the heavy emphasis on these areas diminishes and a more balanced, nonpregnant approach is suitable. Postpartum misalignment is greatest nearest the birth of the baby. However, it is very common to see women past childbearing age whose skeletons still have the look of pregnancy—forward head, increased kyphotic curve, increased lordosis, increased anterior pelvic tilt, increased iliofemoral flexion—and corresponding muscle atrophy and hypertrophy. The biomechanical effects of pregnancy, although they lessen, can easily become the postural problems of midlife and old age.

Therefore, during the extended postpartum period, the essential areas already discussed continue to form the core of strength training. If time is limited, these are the exercises that must be included. But it is also necessary to balance the strength of muscles surrounding each joint. In group classes, new clients may need to work on essentials, while those further removed from birth may need to work on other areas of the body, emphasizing only one or two essential exercises. Hip abduction and adduction, as well as outward rotation and squats in ballet second, are practical to begin around 10 to 12 weeks postpartum.

Guidelines for strength conditioning from ACSM or the National Strength and Conditioning Association may be followed. A minimum consists of 8 to 12 exercises, including all the major muscle groups, performed twice a week. Because the postpartum woman is having to carry an infant whose weight continues to increase, as well as a variety of equipment and supplies, training for power is a desirable goal. This type of training is different from that during pregnancy and places greater stress on the joints, so it is a transition in training focus that women must undertake slowly and gradually over a period of six months to a year.

Flexibility

Muscles of the anterior iliofemoral joint, lumbar spine, chest, and anterior shoulder need extra stretching until the bony levers achieve a nonpregnant alignment. Once again, if not attended to, these areas can remain shortened and can adversely affect posture over the course of the lifetime. Because many women nurse, shortened pectoral muscles can easily be reinforced in the postpartum period. It is helpful for women to open the chest during constructive rest by placing the arms out to the sides with palms up, as well as to do the anterior shoulder stretch used for carpal tunnel release during pregnancy (described in chapter 8).

Alternating sets of strength exercises with their corresponding stretches is a practical way to develop flexibility in all the body areas. Another good tactic is to slowly increase range of motion during the aerobic warm-up by taking steps and making arm and leg gestures that slowly increase in size.

Mind/Body Activities

In the extended postpartum period, mind/body and mother-baby activities require unique consideration. Areas of work that have long-term beneficial effects when sensitively handled by the instructor or trainer are centering techniques; realignment of the skeleton; and the integration of mother-baby activities into cardiovascular, strength, and flexibility components.

Centering

Preparing to move in a biomechanically healthy manner is one of the major functions of centering. Whether the preparation is *sinking chi* in martial arts or *establishing vertical* in ballet, the by-product of this activity is reduced stress on the weight-bearing joints, adjoining nerves, and blood vessels. In the postpartum period, this type of activity is critical to preventing damage due to the variance between the brain's sense of upright, which is not immediately rectified following birth, and the body's shift in actual weight distribution, which does occur at the time of birth. The sooner the brain and body agree on balance, the sooner the damage potential is reduced.

Figure 11.4 shows a postpartum woman standing balanced around her vertical axis, or plumb line, relaxed and focused (refer to description of centering during standing in chapter 8). By actively pressing against the floor, she can stand without tension in the superficial movement muscles. In figure 11.5 she prepares for movement by breathing from her abdomen as she stretches. During pregnancy, her ability to breathe deeply was abridged by the enlarging uterus. Following birth, the deep abdominal muscles need to be tightened and strengthened, and deep abdominal breathing needs to be repatterned.

Realignment

Following birth, the sudden and dramatic shift in the center of gravity—without the accompanying slow changes in bone alignment and neuromuscular adaptations—means that postural re-education in the postpartum period is a major concern. Methods to achieve this include constructive rest position; strengthening abdominals, gluteals (figure 11.6), pelvic floor, and upper back (figure 11.7); stretching the psoas major; stretching the chest and low back; and conscious repetition of healthy alignment patterns in movement.

Because of postpartum hormonal shifts and changes in the center of gravity, postpartum women are susceptible to tendinitis and aching joints of the hands, shoulders, low back, knees, ankles, and feet. Poor techniques

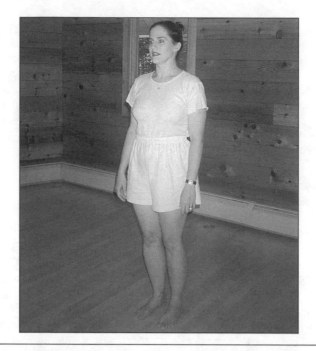

Figure 11.4 Postpartum centering: standing balanced around the central axis. Prior to moving, this postpartum woman has aligned herself vertically. Each leg is aligned so that the ankle and knee are in line with the iliofemoral joint and the entire body is balanced around the vertical axis, or plumb line.

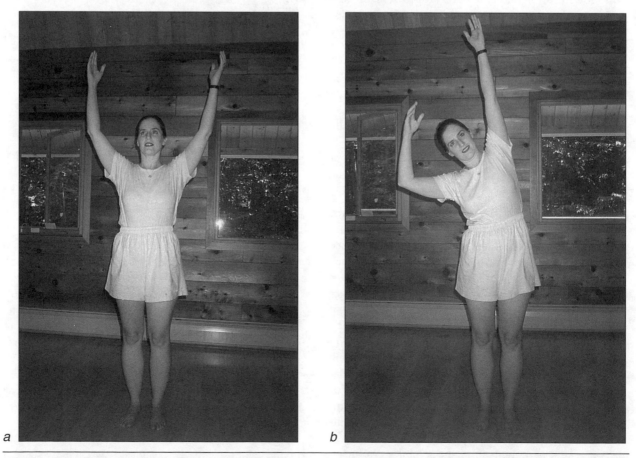

a   b

Figure 11.5 Postpartum centering: abdominal breathing. (a) In preparation for movement, the postpartum woman inhales as she raises her arms, then exhales by hissing and compressing her transverse abdominal muscles. (b) Lengthening one side of her body, she inhales. Then she exhales and returns to the position in (a) and repeats on the other side. Alternating sides, she repeats this action several times before starting her warm-up.

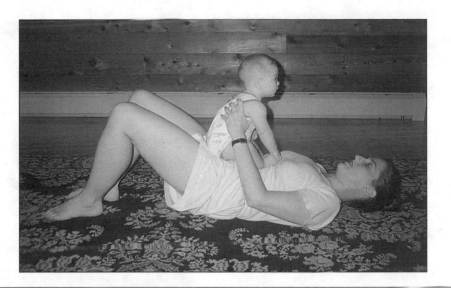

Figure 11.6 Pelvic tilt to strengthen the gluteals. Exhale and hollow the abdomen. Then contract the gluteals and lift the sacral area off the floor a couple of inches, maintaining floor contact with the lumbar spine (back of the waist).

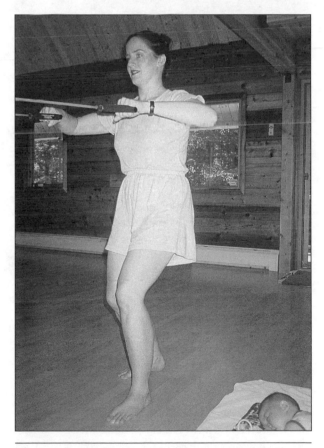

Figure 11.7 Strengthening the upper back. Scapular retraction, horizontal arm extension, and thoracic spine extension all contribute to upper back strength needed to offset the biomechanical effects of pregnancy and nursing. A stable stance, exhaling on the effort and compressing the transverse abdominal muscle produce an effective exercise combining these elements shown here. Tubes, bands, free weights, and machines are all useful.

of carrying and holding their infants exacerbate these conditions. Women can alleviate the conditions somewhat by holding the baby close to the central axis, nursing while seated with pillows under baby, working on ankle proprioception, and not locking knees when standing.

Holding Baby Close. The woman should carry the baby close to the central axis of the body. She needs to use the muscles proximal to the central axis (core stabilizers) to bear the weight, as in the colic carry or frontal carry shown in figure 11.8. She should not carry the baby with the hands, but rather on the forearms, so that the larger, upper arm muscles (biceps and triceps) help support and manipulate the baby. Using the long, small muscle of the lower arm and hand to carry the weight not only is more stressful to the spine, but also can lead to tendinitis in the wrist.

Nursing With Pillows Under Baby. When women are nursing in a seated position, they should support the baby with enough pillows or blankets to bring the baby to the breast. This relieves the weight at the shoulders, reduces kyphosis in the thoracic spine, and frees the arms to manipulate the infant and the environment.

Work on Ankle Proprioception. Postpartum women should wear socks and/or high-top exercise shoes to provide the ankle with cutaneous proprioceptor stimulus in order to help the brain reimage proper alignment in the leg. Simple balances on one leg, skills for direction change, and balance boards are all helpful when used appropriately. Because the foot and ankle play major roles in informing the brain about the upright status, activities that cause the foot and ankle to accommodate are important. Because of looseness, however, care must be taken

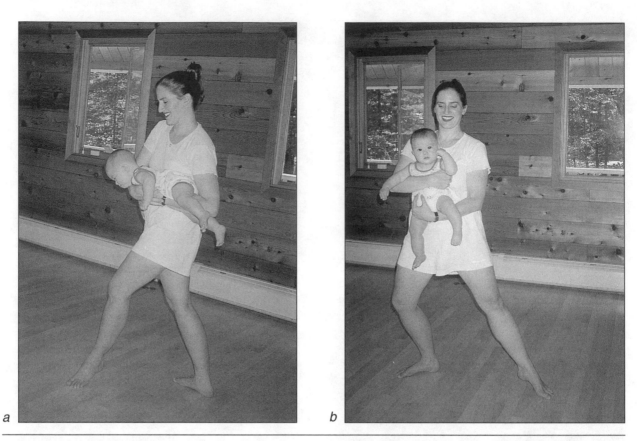

Figure 11.8   Carrying baby close to the central axis. *(a)* The colic carry places the infant's weight over the forearms rather than in the hands. The elbows are kept close to the sides. The heel of one hand can be placed on the solar plexus, which causes a relaxation reflex after a few moments (hence it is often used for colicky babies). *(b)* The frontal carry also places the baby's weight on the forearms and brings the stress toward the mother's core.

to protect the joints. Wearing supportive shoes during aerobic activities and moving at a slow pace when changing direction are helpful precautions.

Not Locking Knees During Standing. Although not locking knees is a standard of practice for fitness in general and many active women are aware of its importance, we frequently see both fit and unfit postpartum women standing with knees locked. Locking knees appears to be a compensation for the discrepancy between brain and body at this time. Even if the new mother stands in an anatomically correct posture, the brain does not accept it as an upright posture immediately. The nervous system needs to be reprogrammed so that the quadriceps do not grip to help maintain upright. Reminding women to keep the hips, knees, and ankles slightly flexed and the legs active during standing provides mechanoreceptor stimulus to the brain and helps prevent an unhealthy postural habit.

Methods of Including Infants

The major ways to include infants in a postpartum program are (1) to bring the babies into the room and involve them with the exercising mothers and (2) to do stroller exercise in a large indoor space or outdoors. A number of popular books published in the 1980s and 1990s present samples of exercise activities to safely include babies in a mother's calisthenics routine [65-68]. These books continue to be excellent resources for people designing mother-baby programs.

Babies in the Room

In a group class, very young infants in car seats or carriages can sleep around the outside edges of a room while moms exercise in the center space. If the space is large, an "island" of babies can be created in the center of the room. Sometimes the babies sleep or play on their own (see figure 11.9) while mothers exercise. At other times, mothers can carry babies in the colic carry or forward carry as shown in figure 11.8. Small babies can be carried at the shoulder when the choreography safely permits, but *both hands should remain on the baby*. Changing position frequently helps prevent discomfort. Babies who are lying down want to change position, too (see figure 11.10)!

Strength activities such as the baby press (as opposed to the bench press!), demonstrated in figure 11.11, are

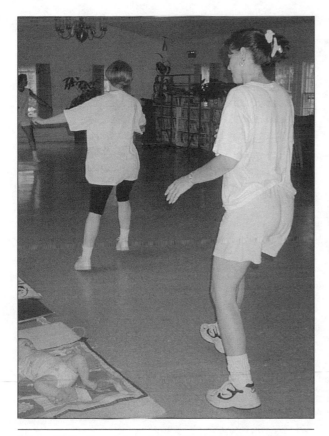

Figure 11.9 Exercising while babies sleep or play. These babies sleep or play while their moms exercise. Note that babies are well within their mothers' line of vision.

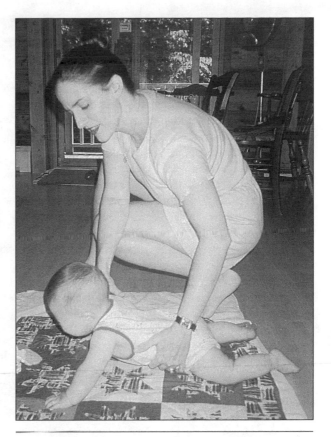

Figure 11.10 Babies who are too young to roll over, sit on their own, or push up onto their hands and knees may need help changing positions. Be sure a mother uses healthy biomechanics to squat (as shown here) rather than bends down while attending to her baby.

fun and are a way for the baby to learn about balance. Another strength activity that babies enjoy is sitting on the mother's abdomen or—if they are very young—lying on their stomachs on top of the mother's abdomen during curl-ups and oblique exercises.

Stretch/strength exercise is another activity the baby can participate in. Figure 11.12 demonstrates both mother and baby stretching their abdomens and strengthening their backs. The baby shown here is also working on rolling over, while the mother observes and encourages. This activity not only is effective for fitness purposes, but also provides an opportunity for mother and baby to interact while the baby works on developing movement skills. All the childhood nursery rhymes, songs, and games are easily adapted to exercise. Books, audio-, and videotapes are helpful for selecting materials. The classic nursery rhyme about Humpty Dumpty allows the baby to experience righting reflexes: "Humpty Dumpty had a great *fall* . . ." becomes a leaning movement to the side followed by a return to upright.

On other occasions, babies may be perfectly happy to rest while mom works, as in figure 11.13. In practice, we find that classes that include babies vary greatly from day to day in the amount of time spent carrying babies,

Safe Baby Reminders

- Always use both hands to hold a baby when moving with a baby.
- Support a baby's head and pelvis when picking her or him up.
- Never shake or toss a baby.
- Don't ignore a crying baby.

exercising with babies, and letting babies sleep, play alone, or play with each other.

Stroller Exercise

Strollers are a wonderful source of inspiration. Walking, lunging (see figure 11.14), steps with gestures, gallops, skips, jogging, grapevines, and all manner of other aerobic steps can be adapted for stroller aerobics. Stroller exercise safety means making sure the equipment is safe, the baby is securely attached, and the environment is safe. After centering and warming up by walking with the strollers, women can pick up the pace for the major portion of

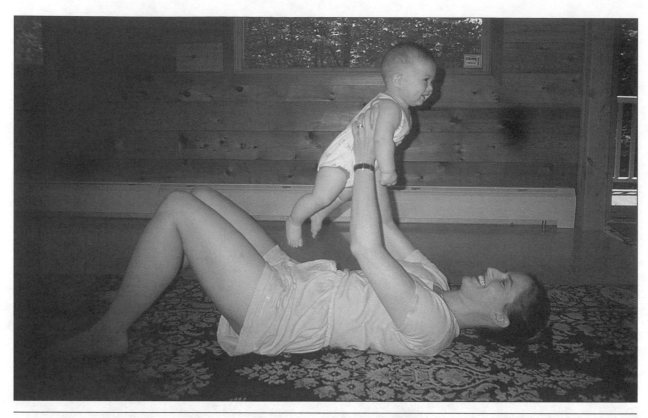

Figure 11.11 The baby press. Pressing the baby instead of weights not only provides resistance for mom, but also teaches the baby about gravity and balance.

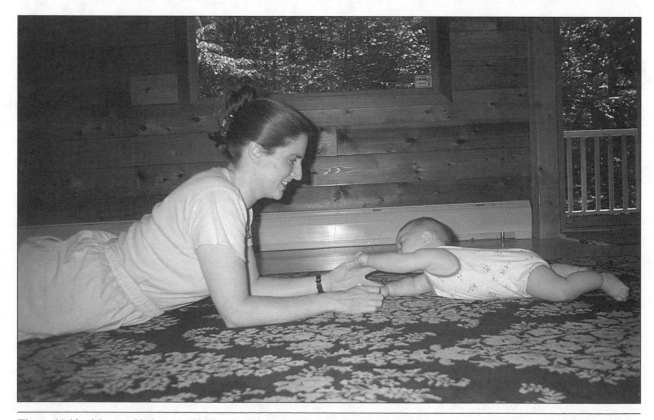

Figure 11.12 Mom and baby stretching their abdomens and strengthening their backs.

234

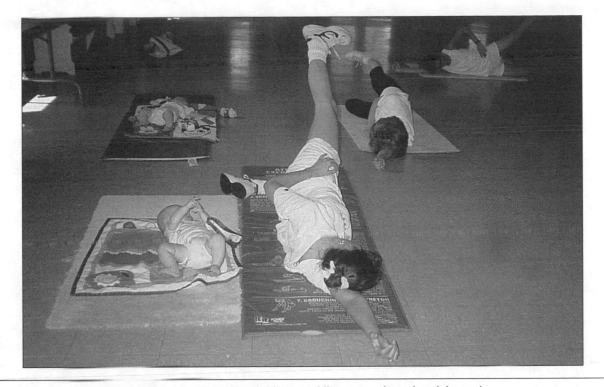

Figure 11.13   Strength work with babies. Sometimes babies rest while mom works on her abductors!

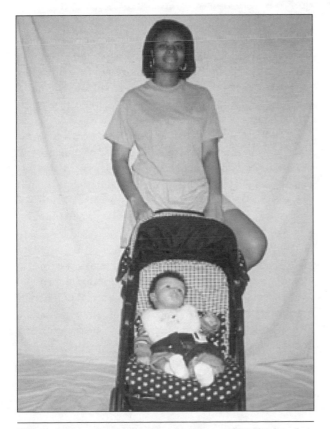

Figure 11.14   Strollers are a great source of inspiration. Locomotor aerobic activities from walking and choreographed steps to lunging or jogging with a stroller, carriage, or jogger, provide an excellent method of achieving postpartum cardiovascular fitness.

the workout. Slowing down for a cool-down period, then stopping and using the handle of the braked stroller for balance to do strength work such as leg lifts, and finishing with some stretching (plus relaxation and a time for mothers and babies to sit together and nurse or play) round out an enjoyable but vigorous activity session.

During a stroller workout, placing strollers in a circle with babies facing out is a way of augmenting variety. Telling stories with movement as a means of entertaining the babies produces a surprisingly intense level of activity. Idea sources include stories from children's books with lots of action or many animals to imitate, accompanied by instrumental music with multiple rhythms (music from the Caribbean, South America, and other cultures often has less demanding beats than the typical American workout sounds). Such activities allow people to move at their own pace and still find a regular beat if they wish. The moms can tell the stories to the babies (sitting in their strollers), who tend to find the whole thing very entertaining. This activity also allows the women to move as gently or strenuously as they prefer, and does not require learning any fixed steps. Focused on entertaining her baby and keeping the story moving, many a mother will work very hard!

In addition to classes in which the entire session is organized around the strollers, mother-baby classes as described earlier can incorporate strollers into just a portion of the session. The strollers provide an alternative to carrying a fussy baby during an aerobic component. On occasion, the same class may involve some mothers jogging by themselves, others carrying babies, and still others jogging behind their carriages. Babies can also be placed in their strollers or car seats in the front of the room and treated to the "mother show."

PROGRAM FORMATS

How much of which elements and in what order depends on the goals and history of the individual woman or the group. Many women are motivated by the desire to lose weight gained in pregnancy, to achieve a firm musculature, to share recreational time with their infants, and to have a chance to meet with other new moms. Consequently, sessions that concentrate primarily on aerobics, strength training, and realignment are effective. Group workouts that can include infants have proven very popular with this population. For women working with a personal trainer, the infant can stay nearby for interaction or for some simple, safe activities—such as curl-ups with the baby on the abdomen.

Facilitating the Transition

The transition from a home exercise routine to a postpartum group fitness program, a nonpregnant program, or a regular personal training regimen can be difficult for many women. Working out how the baby will be integrated into the program, or how the mother will handle separation if the baby is not present, cannot be dismissed as a minor aspect of the process.

Methods of facilitating this transition into a group include making sure the new mother has a "buddy," another mom whose baby is a little older and who can give advice on such matters as what items to be sure to have in the diaper bag, where the good parking spots are, or how to operate the elevator at the gym with a baby car seat on one arm. Another method is to praise the mother for arriving for her first class, even if she is very late or participates less than fully in only a few of the activities, perhaps checking her diastasis, walking through part of the cardiovascular workout, doing curl-ups, and talking with the other moms. Also being sure to complete the screening process helps the instructor know everything she should about each participant, including her preferences and any factors that may affect her exercise prescription. And establishing continuity is important. If the postpartum program flows from a prenatal program, it's an excellent idea to bring soon-to-deliver pregnant women to the postpartum group so they can see how things work after the birth.

Similar methods can be employed with one-on-one clients to facilitate their transition to postpartum workouts. If a trainer works with several women, she or he can arrange for a new mother to have a mentor, a woman who has one or more children. In a corporate setting, postpartum and parenting meetings can be incorporated into the company's wellness program.

Formatting for Various Settings

Readers may refer to the section on program formats in chapter 8 for basic information about the character of an appropriate setting. Additional factors essential to a postpartum program with babies include a location and time of day that are baby friendly and a slightly more permissive attitude about being on time.

There is an apocryphal story of the new mother who fed and cleaned up the baby, got all dressed for her first postpartum exercise class, and was ready to head out the door when the baby spit up all over everything. She changed her own and the baby's clothes, was ready to go again only to discover that the baby was hungry and had to be fed, and in the end arrived for the last 5 minutes of class! When this happens, the class should be encouraged to congratulate the mother for her perseverance and make a positive response to her appearance at the program. Having the support of the group can turn the incident into an exercise program benefit, whereas otherwise such an occurrence could become a barrier to exercise.

Groups

In group settings, a standard 1-hour program format is often too short. Unlike the general population, mothers with babies vary in their arrival time, and they often like to chat following the workout. As a result, an hour and a quarter is a minimum period if 50 to 60 minutes of exercise is a goal.

The format with the broadest appeal consists of an arrival period, followed by centering and warming up, and an aerobic or cardiovascular session with movements that can be executed at various intensities at the same time. If the session starts slowly and progresses steadily in intensity, women who are regulars but are a few minutes late will be able to accommodate.

After the aerobic or cardiovascular portion, strength and stretch activities, a few minutes of relaxation or constructive rest, and some time to nurse or bottle feed and chat provide all the essential components. When babies are present in the room or are integrated into the actual programming, one must keep an eye out for potential dangers, infants who require immediate attention, and the need for appropriate support or assistance of a mother or baby.

One-on-One

A key element in personal training with postpartum mothers is finding the right mix between observation of physical changes due to pregnancy or birth and attention to the rate at which this mother can accomplish her postpartum goals. Each body undergoes experiences and changes that accrue in the childbearing process, some of which may be permanent. It is not always possible at the outset to know how much a postpartum body will change.

Each woman also confronts unique circumstances following birth. Babies adjust to life at their own pace. Mothers have varying levels of intuitive grasp or learned knowledge about infant care. The trainer's job involves perceiving the reality of motherhood and the mother's expectations about fitness, and helping the mother bring reality and expectations into line. Supporting the new mother to stay motivated about caring for herself falls to the trainer when there is no group support.

Tracking the client's participation in various exercise components outside of the private sessions helps the trainer know where to focus during the sessions to be sure she is covering all components. Because some clients work out only when a trainer is present, the trainer has firsthand knowledge of areas that may be less preferable to the client, and can find ways to make them more desirable.

Many issues that face the group fitness instructor are applicable for the personal trainer and vice versa. Care in arranging the setting, the atmosphere of the location, and attitude toward time are all critical. A person who enjoys working with new mothers and infants will find this work tremendously rewarding.

Professional or Competitive Athletes and Dancers

Professional athletes and competitive amateurs form an interesting subgroup in the postpartum population. If such a woman has been able to maintain a high level of readiness for her sport during pregnancy, has little structural adjustment following birth, and makes successful psychological adaptations, she may experience only a mild effect on her physical activities. On the other hand, if she needs realignment or needs time to make the psychological adaptations and does not take the time, she may later experience biomechanical or emotional difficulties. In practice, the time to watch for these problems is generally around three or four months postpartum.

BREASTFEEDING AND EXERCISE

To prevent a new mother from being overwhelmed by the large number of "rules" for breastfeeding, the instructor or trainer may wish to make sure that new mothers know a few basics and where to get help if needed. Some babies have no trouble latching on right from the start, and others—especially premature infants—need help. It is important to be sure that new mothers know they can

get help by contacting a lactation consultant or local La Leche League leader.

Among the basic principles a new mother might find useful are the following:

1. Nurse soon and often after birth.
2. Sucking should be done at the breast, the length and frequency determined by the baby.
3. Position the baby so nursing is comfortable and milk transfer is maximized.
4. Watch the baby's urine and stool output for assurance of supply.
5. Problems have solutions; help is available; know your resources.

It is important to remember that mothers who nurse and exercise need sufficient fluids. Before working out, a nursing mother should be sure to drink an extra 6 or 8 ounces of water. The volume of milk production will not be compromised if the mother is drinking adequately [69, 70]. If the infant of an elite athlete is not gaining weight at an acceptable pace, efforts must be made to see that the care provider is aware of the extent of exercise the nursing mother is doing. Counseling by the care provider of a nursing and exercising mother should include information on increased fluid intake [71].

Another concern of researchers has been the effect of exercise intensity on milk composition. Studies in the late 1980s and early 1990s demonstrated the accumulation of lactic acid and its persistence for 90 minutes in the milk of women exercising at maximal levels [72, 73] and reported problems with infant acceptance of postexercise breast milk [74]. As a result, women who find that their infants have an aversion to postexercise breast milk often express milk prior to exercise to give to their infants afterward, and express and discard postexercise breast milk.

In the later 1990s, several studies on the composition of breast milk of exercising mothers provided more detailed findings. One study looked at the accumulation of lactic acid at various exercise intensities, along with changes in milk pH, lipid, ammonium, and urea levels. The researchers found that although milk lactic acid was significantly elevated through 90 minutes postexercise following a maximal-intensity treadmill session, there was no significant increase following sessions at 50% or 75% $\dot{V}O_2$max, nor were there any significant differences in the other measures at any level of intensity [75].

In another study, researchers found that maximal exercise did not alter concentrations of phosphorus, calcium, magnesium, potassium, or sodium in breast milk at 10, 30, or 60 minutes postexercise [76]. A study of the effects of maximal exercise on immunoglobulin A (IgA) in breast milk showed significantly decreased concentrations of IgA at 10 and 30 minutes postexercise, but levels at 60 minutes were similar to control levels [77]. In addition, levels of IgA1 showed a significant decrease at 10 minutes postexercise but had returned to control concentrations at both 30 and 60 minutes, and no significant changes in IgA2 concentrations were found at any time [77].

Also of interest have been the effects of calorie restriction (as opposed to malnutrition) and maternal weight loss. In reviewing research findings, Dewey concluded that short-term energy deficit in conjunction with exercise and resulting weight loss does not adversely affect lactation, perhaps due to the increase in maternal plasma prolactin concentration associated with a negative energy balance [78]. Little and Clapp compared lactation-induced bone changes between women who participated in self-selected recreational exercise in the early postpartum period and those who did not, and found that exercise had no impact on the bone mineral density loss associated with early postpartum lactation [79].

A related issue is support for the breasts during exercise. Binding them tightly with a jog bra over a nursing bra is one common solution for a nursing mother doing vigorous exercise. Another is a tight-fitting leotard or top, made of synthetic stretch fabric, worn over a bra. A lubricant or pad to protect the nipples from abrasion is also helpful. Any binding should be removed immediately following exercise. A variety of supported positions for nursing, strengthening and stretching the relevant muscles (those of the upper back, shoulders, and chest), and relaxing in constructive rest are all good ways to relieve the discomforts associated with nursing.

RETURN TO A REGULAR EXERCISE PROGRAM

The period of time between joining a postpartum program and returning to a general-population program varies a great deal from one woman to another. Some women wish to stay with a mother-baby group for as long as possible, while others wish to keep the postpartum recovery time as brief as they can. Or one woman may want to work with a personal trainer and expect to resume a nonpregnant routine gradually, while another is impatient.

For some women, mainstreaming soon is a high priority. They may be very active women who want to be away from what they perceive as their exercise peer group for as short a time as possible. Or they may be returning to work and feel they need to be with a similar group for their exercise activities. If they also feel the need for group support, a weekend "stroller aerobics" class or a mothers' support group may be available in the area. Continuing group support during this period is important, especially for first-time mothers.

Assessing Participants' Needs and Concerns

As a program progresses, monitoring a woman's physical recovery, as well as her motivations and goals, allows an instructor or trainer to help each client make a transition at a time that is appropriate for that person. A woman who perceives herself as being in her childbearing stage of life may wish to participate in a postpartum program for a year or more, until her next pregnancy is confirmed and she feels the need to be in a pregnancy program again. As long as such women are healthy and fit as a result of their activities, there is no imperative to push them into a general-population program.

Women who perceive themselves as career women or serious athletes may, on the other hand, be primarily concerned with how quickly they can return to their job or training regimen. Preparing them to work in a competitive or general-population exercise environment may be desirable. In a group with mixed motivations, organizing the session so that one portion allows for choices in activities not only meets multiple needs, but also gives instructors an opportunity to assess unspoken preferences as they observe who chooses what activities.

Participants' responses to nonintrusive questions about the baby's progress ("What new skills has the baby learned?" or "Does the baby enjoy the baby press-up?") provide clues to the woman's sense of security as a mother, as well as her motivations for continuing or discontinuing exercise with her baby. Friendly inquiries into clients' goals help an instructor or trainer determine when to introduce transitional activities, such as step aerobics. Before intense resistance training is introduced, attention should be given to abdominal and pelvic floor integrity.

Assisting Emotional Closure

The emotional, often temporary bond that occurs during the pre/postnatal period between an instructor or trainer and her clients, or among a group of clients, can be the source of some discomfort when the time comes for a woman to leave her postpartum program. Consequently it is helpful to use periodic newsletters, friendly phone calls, or other devices to assist clients with closure. A good carryover technique is to provide a list of special exercises learned as part of the program—such as C-Curves and Kegels—that can be integrated into a woman's nonpregnant regimen.

Sometimes group participants stop attending despite protestations that they plan to continue. As their baby grows and changes, or as their older children develop new needs, their hearts may be with their exercise group, but their life moves on. In practice, we have found it helpful to use a fall and spring newsletter to convey a general (no names are mentioned) well-wishing to those who are "graduating" from the program. Of course, the graduates are invited to visit anytime they wish and to attend the program with a future pregnancy and birth.

PROGRAM EVALUATION

When "graduating" from an extended postpartum program, participants can fill out evaluations using Likert-type scales to indicate their perceived value of the exercise components and how much they enjoyed the program. As with a prenatal program, asking questions that allow new mothers to assess the contribution of the program to their postpartum experience helps an instructor tailor offerings to meet the needs of her population. Instructors should also track injuries and biomechanical discomforts.

Outcomes concerning maternal adaptations and child development were discussed in chapter 10. Many fitness professionals consider maternal and infant psychosocial outcomes outside their scope of practice, but these outcomes are profoundly affected by a woman's lifestyle. Because exercise influences the production of energy by stimulating the adrenals, while late pregnancy and nursing suppress the adrenal energy axis, physical activity is probably a significant factor in counteracting physiological and psychological depression. This is a topic in need of more research. The value of a women's support community—what we sometimes call the *tribal effect*—is another area that needs research in relation to the postpartum period. Fitness professionals working with pre/postnatal populations may find it rewarding to ally themselves with research efforts aimed at evaluating and improving outcomes for postpartum women at risk for depression, child abuse or neglect, as well as physical conditions such as adult-onset diabetes, obesity, or autoimmune disorders.

PROGRAM DESIGN FOR ADOLESCENT MOTHERS

The split view in the U.S. culture of adolescent mothers was discussed in chapter 8. On one hand, efforts to lower the rate of adolescent pregnancy have focused on the negative aspects of this situation, and starting in the late 1990s a reduction in these rates among mid and older teens has been widely reported. On the other hand, the message that the teenage mother receives from this effort is that she is not a desirable person and has a terrible future. For those who work to facilitate these new mothers' transition into healthy, responsible parenthood, this split view creates a formidable challenge.

A full exploration of the realities of adolescent parenting includes examining issues such as the characteristics of this population [80-82], outcomes and consequences of early childbearing [82-90], the impact of living arrangements [91-94], reducing risks for infants of young mothers [95-98], the relationship of demographics to outcomes [99-102], and the need for research and programs for this population [103].

Developmental Conflicts

Girls who give birth during adolescence face serious developmental tasks if they are to become healthy, responsible parents. Adolescence and early parenthood are both periods of major physical, psychological, cognitive, and social growth. The juxtaposition of these two stages, with goals that are often in opposition, creates the potential for crisis in the life of the new adolescent mother. Sadler and Catrone [104] developed the conceptual framework for describing this phenomenon and identified the components of developmental conflict for inner-city adolescent mothers—a significant population at high risk for experiencing these problems of off-time parenting.

Reviewing existing models of adolescence and early parenting, Sadler and Catrone developed their model in relation to observed behaviors in adolescent parents and established that there are developmental conflicts in the following areas:

1. Identity issues
2. Independence and individuation
3. Cognitive development
4. Sexual identity

Table 11.1 lists the specific issues within each area. These issues provide themes for developing an active curriculum to facilitate positive growth experiences for this population.

Major Health Issues

Pregnant adolescents are at risk for preterm delivery and pregnancy-induced hypertension, while their infants are at risk of low birth weight. Prenatal care is a major factor in preventing these problems (see chapter 8). Following birth, young mothers are at risk for depression and poor long-term outcomes. If their diet has been poor, anemia or other conditions can occur. Having unprotected sex puts girls at risk of repeat pregnancy, sexually transmitted diseases, and HIV (human immunodeficiency virus).

Their children are at risk, as well. Those born early or with low birth weight may have developmental delays or restrictions. If the adolescent mother comes from a dysfunctional environment or does not receive parent

Table 11.1   Developmental Conflicts of Adolescent Motherhood

Adolescence	Motherhood
Identity issues	
Trying on different roles	Parenting has specific roles
Time with peers	24-hour-a-day job
Independence and individuation	
Loosening dependent ties with parents	Increased dependence on family for economic and child care support
Desire for more mobility and time with friends	Tied to home more because of baby
Cognitive development	
Concrete thought and reasoning	Maternal role requires future planning
Egocentric	Thinking about consequences; safety
	Anticipating child's behavior
	Perceiving child as separate
Sexual identity	
Adjustment to physical changes of adolescence	Physical changes of pregnancy and postpartum
May be uncomfortable with sexuality despite sexual activity	Breastfeeding issues

Sadler, L.S., and Catrone, C., 1983, "The adolescent parent: A dual developmental crisis," *Journal of Adolescent Health Care* 4(2):100-105; Sadler, L.S., and Cowlin, A.F., 1998, *Moving into parenthood*, presented at the NOAPPP 1998 Conference, Denver, CO.

training, her offspring may be at risk for child abuse or suffer interruption in the attachment process.

Interventions That Produce Positive Results for Adolescent Mothers

School-based interventions can help reduce the incidence of low birth weight [105] and repeat pregnancies [106], as well as provide an appropriate setting for learning parenting skills. Staying in school is a critical issue for young mothers if they are to achieve positive long-term outcomes. Bringing nurturing programs into the schools and providing follow-up for as long as two years [80] make it possible to achieve optimal results.

Parenting education, nutrition, exercise, and creative coping skills form the bases of the Parallel Curriculum for Parent Education and Creative Physical Activity developed by Sadler and Cowlin at the Polly T. McCabe Center in New Haven. Major topics, covered both as cognitive and behavioral material, include the following:

1. Beginnings: introducing class members, listening to birth stories, screening, introduction of life fitness goals, fitness testing, and fitness skills

2. The many roles of new mothers: getting to know the newborn, "Who Am I?" creative arts project (see figure 11.15)

3. Juggling and coping: negotiating day care and other help, juggling games and activities

4. Nutrition for babies and mothers

5. Fitness, inside and out: postpartum health care, contraception, fitness activities

6. Babies and mothers growing and changing: infant growth and development, training effects, creative movement

7. Safety for mothers and babies

8. Health and health care: infant illness and routine health visits, self-expression through movement and art

9. Program evaluation: parenting Jeopardy game, fitness posttest, exam

Parenting Education

Active rather than passive learning, student questions, and "teachable moments" provide young mothers with the opportunity to direct their own knowledge gain. One can cover basic information concerning infant care and maternal adjustment by gently guiding the discussion and

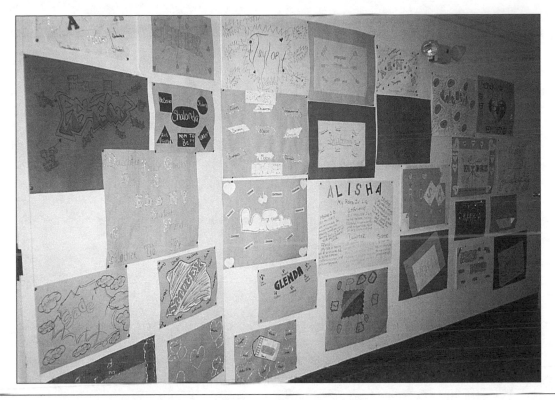

Figure 11.15 Who Am I? An art project for new adolescent mothers. Surrounding their names with their many roles in life — mother, daughter, student, athlete, singer, cousin, friend, niece, girlfriend, etc.—helps new adolescent mothers see what a complex person they have become. Treating this project as an activity of self-discovery produces surprising results, as these examples illustrate.

designing fitness activities that demonstrate fundamental parenting skills, such as safely lifting and carrying an infant. It is important to keep in mind that parent education for this group must take into account the special physical, social, psychological, and cognitive aspects of adolescence. Doing so requires the educator to combine characteristics of adult learners, who like to control their learning and learn from each other, with the drive for skill acquisition that characterizes adolescents. Handling many of the needed skills of parenting as new skills to be acquired through games and activities, and fostering peer mentoring, are two strong methods of bringing the material to life for young mothers.

Nutrition

At a time when it is critical for new mothers to take responsibility for the nutrition of their infants, adolescents themselves rarely have much accurate information about nutrition and often have terrible food habits. The author evaluated the food diaries of postpartum adolescents enrolled in the McCabe program during the 1992-1993 school year and found that they averaged 16% protein, 40% carbohydrate, and 44% fat [107]. Simply learning about food and its nutritional content can be a revelation for this population. Since instituting a nutrition compo-

nent, we have seen dramatic changes in the diets of our students. A number of excellent teaching tools are commercially available for this purpose. Keeping food diaries and analyzing nutritional content are first steps in helping the girls to become educated about nutrition.

Exercise

There are no studies evaluating the impact of exercise programs on the well-being of adolescent mothers and their offspring. However, information from related areas on three important issues helps us form procedures and guidelines for vigorous physical activity:

1. Health screening and prior exercise experience
2. Exercise as a means to parenting and life skill acquisition
3. Exercise as an aid in alleviating depression

It is clearly imperative that young mothers be introduced to postpartum exercise in an appropriate manner. Our experience in screening postpartum girls helped us discover that many had been highly physically active prior to pregnancy, in a variety of activities. The form "Exercise Screening Form for New Adolescent Mothers" can be used to determine the type and extent of prior activity

Exercise Screening Form for New Adolescent Mothers

Name:_____ Age:_____ years

Ethnic background: ☐ White ☐ African American ☐ Hispanic/African American ☐ Hispanic ☐ Asian

Today's date:_____ Grade:_____ (in school)

Baby's name:_____ Check: Boy __ Girl __

Baby's birth date:_____ Weight:___ lbs. ___ oz. Length:___ inches

Baby's gestational age:_____ weeks   Baby's age now:_____ weeks

A. Did your doctor, midwife, or nurse tell you to wait a certain amount of time before starting exercise? ☐ Yes ☐ No
   If yes, how long? _____ weeks

B. Do you have any of these diseases that require constant medical attention?

   Asthma   ☐ Yes ☐ No
   Diabetes   ☐ Yes ☐ No
   Heart disease   ☐ Yes ☐ No
   Severe anemia   ☐ Yes ☐ No
   Thyroid disease   ☐ Yes ☐ No
   Other   ☐ Yes ☐ No If yes, name:_____

C. Do you have any injuries or broken bones? ☐ Yes ☐ No If yes, check all that apply.

   1. Spine ☐   8. Thigh ☐

   2. Neck ☐   9. Knee ☐

   3. Shoulder ☐   10. Lower leg ☐

   4. Upper arm ☐   11. Ankle ☐

   5. Lower arm/elbow ☐   12. Foot ☐

   6. Hand/wrist ☐   13. Head ☐

   7. Pelvis/hip/buttocks ☐

D. In the year before you were pregnant, how many days per week did you participate in sports, dance, cheerleading, gym class, exercise, or other physical activity? ☐ 0 ☐ 1 ☐ 2 ☐ 3 ☐ more than 3

E. Which of these activities did you do regularly?

   1. Aerobics or aerobic dancing ☐   8. Swimming ☐

   2. Running (cross country/track) ☐   9. Jump rope ☐

   3. Walking ☐   10. Dancing or creative movement ☐

   4. Basketball ☐   11. Weightlifting ☐

   5. Softball ☐   12. Cheerleading ☐

   6. Volleyball ☐   13. Drill team ☐

   7. Bicycling ☐   14. Other ☐ name:_____

F. While you were pregnant, how many times per week did you do physical activity or exercise?
   ☐ 1 ☐ 2 ☐ 3 ☐ more than 3

G. Which of these activities did you do regularly?

1. Aerobics or aerobic dancing ☐	8. Swimming ☐
2. Running (cross country/track) ☐	9. Jump rope ☐
3. Walking ☐	10. Dancing or creative movement ☐
4. Basketball ☐	11. Weightlifting ☐
5. Softball ☐	12. Cheerleading ☐
6. Volleyball ☐	13. Drill team ☐
7. Bicycling ☐	14. Other ☐ name:_____

H. Did you continue exercise until your delivery? ☐ Yes ☐ No

I. Did you ever belong to a school sports team? ☐ Yes ☐ No   If yes, which sports? _____

_____

If yes, what grade were you in?
☐ before 7th grade
☐ 7th grade
☐ 8th grade
☐ 9th grade
☐ 10th grade
☐ 11th grade
☐ 12th grade

J. Did you ever belong to a cheerleading squad, drill team, or pep squad? ☐ Yes ☐ No
If yes, what grade were you in?
☐ before 7th grade
☐ 7th grade
☐ 8th grade
☐ 9th grade
☐ 10th grade
☐ 11th grade
☐ 12th grade

K. Did you ever belong to a dance group? ☐ Yes ☐ No   If yes, what grade were you in?
☐ before 7th grade
☐ 7th grade
☐ 8th grade
☐ 9th grade
☐ 10th grade
☐ 11th grade
☐ 12th grade

BMI:_____

A.F. Cowlin, 2002, *Women's fitness program development* (Champaign, IL: Human Kinetics).

in postpartum adolescents, based on our findings of the activities often engaged in by the population served at the McCabe Center. We use these activities as a way of keeping exercise vital in the girls' lives. There are also important teamwork, competition, and negotiation skills that girls can become aware of through games and sports. In addition, they learn kinesthesia, motor skills, and aesthetic sensibilities that contribute to self-image through creative movement, aerobic dancing, resistance training, and flexibility activities. In the same way that students learn to observe a teammate or opponent in the field, they learn to observe their infant as he or she struggles to master the environment.

The other important functions of screening are to ensure that the new mother is not at risk of injury or illness and to assess her emotional state. This is accomplished in the interview process that accompanies the screening. Allowing girls to tell their birth stories, and discretely inquiring into whether they have done Kegel exercises or how their stitches are doing (if they have had surgical procedures), provide a line into their assessment of their experience and the effect on their well-being. Birth is a dramatic physical embarkment point in any woman's life, no less so for an adolescent. We know that both nurturing the new mother and encouraging her to be active provide support and physiological stimulus that may help her make a healthy transition to motherhood.

Creative Coping

Dance movement therapy has been shown to be effective with mothers and young children at risk of abuse when the pair have suffered an interruption in the attachment process but other mother-child relationships in the family system are functioning normally [108]. Creative activities can function in mothers' lives to crystallize real-life issues and provide ways to deal with them in real time. Creative coping is the term used by Sadler and Cowlin to describe their method of assessing critical developmental issues and finding activity structures through which new adolescent mothers can seek ways of coping. Game invention, relaxation techniques, and adapting appropriate youth trends are among the means one can use to accomplish this end. For example, when a girl is learning how to gain control of her abdominal muscles following birth, another young mom who has already learned the techniques is her peer teacher (see figure 11.16). Apart from being a physical activity that engages the attention of both young women, this fosters community and helps the young teacher acquire communications skills. Other examples are playing the Jeopardy game and creating songs or entertainment using information learned about baby safety.

So little attention and so few resources are allocated to adolescent mothers that any effort by health and fit-

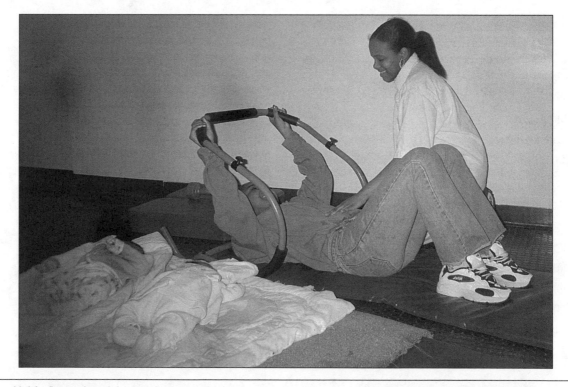

Figure 11.16 Inner-city adolescent mothers participating in a physical activity program. Social support, peer leadership, not being separated from their infants, and being in a safe environment that encourages self-efficacy may allow these young mothers an opportunity to establish healthy habits.

ness professionals willing to invest themselves in improved outcomes is a welcome addition. We are just beginning to find out what works best [109]; more people developing interventions are needed in the field.

LOOKING AHEAD

This part of the text has described giving birth and becoming a mother, powerful identity-forming experiences in a woman's life. In addition, it has presented suggestions about how the fitness field can tap into this powerful phenomenon to create meaningful formats for women's fitness programs and new strategies for assessing fitness benefits. Assisting women in their recovery from pregnancy and birth, helping them develop capabilities needed for parenting, and providing arenas in which they can become both attentive mothers and self-efficacious individuals are goals that truly reflect gender-based fitness programming. The next and last section of the text addresses the process during which women lose their reproductive capacity and face another transition in physical and psychosocial identity: menopause.

REFERENCES

1. Ware, J.R., Jr., and Serbourne, C.D. 1992. The MOS 36-item Short Form Survey (SF-36). Conceptual framework and item selection. *Medical Care* 30:473-483.
2. Shephard, R.J., Thomas, S., and Weller, I. 1991. The Canadian Home Fitness Test: 1991 Update. *Sports Medicine* 11:356-366.
3. American College of Sports Medicine and American Heart Association. 1998. Recommendations for cardiovascular screening, staffing and emergency policies at health/fitness facilities. *Medicine and Science in Sports and Exercise* 30:1009-1018.
4. American College of Sports Medicine. 2000. *ACSM's guidelines for graded exercise testing and prescription*, 6th ed. Baltimore: Lippincott Williams and Wilkins.
5. Tulman, L., and Fawcett, J. 1988. Return of functional ability after childbirth. *Nursing Research* 37:77-81.
6. Varney, H. 1996. *Varney's midwifery*, 3rd ed. Boston: Jones & Bartlett, p. 769.
7. Vullo, U.J., Richardson, J.K., and Hurvitz, E.A. 1996. Hip, knee and foot pain during pregnancy and the postpartum period. *Journal of Family Practice* 43(1):63-68.
8. Dumas, G.A., and Reid, J.G. 1997. Laxity of knee cruciate ligaments during pregnancy. *The Journal of Orthopaedic and Sports Physical Therapy* 26(1):2-6.
9. Huston, L.J., and Wojtys, E.M. 1996. Neuromuscular performance characteristics in elite female athletes. *American Journal of Sports Medicine* 24(4):427-436.
10. Kyman, W. 1991. Maternal satisfaction with the birth experience. *Journal of Social Behavior and Personality* 6:57-70.
11. Campbell, S.B., and Cohn, J.F. 1991. Prevalence and correlates of postpartum depression in first-time mothers. *Journal of Abnormal Psychology* 100:594-599.
12. Hill, P.D., Ledbetter, R.J., and Kavanaugh, K.L. 1997. Breastfeeding patterns of low-birth-weight infants after hospital discharge. *Journal of Obstetric, Gynecologic, and Neonatal Nursing* 26:187-197.
13. Lederman, R.P., Weingarten, C.T., and Lederman, E. 1981. Postpartum self-evaluation questionnaire: Measures of maternal adaptation. In R.P. Lederman, B.S. Raff, and P. Carrol (eds.), *Perinatal parental behavior: Nursing research and implications for newborn health*. NY: Alan R. Liss, Inc.
14. Halman, L.J., Oakley, D., and Lederman, R. 1995. Adaptation to pregnancy and motherhood among subfecund and fecund primiparous women. *Maternal-Child Nursing Journal* 23:90-100.
15. Reece, S.M. 1995. Stress and maternal adaptation in first-time mothers more than 35 years old. *Applied Nursing Research* 8:61-66.
16. Cohler, B.J., Weiss, J.L., and Grunebaum, H. In J. Touliatos, B.F. Perlmutter, and M.A. Straus (eds.). 1990. *Handbook of family measurement techniques*. Newbury Park, CA: Sage.
17. Kamarck, T.W., Shiffman, S.M., Smithline, L., Goodie, J.L., Paty, J.A., Gnys, M., and Jong, J.Y. 1998. Effects of task strain social conflict, and emotional activation on ambulatory cardiovascular activity: Daily life consequences of recurring stress in a multiethnic adult sample. *Health Psychology* 17:17-29.
18. Sampselle, C.M., Miller, J.M., Mims, B.L., DeLancey, J.O., Ashton-Miller, J.A., and Antonakos, C.L. 1998. Effect of pelvic muscle exercise on transient incontinence during pregnancy and after birth. *Obstetrics and Gynecology* 91(3):406-412.
19. Levine, D., and Whittle, M.W. 1996. The effects of pelvic movement on lumbar lordosis in the standing position. *The Journal of Orthopaedic and Sports Physical Therapy* 24(3):130-135.
20. Van der Net, J., van der Hoeven, H., Esseveld, F., de Wilde, E.J., Kuis, W., and Holders, P.J. 1995. Musculoskeletal disorders in juvenile onset mixed connective tissue disease. *Journal of Rheumatology* 22:751-757.
21. Fawcett, J., and York, R. 1986. Spouses' physical and psychological symptoms during pregnancy and the postpartum period. *Nursing Research* 35:144-148.
22. Richards, J.S., Nepomuceno, C., Riles, M., and Suer, Z. 1982. Assessing pain behavior: The UAB Pain Behavior Scale. *Pain* 14:393-396.
23. Sweigard, L. 1974. Skeletal deviations identified in postural alignment. Chapter 17 in *Human movement potential*. NY: UPA.
24. Beck, C.T. 1995. Perceptions of nurses' caring by mothers experiencing postpartum depression. *Journal of Obstetric, Gynecologic, and Neonatal Nursing* 24:819-825.
25. Beck, C.T. 1995. Screening methods for postpartum depression. *Journal of Obstetric, Gynecologic, and Neonatal Nursing* 24:308-312.
26. Cramer, B. 1994. Are postpartum depressions a mother-infant relationship disorder? *Infant Mental Health Journal* 14(4):283-297.
27. Campbell, S.B., and Cohn, J.F. 1991. Prevalence and correlates of postpartum depression in first-time mothers. *Journal of Abnormal Psychology* 100:594-599.
28. Chalmers, B. 1991. Changing childbirth custom. *Pre- and Peri-Natal Psychology* 5:221-232.
29. Bucks, R.S., Williams, A., Whitfield, M.J., and Routh, D.A. 1990. Towards a typology of general practitioners' attitudes toward general practice. *Social Science and Medicine* 30:537-547.
30. Nowak, K.M. 1989. Coping style, cognitive hardiness, and health status. *Journal of Behavioral Medicine* 12:145-158.
31. Chalmers, B. 1987. Black women's birth experiences: Changing traditions. *Journal of Psychosomatic Obstetrics and Gynecology* 6:211-224.
32. Chalmers, B. 1987. The Pedi woman's experiences of childbirth and early parenthood: A summary of major findings. *Curations* 11:12-19.
33. Like, R., and Zyzanski, S.J. 1987. Patient satisfaction with the clinical encounter: Social psychological determinants. *Social Science and Medicine* 24:351-357.
34. Sechrist, K.R., Walker, S.N., and Pender, N.J. 1987. Development and psychometric evaluation of the exercise benefits/barriers scale. *Research in Nursing & Health* 10:357-365.

35. Shimizu, Y.M., and Kaplan, B.J. 1987. Postpartum depression in the United States and Japan. *Journal of Cross-Cultural Psychology* 18:15-30.

36. Murdaugh, C., and Hinshaw, A.S. 1986. Theoretical model testing to identify personality variables effecting preventive behaviors. *Nursing Research* 35:19-23.

37. Good, M.J.D., Bood, B.J., and Nassi, A.J. 1983. Patient requests in primary health care settings: Development and validation of a research instrument. *Journal of Behavioral Medicine* 6:151.

38. Fishwick, N.J. 1998. Assessment of women for partner abuse. *Journal of Obstetric, Gynecologic, and Neonatal Nursing* 27:661-670.

39. Ragozine, J.E. 1998. Abuse during pregnancy. The role of the nurse practitioner. *Contemporary Nurse Practitioner* 3(1):3-10.

40. Feldhaus, K.M., Kosiol-McLain, J., Amsbury, H.L., Norton, I.M., Lowenstein, S.R., and Abbott, J.T. 1997. Accuracy of 3 brief screening questions for detecting partner violence in the emergency department. *Journal of the American Medical Association* 277:1357-1361.

41. Furniss, K. 1993. Screening for abuse in the clinical setting. *AWHONN's Clinical Issues* 14:402-405.

42. American Medical Association. 1992. A.M.A. diagnostic and treatment guidelines on domestic violence. *Archives of Family Medicine* 1:39-47.

43. McCoy, D.L. (n.d.). *Sexual abuse screening inventory.* Odessa, FL: Psychological Assessment Resources.

44. Hardy, H.M., and Boyer, B.J. 1993. Gender differences in attributions for triathlon performance. *Sex Roles* 29:527-543.

45. Pridham, K.F., Lytton, D., Chang, A.S., and Rutledge, D. 1991. Early postpartum transition: Progress in maternal identity and role attainment. *Research in Nursing & Health* 14:21-31.

46. O'Hara, M.W., Varner, M.W., and Johnson, S.R. 1986. Assessing stressful life events associated with childbearing: The peripartum events scale. *Journal of Reproductive and Infant Psychology* 4:85-98.

47. Pridham, K.F., and Schutz, M.E. 1983. Parental goals and the birthing experience. *Journal of Obstetric, Gynecologic, and Neonatal Nursing* 12:50-55.

48. Simer, M.M. 1983. Effects of information on postsurgical coping. *Nursing Research* 32:282-287.

49. Hodnett, E. 1982. Patient control during labor: Effects of two types of fetal monitors. *Journal of Obstetric, Gynecologic, and Neonatal Nursing* 2:94-99.

50. Lundy, B., Field, T., McBride, C., Abrams, S., and Carraway, K. 1997. Child psychiatric patients' interactions with their mothers. *Child Psychiatry and Human Development* 27:231-240.

51. Kim, M.M., O'Connor, K.S., McLean, J., Robson, A., and Chance, G. 1996. Do parents and professionals agree on the developmental status of high-risk infants? *Pediatrics* 97:676-681.

52. Campbell, S.B., Cohn, J.F., and Meyers, T. 1995. Depression in first-time mothers: Mother-infant interaction and depression chronicity. *Developmental Psychology* 31:349-357.

53. Catalano, P.M., Thomas, A.J., Availone, D.A., and Amini, S.B. 1995. Anthropometric estimation of neonatal body composition. *American Journal of Obstetrics and Gynecology* 173:1176-1181.

54. Newcomb, P.A., Storer, B.E., Longnecker, M.P., Mittendorf, R., Greenberg, E.R., Clapp, R.W., Burke, K.P., Willett, W.C., and MacMahon, B. 1994. Lactation and a reduced risk of premenopausal breast cancer. *New England Journal of Medicine* 330:81-87.

55. DePietro, J.A., Porges, S.W., and Uhly, B. 1992. Reactivity and developmental competence in preterm and full-term infants. *Developmental Psychology* 28:831-841.

56. Matthews, M.K. 1988. Developing an instrument to assess infant breastfeeding behaviour in the early neonatal period. *Midwifery* 4:154-165.

57. Seefeldt, V.D., and Harrison, G.G. 1988. Infants, children and youth. In T.G. Lohman, A.F. Roche, and R. Martorell (eds.), *An-thropometric standardization reference manual.* Champaign, IL: Human Kinetics, pp. 111-114.

58. Aberman, S., and Kirchhoff, K.T. 1985. Infant-feeding practices. *Journal of Obstetric, Gynecologic, and Neonatal Nursing* 14:394-398.

59. Mandl, K.D., Brennan, T.A., Wise, P.H., Tronick, E.Z., and Homer, C.J. 1997. Maternal and infant health. *Archives of Pediatrics and Adolescent Medicine* 151:915-921.

60. Koniak-Griffin, D., Ludington-Hoe, S., and Verzemnieks, I. 1995. Longitudinal effects of unimodal and multimodal stimulation on development and interaction of healthy infants. *Research in Nursing & Health* 18:27-38.

61. Seidman, E., LaRue, A., Aber, J.L., Mitchell, C., Feinman, J., Yoshikawa, H., Comtois, K.A., Golz, J., Miller, R.L., and Ortiz-Torres, B. 1995. Development and validation of adolescent-perceived microsystem scales: Social support, daily hassles, and involvement. *American Journal of Community Psychology* 23(3):355-388.

62. Spieker, S.J., and Bensley, L. 1994. Roles of living arrangements and grandmother social support in adolescent mothering and infant attachment. *Developmental Psychology* 30:102-111.

63. Ray, J. 1993. Survival methods of young street mothers. *Child and Adolescent Social Work Journal* 10:189-205.

64. Elsen, M., Zellman, G.L., and McAlister, A.L. 1992. A health belief model-social learning theory approach to adolescents' fertility control: Findings from a controlled field trial. *Health Education Quarterly* 19:249-262.

65. Fienup-Riordan, A. 1980. *Shape up with baby.* Seattle: the pennypress.

66. Olkin, S.K. 1992. *Positive parenting fitness.* Garden City Park, NY: Avery.

67. Whiteford, B., and Polden, M. 1984. *The postnatal exercise book.* NY: Pantheon.

68. Young, K. 1984. *Exercise can be child's play.* NY: Thomas Nelson Pub.

69. Dewey, K.G., Lovelady, C.A., Nommsen-Rivers, L.A., McCrory, M.A., and Lonnerdal, B. 1994. A randomized study of the effects of aerobic exercise by lactating women on breast milk volume and composition. *New England Journal of Medicine* 330(7):449-453.

70. Lovelady, C.A., Lonnerdal, B., and Dewey, K.B. 1990. Lactation performance of exercising women. *American Journal of Clinical Nutrition* 52:103-109.

71. Hale, R.W., and Milne, L. 1996. The elite athlete and exercise in pregnancy. *Seminars in Perinatology* 20(4):277-284.

72. Wallace, J.P., and Rabin, J. 1991. The concentration of lactic acid in breast milk following maximal exercise. *International Journal of Sports Medicine* 3:328-331.

73. Wallace, J.P., and Rabin, J. 1986. The accumulation of lactic acid in mother's milk following maximal exercise. *Medicine and Science in Sports and Exercise* 18:S47.

74. Wallace, J.P., Inbart, G., and Ernsthausen, K. 1992. Infant acceptance of postexercise breast milk. *Pediatrics* 89(6):1245-1247.

75. Carey, G.B., Quinn, T.J., and Goodwin, S.E. 1997. Breast milk composition after exercise of different intensities. *Journal of Human Lactation* 13(2):115-120.

76. Fly, A.D., Uhlin, K.L., and Wallace, J.P. 1998. Major mineral concentrations in human milk do not change after maximal exercise testing. *American Journal of Clinical Nutrition* 68(2):345-349.

77. Gregory, R.L., Wallace, J.P., Gfell, L.E., Marks, J., and King, B.A. 1997. Effect of exercise on milk immunoglobin A. *Medicine and Science in Sports and Exercise* 29(12):1596-1601.

78. Dewey, K.G. 1998. Effects of maternal caloric restriction and exercise during lactation. *Journal of Nutrition* 128(2 Suppl):386S-389S.

79. Little, K.D., and Clapp, J.F., 3rd. 1998. Self-selected recreational exercise has no impact on early postpartum lactation-induced bone

loss. *Medicine and Science in Sports and Exercise* 30(6):831-836.

80. East, P., and Felice, M. 1996. *Adolescent pregnancy and parenting*. Mahwah, NJ: Lawrence Erlbaum.

81. Brooks-Gunn, J., and Chase Lansdale, P.L. 1995. Adolescent parenthood. In M.H. Bornstein (ed.), *Handbook of parenting: Status and social conditions of parenting*, Vol. 3. Mahwah, NJ: Lawrence Erlbaum.

82. Sadler, L.S. 1988. The adolescent parent. In M.-A. Corbett and J.H. Meyer (eds.), *The adolescent and pregnancy*. Boston: Blackwell Scientific.

83. Bachrach, C.A., Clogg, C.C., and Carber, K. 1993. Outcomes of early childbearing. *Journal of Research on Adolescence* 3(4):337-349.

84. Baldwin, W. 1993. The consequences of early childbearing: A perspective. *Journal of Research on Adolescence* 3(4):349-353.

85. Geronimus, A., and Korenman, S. 1992. The socioeconomic consequences of teen childbearing reconsidered. *Quarterly Journal of Economics* 107.1187-1214.

86. Horwitz, S.M., Klerman, L.V., Kuo, H.S., and Jekel, J.F. 1991. School-age mothers: Predictors of long-term educational and economic outcomes. *Pediatrics* 87(6):862-867.

87. Upchurch, D.M., and McCarthy, J. 1990. The timing of first birth and high school completion. *American Sociological Review* 55(2):224-234.

88. Furstenberg, F.F., Jr., Brooks-Gunn, J., and Morgan, P. 1987. *Adolescent mothers in later life*. NY: Cambridge University Press.

89. Brooks-Gunn, J., and Furstenberg, F.F., Jr. 1986. Antecedents and consequences of parenting: The case of adolescent motherhood. In A. Fogel and G.F. Melson (eds.), *Origins of nurturance: Developmental, biological and cultural perspectives on caregiving*. Hillsdale, NJ: Lawrence Erlbaum.

90. Coll, C.G., Vohr, B.R., Hoffman, J., and Oh, W. 1986. Maternal and environmental factors affecting developmental outcomes of infants of adolescent mothers. *Journal of Developmental and Behavioral Pediatrics* 7:230-236.

91. Sadler, L.S. 1997. *The process of intergenerational child rearing among urban African American adolescent mothers and grandmothers during the transition to parenthood*. Unpublished Doctoral Dissertation, University of Connecticut, Storrs, CT.

92. Baydar, N., and Brooks-Gunn, J. 1998. Profiles of grandmothers who help care for their grandchildren in the United States. *Family Relations* 47(4):385-393.

93. Pope, S., Casey, P., Bradley, R., and Brooks-Gunn, J. 1993. The effect of intergenerational factors on the development of low birth weight infants born to adolescent mothers. *Journal of the American Medical Association* 269(11):1396-1400.

94. Apfel, N., and Seitz, V. 1991. Four models of adolescent mother-grandmother relationships in black inner city families. *Family Relations* 40:421-429.

95. Osofsky, J.D., Eberhart-Wright, A., and Ware, L.M. 1992. Children of adolescent mothers: A group at risk for psychopathology. *Infant Mental Health Journal* 13(2):119-131.

96. Carter, S.L., Osofsky, J.D., and Hann, D.M. 1991. Speaking for the baby: A therapeutic intervention with adolescent mothers and their infants. *Infant Mental Health Journal* 12(4):291-301.

97. Luster, T., and Dubow, E. 1990. Predictors of the quality of the home environment that adolescent mothers provide for their school-aged children. *Journal of Youth and Adolescence* 19(5):475-495.

98. Van Cleve, S.N., and Sadler, L.S. 1990. Adolescent parents and toddlers: Strategies for intervention. *Public Health Nursing* 7(1):22-27.

99. Leadbeater, B.J., and Linares, O. 1992. Depressive symptoms in Black and Puerto Rican adolescent mothers in the first 3 years postpartum. *Development and Psychopathology* 4(3):451-468.

100. Gutierrez, J. and Sameroff, A. 1990. Determinants of complexity in Mexican-American and Anglo-American mothers' conceptions of child development. *Child Development* 61:384-394.

101. Garcia Coll, C.T. 1989. The consequences of teenage childbearing in traditional Puerto Rican culture. In J.K. Nugent, B.M. Lester, and T.B. Brazelton (eds.), *The cultural context of infancy: Biology, culture and infant development*, Vol. 1. Norwood, NJ: Ablex.

102. Field, T., Widmayer, S.M., Stringer, S., and Ignatoff, E. 1980. Teenage, lower-class, Black mothers and their preterm infants: An intervention and developmental follow-up. *Child Development* 51:426-436.

103. Chase-Lansdale, P.L., Brooks-Gunn, J., and Paikoff, R.L. 1991. Research and programs for adolescent mothers: Missing links and future promises. *Family Relations* 40(4):396-404.

104. Sadler, L.S., and Catrone, C. 1983. The Adolescent parent: A dual developmental crisis. *Journal of Adolescent Health Care* 4(2):100-105.

105. Seitz, V., and Apfel, N. 1994. Effects of a school for pregnant students on the incidence of low birthweight deliveries. *Child Development* 65:666-676.

106. Seitz, V., and Apfel, N. 1993. Adolescent mothers and repeated childbearing: Effects of a school-based intervention program. *American Journal of Orthopsychiatry* 63:572-581.

107. Cowlin, A.F. 1994. Nutritional intake of new adolescent mothers. Data presented at the NOAPPP 1998 Conference. Denver, CO.

108. Meekums, B. 1991. Dance/movement therapy with mothers and young children at risk of abuse. *Arts in Psychotherapy* 18(3):223-230.

109. Seitz, V., and Apfel, N. 1999. Effective interventions for adolescent mothers. *Clinical Psychology: Science and Practice* 6(1)50-66.

PART IV

MENOPAUSE

Some women have been physically active all their lives, have eaten well, have cared for themselves (physically, fiscally, mentally, and spiritually), and thus arrive in midlife with many resources to undergo yet another change in form and identity. At the other end of the spectrum, some women arrive with few resources. Of course, most women arrive somewhere in between. Some women are protected from certain diseases by their exercise history; others are threatened. Some understand the physiological issues, and others know only their emotional responses. Some seek a magic bullet; others choose a more complex path. Some spend time and money on this phenomenon while others do not; some seek assistance in the counsel of women while others are stoic. In addition, all have been bombarded by cultural images and power structures that affect their outlook on this time. And all of the factors are profoundly affected by heredity.

This part of the book consists of three chapters. The first considers menopause from cultural, physiological, and psychosocial perspectives, as well as the ways in which physical activity affects the forces acting on women beginning in midlife. The second chapter establishes goals and priorities of fitness programs for this population. The final chapter makes suggestions about program design, provides a sample midlife program format, and concludes by looking ahead to the challenge of creating new fitness programs for women.

CHAPTER 12

UNDERSTANDING MENOPAUSE

This chapter starts by describing menopause from the medical and anthropological points of view, then defines the biological phases of menopause. Next, it reviews the major physiological changes that occur, as well as signs, symptoms, and conditions associated with the midlife change in reproductive status. Following a discussion of psychosocial considerations, the chapter concludes by presenting approaches commonly used in dealing with the changes associated with menopause.

Except for the human species, female mammals are fertile throughout their life span. Does human menopause occur as a sign of impending death? Is the job of estrogen that of protecting the eggs by protecting their vehicle, the female? Once there are no more eggs, is there no reason for estrogen to continue protecting the female? Is the postmenopausal woman merely the result of an increasing life span in humans? Is menopause a disorder, something to be treated as an illness? Is it logical to replace the missing estrogens, progesterones, and androgens in order to maintain the female as though she were still fertile?

On the other hand, could postmenopausal women have evolved for a reason? Pregnancy in the fifth decade means dependent children through the sixth and seventh decades, or the possibility of orphans. Can the human animal have adapted to prevent this? What evolutionary function might postmenopausal women serve? Might postmenopausal women be a benefit to the survival of the species?

Medicine asks the question: How shall we best *treat* menopause? Anthropology asks the question: What *func-tion* does postmenopause serve? Matters are complicated by the fact that different cultures define and experience a midlife change differently (some don't recognize it as a separate event), and women within a given culture have varying experiences. Beyond the cessation of ovulation and menstruation, the idea that there is one definition of Menopause, the Event and the Experience, is not workable [1-5]. However, as in all the stages of a woman's life, there are landmarks—feelings and events we often call symptoms—that many women experience and talk about.

DEFINING MENOPAUSE

Mary Ellen Rousseau points out that the only universal change associated with women's midlife period is the cessation of menstruation [6]. Studies of gynecological status, health behaviors, well-being, and somatic symptoms conducted in Sweden [7], Australia [8], and Great Britain [9] each demonstrated that there is very little correlation among these factors in midlife women. The clinical changes that occur can be quite remarkable, but it is important to see them in a cultural and personal context [2, 3, 10, 11]. In Western medicine, the process is considered to have three major phases: perimenopause, menopause, and postmenopause. Before a woman becomes perimenopausal, she is considered premenopausal, or "normal."

Perimenopause

Various terms are used in conjunction with the changing gynecological status. The term *climacteric,* taken from the Greek, refers to the process of climbing the rungs of a ladder and finishing with the cessation of menstruation altogether, the whole process taking about 10 years. It is an interesting concept, but as sometimes happens with constructs coming from the medical model, it does not always harmonize with women's experience. It is simply too linear. In the later decades of the 20th century, the term *perimenopause* found its way into the medical and popular vernaculars, and it seems to have caught on as a way of delineating the time in which women and their care providers identify changes.

A woman is born with a few million follicles but will ovulate only about 400 to 500 times during her reproductive years. In her late 30s, the development of fewer follicles leads to anovulatory cycles and elongated periods, and by her 40s, anovulatory cycles occur more often [12]. Hormonally, elevations in follicle stimulating hormone (FSH) and decreases in inhibin occur as follicle ripening and ovulation become less frequent. Changes in receptor sites—including those in the cardiovasculature and skeleton—also accompany endocrine changes. As estrogen and progesterone decrease, shortened luteal phases and other menstrual irregularities increase. In addition, gonadotropin production is no longer inhibited, so luteinizing hormone (LH) and FSH rise dramatically, FSH to higher levels than LH. At this point women are technically considered *perimenopausal.* Levels of FSH and LH remain high for some time and stabilize after the cessation of menstruation.

Menopause

The depletion of productive follicles means that ovulation can no longer take place. Although anovulatory cycles may proceed for a while, there is generally a lessening of menstrual flow *(hypomenorrhea)* and then cessation [13]. Frequent or heavier periods *(hypermenorrhea)* are experienced for a while by some women when follicular estrogen production continues, but this should be monitored for possible endometrial hyperplasia, an indication that there is a potential for cancer to develop. The exact pattern varies greatly from individual to individual. But at some point, a woman becomes amenorrheic—that is, without menses.

Once a woman has been amenorrheic for a full year, she is considered to have attained menopause. For some time, the mean age for natural menopause in the West has been around 51 years of age [14-18]. However, the ages at which women stop menstruating for good cover a wide span. It is common to stop from age 45 to age 55, but some women cease menses as early as the late 30s or as late as the early 60s.

Although the reactions of Western women to this process of change can be profound, the experience was not perceived as negative by most women in at least one large longitudinal study, the Massachusetts Women's Health Study [14]. The impression that menopause causes mental distress and depression may be an artifact because the population that seeks help for difficulties has been studied more than the population that does not seek help. The idea that menopause is a negative experience does not coincide with information from the general population [1, 19, 20]. It is important to remind ourselves that change is a process with which women are familiar.

Surgical menopause results from a *complete* or *radical hysterectomy,* in which a woman's ovaries *(oophorectomy)* and cervix, as well as her uterus, have been removed; as a result she becomes menopausal. In general, she will be treated with hormone replacement therapy (HRT) unless there is a high risk of estrogen-dependent cancer. If a woman undergoes a *partial hysterectomy,* she has lost her uterus but not her ovaries, or perhaps only one ovary. In this case, treatment will vary, as she still has a source of the endogenous gonadal hormones, estrogen and progesterone.

Postmenopause

In the years after menopause, a woman's body continues to make adjustments. The concept of menopause as reproductive aging in women, or the physiological decline in the function of the hypothalamic-pituitary-ovarian axis, is a product of 20th-century medicine. From this perspective, once a woman is no longer a viable receptacle for the male's DNA, she is viewed as aging or declining, and all of the somatic consequences are seen as deteriorations. The idea that this condition can be cured or treated through medical intervention—much like type 1 diabetes—has been a popular medical perspective since at least the 1960s when Wilson published *Feminine Forever* [21]. However, as evidence about the nature of aging in both women and men is gathered, new questions are being raised about the relationship between menopause and aging: Does one cause the other? Are they aspects of the same biological phenomenon?

The anthropological perspective that menopause is an evolutionary adaptation with advantages for women, their offspring, and the community has been difficult to demonstrate. Early attempts to demonstrate such an effect were tied to the benefit for children in the direct lineage. However, in 1997 Hawkes, O'Connell, and Blurton Jones published their work on postmenopausal women of the Hadza tribe in Tanzania, giving impetus to the idea that senior females who are not fertile provide a hunter-gatherer community with a desirable evolutionary advantage for offspring survival. By not tying the grandmother's contribution to the children in her direct line, the authors showed that the superior ability of postmenopausal women to gather edible food, as well as to maintain information that is useful over the long run (wisdom), benefited children in the extended family and the larger community [22].

One of the researchers' observations involved the ability of the older women to spend 7 or 8 hours a day in the strenuous job of gathering food. Once children become independent, if life is vigorous, might the protection that estrogen provides during the childbearing and nurturing years (when physical activity decreases as women nurse and oversee children's welfare) be unnecessary? Given the trend toward contemporary sedentary existence, one is forced to ask about the nature of postmenopausal disorders such as heart disease, loss of muscle mass, osteoporosis, and diabetes. Can these be as much disorders of aging in an unhealthy, sedentary population as the result of a change in reproductive status?

PHYSIOLOGICAL CHANGES ASSOCIATED WITH MENOPAUSE

Whatever a woman elects to do in response to the changes that occur in her midlife period, the more information she has about the generic process, about individual variations, and about methods for dealing with symptoms, the more control she can exert over the quality of her life. Given the profound influence that culture has on the way the menopausal process is perceived and experienced, it is no surprise that in the West the biological aspects of the midlife process have been dissected, researched, and analyzed and that the odds have been determined for a multitude of events. Consequently, these findings form a large portion of the information we use to screen clients, develop appropriate exercise programs, and create support structures for midlife clients.

Changes in Hormone Production

In addition to the previously outlined changes in LH and FSH during the perimenopausal period, the levels of estrogen and progesterone produced by the ovaries decrease, while androstenedione and testosterone production is maintained for a further period of time before decreasing [23]. These hormonal changes mean that androgens are present in a much higher proportion in relation to female hormones than previously. Androgens are responsible for maintaining the libido, which women may find reassuring. This change in proportion may also be responsible for some change in mental state and emotional tone. At this time, organs other than the ovaries increase their production of the weaker estrogens, which have important functions of their own and in large quantities can form building blocks for stronger estrogens. The adrenal glands, skin, muscles, brain, pineal gland, hair follicles, and body fat are all involved in taking over the role of hormone production.

Of the three types of estrogens (estrone or E1, estradiol or E2, and estriol or E3), the estradiols—which predominate in premenopausal women—are the strongest and carry the greatest heart and bone protection characteristics (particularly 17-beta estradiol). The loss of estradiol is generally considered responsible for many of the effects associated with menopause. Prior to menopause, in addition to being produced by the ovaries, estradiol is produced by the corpus luteum and by the placenta in pregnancy. Estradiol can be metabolized from estrone (and vice versa), the estrogen associated with postmenopause. Converted from androstenedione in the fat cells, estrone is derived with greater efficiency as weight [24, 25] and age [26] increase.

Increased rates of heart disease, osteoporosis, autoimmune disorders, Alzheimer's, and other conditions have been attributed to the loss of estrogen during the perimenopausal process, and a degree of protection from these conditions has been attributed to HRT. But the situation is not as simple as direct cause and effect. Midlife brings with it a cascade of metabolic events, any one of which may have a number of innervations and can be altered at many stages.

A complex of mechanisms is in motion in the female body during menopause. In coronary artery disease (CAD), for example, adverse effects of dyslipidemia—independent of the loss of estrogen protection—have been demonstrated through research explicating the role of diabetes in causing CAD in premenopausal women [27]. To elevate high-density lipoprotein (HDL) and lose central obesity (two risk factors for CAD associated with dyslipidemia), women require exercise, unlike men, who require only a proper diet [28]. During menopause, if we add estrogen in order to elevate HDL, the risk of uterine cancer increases, so we must also add progesterone. But, whereas estrogen is protective of HDL, progesterone has the opposite effect. Complexities are also apparent for hormone replacement and cancer, as well as other conditions. And, until studies involve large numbers of healthy, active women who have proceeded through menopause with a variety of hormone strategies and even without hormone therapy, the picture will continue to be incomplete.

Progesterones, which often act as modulators or antagonists of estrogens—as well as stimulating secretions of their own and providing their own benefits and detriments—also decrease in the perimenopausal and postmenopausal periods. The shortened luteal phase associated with anovulation may actually cause decreased progesterone levels, and resulting menstrual irregularities can be one of the first signals that reproductive status is changing.

Aging and Menopause

Interestingly, the effects of spaceflight on hormone function provide insight into the relationship between aging and changes in reproductive status, as well as helping us understand why weight-bearing and resistance exercise play critical roles in lessening the effects of aging and menopause. The operational factor influencing endocrine function during spaceflight appears to be the absence of the force of gravity. This factor affects a number of endocrine subsystems (including the hypothalamic-pituitary-gonadal axis, the hypothalamic-pituitary-adrenal axis, the hypothalamic-pituitary-somatomammotrophic axis, the hypothalamic-pituitary-thyroid axis, and the renin-angiotensin-aldosterone axis [regulating water and electrolytes]), as well as bone demineralization, anemia, insulin resistance, and the sympathetic system [29]. In space, some endocrine systems—particularly those regulating bone and muscle metabolism and reproduction—undergo changes that resemble functional aging, but recovery always occurs within weeks or months of the return to gravity [29]. Malfunction also occurs in space with immune, neurosensory, and cardiovascular systems [29]. The human body has adapted over many thousands of years to function in the force field of gravity. Antigravity exertion affects biochemical and biomechanical functions, playing a mitigating role in the development of symptoms associated with aging and menopause.

Does this mean we should see later menopause in women who have done weight-bearing exercise regularly for most of their lives up to this point? In at least one study on the effects of exercise in various life stages, no significant relationship was found between the degree of exercise in life stages and the age at menopause [30]. We know from evidence presented in previous chapters that, actually, large doses of strenuous exercise at a young age may result in premature menopause and accelerations of aging symptoms such as osteoporosis.

On the other hand, the degree of a woman's psychosomatic symptoms in perimenopause has been found to be inversely related to the degree of exercise from her 30s on (less exercise produced greater feelings of "weakness") and from her 40s on ("nervousness" and "melancholia") [30]. The researchers also concluded that the greater the degree of exercise from her 40s on, the lesser the degree of a woman's symptoms after menopause, and that exercising moderately from the subjective point of view in the perimenopausal period may alleviate symptoms [30]. The first menstrual irregularities frequently appear when a woman is in her late 40s, but asymptomatic hormonal fluctuations and anovulatory cycles begin sooner, often in the 30s. By perimenopause, a woman may be well into the period that triggers the need for concerted antigravity exertion to fend off the effects of menopause and aging.

But what about underlying biological mechanisms? Navarro et al. have put forth the notion that the basic muscle cell aging processes and cell adaptive mechanisms that result in sarcopenia (age-related loss of muscle mass caused by the decline in protein turnover)—especially mitochondrial production of free radicals and their secondary effects—may help explain other adverse cellular changes [31]. Basic cell aging results from intrinsic changes in the cell, but also from shifts in hormonal and neurotransmitter signals, affecting the response of skeletal muscle to exercise [31]. Both exercise and hormone replacement may be important mechanisms for slowing the age-related decline in protein turnover [32, 33].

The relationship among aging, menopause, and disease is a complex tangle of interrelated processes. Myriad questions about aging itself remain to be answered, as well as about how aging relates to menopause and disease. As we learn more about human biology, the questions become more convoluted. Is aging a process separate from disease? Is the underlying rate of aging a phenomenon distinct from the effects of disease, and does it begin in the 30s, as has been suggested [34]? What do sex differences tell us about aging and menopause? Research on macronutrient self-selection in aging mice, for example, shows that females increase protein intake during and after exercise [35]. What does this mean to our understanding of the role of nutrition in menopause? Is research separating disorders associated with aging, disease, and menopause, or is it driving them together? What does it mean that neuronal-type glutamate receptors in bone have been identified, and that communication within the bony system is similar and/or connected to that within the central nervous system [36]? Could the loss of estrogen cause or contribute to osteoporosis and Alzheimer's disease as part of the same mechanism? Are they separate diseases related to aging? Is it possible both things are true?

Technology is helping drive knowledge and systematic thinking about the human body into a realm women find easy to accept: the addition of horizontal connections of phenomena to the vertical or hierarchical structure that has long been the underpinning of science. As women, we are prepared to accept yet another complicated network of meaning. We understand that menopause is one more transition phase during which we move into another body. It is interesting to step back from the details and look at the emerging large picture. The striking feature that comes into focus as we step back is the fact that resisting inertia helps keep us alive, both literally (e.g., lifting weights) and figuratively (e.g., reaching out to horizontal sources of information such as sisters, friends, or the Internet for new information about breast cancer, then taking that information up the chain of health care).

SIGNS, SYMPTOMS, AND DISORDERS

Family history, genetics, lifestyle, and individual responses play roles in how a woman's hormonal changes proceed. Even though there is no universal pattern of experience, there are a number identifiable characteristics that many women experience in response to changing hormones. The particular signs, symptoms, and disorders a woman reports can be a window into her hormonal process. Phenomena commonly reported include menstrual irregularities, vasomotor symptoms (hot flashes), vaginal thinning and discomfort, bladder thinning and incontinence, urogenital prolapse, osteoporosis, mental changes, and heart disease. These are described further on in this section. Diabetes is discussed in relation to heart disease. While a number of cancers are associated with midlife, the interactions that occur in relation to the treatment of menopause with hormone replacement are covered in the discussion of *hormone replacement therapy.*

Menstrual Irregularities

The premenopausal period can be marked by menstrual irregularities. Missed cycles, unusually long or short cycles, continuous bleeding, and unusual bleeding patterns are common signs. Both hypomenorrhea and hypermenorrhea symptoms are remarked on with frequency. Their causes have already been outlined. When one catalogues women's experiences, it is striking how different the pattern of changes can be from person to person. Table 12.1 demonstrates these differences, as well as how variously women define their self-assessed stage at similar ages and how they describe their situations, some with the briefest comment and others with detailed characterizations.

Vasomotor Symptoms, or Hot Flashes

Vasomotor symptoms, also called *hot flashes, hot flushes,* or *night sweats,* are probably the most common symptom of a changing gynecological status in Western women. Many women—perhaps 80% or 90%—experience them at some point [37-39]. Temperature regulation requires integration of autonomic, endocrine, and skeletomotor responses in the hypothalamus [40]. The sensation of being overheated is related to the metabolism of the neurotransmitter norepinephrine. Because norepinephrine metabolism is mediated by estrogen in the hypothalamus, and estrogen is at a low ebb, malfunctions in the body's thermostat occur. The condition is aggravated by stress, which results in increased norepinephrine, and generally abates postmenopausally. In addition, the increasing levels of FSH cause altered signals concerning the internal temperature set-point.

Table 12.1 **The Varied Experiences of Menstruation Associated With Midlife**

Case	Age and self-assessed status	Description of menstrual cycles
1	51 and menopausal	8 years of long, heavy periods lasting 2-4 months, then skip a month or two; Provera would organize them for a while. Then at 49, 1 regular period, followed by 22 months of amenorrhea, then 1 regular period (had endometrial biopsy, no problem; probably ovulated), then amenorrhea since
2	49 and almost perimenopausal	Severe headaches since early 40s; heavy flows; then light flows
3	52 and normal, but hot flashes	Regular
4	50 and perimenopausal	Lighter flows; gained a little weight in the abdomen and can't stand it; stopped a couple months ago; has a feeling that's it
5	50 and perimenopausal	Irregular periods, headaches, tiredness, feet hurt, dry skin

Cowlin, unpublished data.

Waking at night in a heavy sweat can be uncomfortable and annoying. Changing one's clothes and practicing a relaxation technique can have a soothing effect, however. Facial flushing or general feelings of being warm are also common experiences. When one is working with clients who experience these symptoms, it is important to acknowledge that the symptoms are real, that they have a variety of underlying causes, and that a woman can help herself deal with them in several ways.

Hot flashes can be helped by estrogen replacement and/or a diet high in *phytoestrogens* (plant compounds that are weak estrogen precursors, discussed near the end of chapter 14), exercise, and stress management. Black cohosh, the underground roots of the Native American plant, *Cimicifuga racemosa,* has been evaluated in clinical studies and shown to be effective and well tolerated for treatment of hot flashes, sleep disturbances, and depression related to menopause [41, 42]. Susan Cohen, who has conducted research on black cohosh, makes the following observations: placebo-intervention comparison studies have demonstrated that this substance is effective in alleviating symptoms of vaginal atrophy as well as hot flashes and sleep disturbances; black cohosh has been shown to be safe when used for periods of six months; and it is necessary to use a preparation of standardized ethanolic extract of the rhizome to assure the presence of the active ingredient [43, 44]. Vitamin E may also be prescribed by a care provider. Any use of chemical substances, including herbs, must be directed by a qualified professional, and exercise instructors and trainers must take care not to prescribe medicinal substances. Other conditions that may exacerbate hot flashes include hyperthyroidism, alcoholism, diabetes, pregnancy, and premenstrual syndrome.

Vaginal Thinning

Associated with decreased estrogen are changes in the female reproductive tract [13]. The thinning of the vaginal epithelium and an increasingly sparse capillary bed contribute to a change in appearance and reduction of mucus production. Symptoms vary greatly and can be subjective. Some women develop discomfort with sexual intercourse and find topical estrogen and/or progesterone creams or vaginal lubricants helpful. Because sexual activity brings blood to the pelvis and vaginal tissues, sexually active women experience less atrophy than those only using estrogen [6]. It is helpful to remind women that they should use plant-based and not petroleum-based lubricants, as petroleum-based products can prevent the release of natural secretions.

Changes in the vagina can also include susceptibility to opportunistic pathogenic organisms. The decrease in estrogen, exposure to antibiotics, nature and number of an individual's epithelial sites to which various flora may bind, and exposure to pathogens affect the infections that a woman may be subject to [45]. Whether douching represents an actual cause of increased risk for various infections, or instead an association with unsafe sexual practices that are the cause of risk, is uncertain [46]. Nonetheless, douching is associated with increased risk for various disorders, including cervical cancer [46, 47].

Bladder Thinning and Incontinence

Another change that can occur is thinning of the bladder, including the ureter, as well as urinary tract dryness. Urinary urgency and incontinence are also experienced. Detrusor instability—a condition in which the muscle that controls the ureter contracts erratically—is responsible for a high percentage of incontinence and is effectively treated with calcium channel blockers [46]. Urgency can be treated with behavior modification, by having women practice Kegels and wait a few more minutes before heading for the bathroom. Many physical therapy facilities have behavioral modification programs employing this procedure. Stress incontinence is effectively treated by strengthening the muscles of the pelvic floor.

Seeking advice on managing incontinence is difficult for many women. A study of the issue among Australian women indicated that the difficulty may result from women's perception that the incontinence is an inevitable part of being female; the study also showed that women explained the phenomenon in terms of personal history and their own failings [48]. They saw childbirth, menopause, and aging as causes, and saw being overweight or not exercising as personal failings linked to incontinence [48].

Urogenital Prolapse

Problems associated with bladder or uterine prolapse—the bladder or uterus falling through weakened pelvic floor muscles—are not directly related to the reduction in estrogen. Strengthening the pelvic floor muscles may be effective and is almost universally indicated to help improve the situation. Findings in one study showed low levels of collagen in the urogenital organs and skin of women with genital prolapse [49]. Because collagen is responsible for the elastic quality of connective tissue in muscles and tendons, persons with low levels are subject to connective tissue plasticity due to forced stretching, as well as reduced flexibility due to tightness. The researchers found that postmenopausal women with prolapse also had impairment of pulmonary function and concluded that the associating factor may be lack of collagen, as the lungs depend on abundant connective tissue for their capacity to expand and contract [49]. Another study concerned endurance exercise lessening passive stiffness in older mice via the alteration of elastic properties of collagen [50]. Our understanding of these factors is sufficient to make us aware that extreme stiffness, tightness, or damage from overstretching may be an indication to check for prolapse and to refer appropriate cases to physical therapy. In any case, pelvic floor exercises and aerobic exercise are indicated for midlife and older women, but high-impact weight-bearing activities may not be.

Osteoporosis

Progressive loss of bone mineral density (BMD) associated with falls, fractures, and deformities has become epidemic in the United States, due to an increasingly sedentary lifestyle, decreasing parity (number of births per woman), effects of smoking, adverse dietary changes, and the increasing life expectancy [51]. Bone mineral density loss is greatest in the perimenopausal period, and women may incur nearly half their bone loss before menopause actually happens [37]. The rate of fracture of the proximal femur for white women in the United States begins an abrupt rise between ages 40 and 44 [52]. White women have a lifetime risk rate of 15% for what is usually termed a *hip fracture*, but is actually a fracture of the proximal femur (the neck and trochanters) [53], while Asian and Black women have much lower risk rates.

The skeleton is made up predominantly of *cortical bone*, with the remainder—the spine, proximal femur, and radial bones—being *trabecular bone*. Osteoporosis is defined as loss of the quantity of all bone to a level two standard deviations below peak age-matched maximum, but the major loss is in trabecular bone—hence the association of osteoporosis with fractures of the femoral head and distal arm and with deformities of the spine. Building BMD through good nutrition and weight-bearing exercise from childhood through the mid-30s is vital to providing the highest density at the start of the period of major bone loss. It is well documented that the strongest impact of exercise is its capacity to facilitate optimal peak development of BMD during the premenopausal years as a preventive measure for osteoporosis [54-63]. There is evidence that participation in high-impact activities in young, healthy athletes results in the highest peak BMD [64, 65].

The effect of exercise on BMD in the perimenopausal and postmenopausal periods has been more difficult to assess. It appears that loading the bone(s) in question through strength conditioning exercises can help delay bone loss or, in postmenopausal women, produce small increases over time, as well as reducing the risk of fractures by lowering the incidence of falls [66-69]. Some research shows site-specific (shoulder) increases in BMD in the postmenopausal period with swimming [70]. Another group of researchers found that habitual volleyball exercise for pre-, peri-, and postmenopausal Japanese women did not alleviate menopause-related bone loss in the lumbar spine [71]. Still other researchers find no relationship between aerobic exercise and BMD [72] or no relationship of fitness level to BMD [73]. One study showing no relationship presented the conclusion that poor compliance among the untrained women involved in the study was the reason [74].

Mechanisms of Bone Loss

The metabolism of calcium is regulated by three hormones [75]. Parathyroid hormone (PTH) is secreted in response to a decrease in blood calcium levels and causes bone cells to *resorb* (dissolve) so that calcium salts stored as bone can enter the blood. Calcitonin is secreted by the thyroid and stimulates calcium deposition into the bones. Dihydroxycholecalciferol, a derivative of vitamin D, facilitates the absorption of dietary calcium in the intestines. Parathyroid hormone is active mainly in the kidneys to conserve calcium, as long as sufficient calcitonin and calcium are provided through the diet. If these latter two are insufficient, additional PTH is released and bone and teeth are resorbed.

As a woman ages, her ability to absorb calcium decreases and she loses more calcium through her urine than previously. In menopause, the lack of estrogen results in increased secretion of PTH, and bone is resorbed to maintain blood calcium levels. Consequently, loading the bone through weight-bearing exercise and resistance training, calcium and vitamin D supplementation, and often estrogen are required to reestablish calcium absorption and deposition.

Another factor in bone calcium loss is its depletion as an alkaline salt. Such salts are necessary to balance the endogenous acid generated from normal dietary precursors [76], especially protein. Blood pH and bicarbonate concentrations are reduced as endogenous acid production increases within a normal range [77, 78]. These factors are independent markers for bone resorption and inhibition of bone formation [79-81]. On the basis of this information, Sebastian et al. examined the hypothesis that oral administration of alkali could reduce bone loss. They found that short-term administration of potassium bicarbonate improved calcium and phosphorus balance, reduced bone resorption, and increased the rate of bone formation in postmenopausal women [82].

There are more obscure mechanisms that may contribute to the marked decrease in bone mass in midlife and older women. These include a latent hypo-androgenism that becomes apparent only after menopause, lowered calcium uptake in the gut due to genetic defects in dihydroxycholecalciferol receptors, and the effect of hormone loss on mechanoreceptors whose job it is to transfer physical stress into bone-building biochemical signals and whose effect increases in the presence of sex hormones [83].

Risk Factors

Risk factors for osteoporosis include lack of weight-bearing exercise; a high-fat, high-protein diet (particularly red meat, the metabolism of which draws calcium from the bones to offset the high levels of phosphorus in the meat); smoking; alcoholism; high levels of antibiotic use; hormone deficiencies; mineral deficiencies; null parity (not having borne children); and a history of amenorrhea due to an activity-nutrition imbalance. There are other interesting associations: spinal bone loss is greater among women with surgical menopause [84], and hyper-insulinemia may contribute to increased BMD in women who later develop obesity and diabetes [85].

The relationship between body composition and bone turnover is an interesting topic. Studying markers for bone formation (serum osteocalcin) and resorption (urinary type 1 collagen cross-linked N-telopeptides) in early-post-menopausal women, researchers concluded that associations were suggested for fat mass and whole-body bone mineral content with decreased bone turnover, and for muscle strength and height with increased bone turnover in early-postmenopausal women [86]. In examining the effect of self-reported activity level and type on kyphosis (the outward curve of the upper spine) in postmeno-pausal women, researchers found that body fat was the best single predictor of kyphosis in both the active and sedentary cohorts [87]. That is, women with higher levels of body fat were more likely to experience increased kyphosis than were women with lower levels of body fat.

While women of African and Asian descent are generally considered to be at lower risk for osteoporosis, there are intriguing findings regarding Asian women. One research group, studying Australian women of Asian descent, concluded that ethnicity was not related to BMD in this group but that clinical and lifestyle factors were related [88]. Reinforcing the finding that lifestyle is a factor for Asian women, a study of postmenopausal Taiwanese women concluded that physical activity played a major role in BMD levels [89].

Determining Bone Mineral Density

Two technologies are used to determine BMD. One is ultrasound bone densitometry, and the other is dual-energy X-ray absorptiometry (DEXA), which is consid-ered more accurate. A comparison of the two methods for accuracy indicated that it is important to take the exercise history of postmenopausal women into consideration when estimating lumbar spine BMD from ultrasound bone densitometer results for the calcaneus, a standard measurement [90]. A history of high levels of chronic exercise may indicate greater lumbar BMD than normal. As DEXA becomes more portable and less expensive, women are increasingly able to obtain accurate information about their bone density.

Strategies for Dealing With Osteoporosis

With osteoporosis affecting 20 million women in the United States and the cost of treating its complications running over $10 billion per year, strategies to prevent the disorder are obviously important. These include developing peak bone mass through proper nutrition, exercise, and hormone sufficiency in youth and maintaining bone mass through similar measures as women age [91]. In a number of cultural settings, exercise has a positive association with the BMD level of women in midlife and older years [92-96]. However, the American College of Sports Medicine (ACSM) warns against making the false assumption that exercise, or exercise and diet, can substitute for hormone replacement in the menopausal period [97]. Although a decline in activity level clearly results in profound loss of bone mass, the results of increased activity accrue more slowly and are less clear. According to ACSM, cross-sectional studies have demonstrated a more positive effect of exercise on bone than prospective studies [97].

A large study of cost-effectiveness in Australian nursing homes showed that the lifestyle intervention employing exercise—while effective—was the most costly of various interventions, including estrogen replacement at varying ages and bone-building medications [98]. But the authors remarked on the need to distribute the cost of exercise over other conditions and diseases that also benefit from ongoing participation in exercise, such as cardiovascular disease. Although estrogen replacement is effective in some situations for women at risk of cardiovascular disease, exercise and other lifestyle factors are also necessary for optimal outcomes [99]. In cases in which the risk of cancer is high, exercise may become the preferred treatment. Because exercise is also a prevention and treatment for obesity and diabetes and because it improves psychological well-being, its cost is further reduced if these conditions are part of the factoring process.

Heart Disease

The various *cardiovascular diseases* (CVDs) that are gathered under the term *heart disease* are explained in detail in many other texts, as are the responses of these disorders to cardiovascular conditioning exercise as prevention and treatment, primarily in men. Here we very briefly review these disorders; the impact of menopause on the female cardiovasculature; and pertinent findings regarding exercise, perimenopausal and postmenopausal women, and heart disease.

Included in the category of cardiovascular diseases is *coronary heart disease* (CHD), also called *coronary artery disease* (CAD) or *ischemic heart disease,* which can lead to *heart attack* or *myocardial infarction* (necrosis of heart tissue) due to reduced blood flow. The primary cause of these diseases is coronary *atherosclerosis,* or deposits of fat and calcium in the coronary arteries. The disorder begins in childhood and results largely from a combination of genetics and lifestyle. Other CVDs are *hypertension, stroke, congestive heart failure, peripheral vascular disease,* and diseases of the heart—*valvular, rheumatic,* and *congenital heart disease.* Hypertension, or high blood pressure, is more prevalent in African American and Hispanic women than in white women [100].

In the United States, half a million women—primarily postmenopausal women—die of CVD (with CAD the leading cause) each year, twice as many as the number who die from all cancers combined [28, 101-103]. Hormone replacement may reduce the risk of CVD somewhere between 20% and 45%, perhaps by helping to maintain high levels of HDL and low levels of low-density lipoprotein and triglycerides in certain combinations [28, 104], although risk of heart disease varies greatly from population to population [105]. For instance, in nations such as Italy, the cancer risk is much higher and heart disease risk lower than in the United States. While American women appear to be protected by hormone-associated HDL levels, no such protection appears to occur for Russian women [106].

Lipids and Other Blood Factors

The extent to which cholesterols, triglycerides, fibrinogen, and blood pressure are affected by endogenous sex hormones at menopause, and the extent to which these factors are predictors of CVD in women as compared to men, are not agreed on in the literature [6, 28, 104, 107-109]. There is a complex association between the use of estrogen as part of HRT and reduced risk of CVD in the United States [110-121]. We need more study of women who pass through menopause without HRT or heart disease. Also complicating matters are effective pharmaceuticals such as statins to lower cholesterol and blood pressure medications taken with or without HRT. The relationship of the amino acid homocysteine to cholesterol and subsequent damage to the cardiovasculature has to be delineated in women as well.

High levels of Lp(a) lipoprotein are an independent risk factor for recurrent atherosclerosis in both males and postmenopausal women, and are seen more often in populations of African and Asian descent [122]. Because Lp(a) is not generally reported in the standard lipid profile, clients with these ethnic backgrounds may wish to request this measurement, especially if there is a family history of atherosclerosis. Although genetics is a critical factor in the potential for developing atherosclerosis and other CVDs, lifestyle factors are critical in the actual development of disease. Not smoking, a healthy diet, and regular aerobic exercise are measures for prevention, as well as for treatment [6, 107, 122].

Diabetes

Diabetes also has an impact on heart disease. Eighty percent of diabetic patients die of CVD, of which 75% is CAD [123]. Postmenopausal women are more insulin resistant than premenopausal women [124], and a relationship among obesity (increased body mass index), insulin resistance, dyslipidemia, and uric acid (a likely link to CAD) has been established [27, 123]. This provides more evidence that it is in the best interest of menopausal and postmenopausal women to eat healthy diets (including foods with a low glycemic index) and to exercise regularly.

Features of the Female Heart

The female heart exhibits dramatic differences from the male heart, especially from puberty on. Legato [28] details much of what we know about women's hearts, including findings showing that the female heart is about two-thirds the size of a man's, has a longer QT interval, and has more frequent incidence of palpitations; there are conflicting findings on whether or not women have more common premature supraventricular ectopy and runs of supraventricular contractions (this appears to abate as women age). Also, there is increased incidence of premature ventricular beats (with a greater increase if women are taking oral contraceptives or thyroid hormone), and resting heart rates are higher in nonathletic women than in nonathletic men. Lev et al. found that aortic flow parameters, during rest and both isometric and dynamic exercise, were significantly higher in early-postmenopausal women (55 ± 5 years) than in middle-aged men (52 ± 4 years), and that women showed higher hemodynamic parameters during exercise, with most values approaching significance [125].

Hormone Replacement, Medication, Exercise, and Heart Disease

Whether or not an adequate and ongoing exercise history obviates the need for HRT, statins or blood pressure medication, is controversial. Women must make decisions on an individual basis, in consultation with their care providers and support systems, about how to proceed. In addition to those factors described so far, there are others; two of these are employment history and iron metabolism. Ickovics et al. looked at a cohort of 541 Pennsylvania women aged 42 to 50 years, recording employment, health-related variables, and cholesterol at baseline and three years later. Although there was no difference in cholesterol or health behaviors at baseline, the women who were employed at baseline showed a significant decrease in total HDL at follow-up [126]. Those employed both at baseline and at follow-up had the lowest HDL profile at follow-up, and those employed at baseline were less likely to have increased exercise and more likely to have gained weight than those who were not employed at baseline [126]. It has not been determined whether employment leads to less time for physical activity or more sedentary activities of daily living due to job-related factors, whether work produces more stresses that predispose one against exercise, or whether other factors related to employment might cause changes in cholesterol in the perimenopausal years [126]. In another study, Naimark et al. found that sufficient levels of walking (five sessions per week) provided a dose effect that reduced levels of excess stored iron in previously sedentary postmenopausal women (significant increases of stored iron following menopause and excess stored iron are risk factors for CAD) [127].

Various studies have addressed the relationships between exercise and heart disease and those between HRT and heart disease in women. To test the hypothesis that a group of physically active postmenopausal women and a group of women on HRT would each have more favorable blood pressure (BP)-related risk factors for CVD than otherwise healthy controls, Stevenson et al. measured maximum oxygen consumption, waist-to-hip ratio (central obesity), waist circumference, casual and 24-hour BP, and daytime and nighttime systolic and diastolic BPs. Results showed that in the active women compared to the controls $\dot{V}O_2$max was higher, and waist-to-hip ratio and waist circumference were lower. The active women had lower levels of casual, 24-hour, and daytime systolic BP; lower daytime systolic BP loads (% recordings > 140/90); lower daytime and nighttime BP variabilities; and a reduced systolic BP response to submaximal exercise [128]. Women on HRT tended to have lower levels of 24-hour and nighttime diastolic BP and smaller daytime and 24-hour diastolic BP loads than the controls [128]. After stepwise multiple regression analysis, the researchers found that waist circumference was the primary predictor of most of the systolic BP-related CVD risk factors and that HRT was the best pre-

dictor for diastolic BP loads [128].Other research has shown either no decrease or a small but statistically significant decrease in BP in women on HRT [117, 119], and one study demonstrated that a few women on HRT experienced increased BP [15]. Green et al. concluded that estrogen supplementation (vs. non-estrogen supplementation) may be associated with higher peak cardiac outputs in exercise-trained postmenopausal women [129]. Peak oxygen consumptions in the two groups were almost identical, but the supplementation group had higher peak cardiac index (QI peak) in conjunction with less difference in arterial and venous O_2 levels (lower a-$\bar{v}O_2$ difference) and lower peripheral resistance [129]. The significance of these outcomes in relation to heart disease has not been assessed; however, they are all in the direction we recognize as indicating a healthy cardiovasculature.

Research on the causes and mechanisms of CVD in relation to menopause, as well as the markers and associations, has really just begun. For now, one way health and fitness professionals can help is to make as much reliable information as possible available to perimenopausal, menopausal, and postmenopausal women, including research articles and reports.

PSYCHOSOCIAL CONSIDERATIONS

A woman's health has an impact on her mental and emotional well-being. Physical changes in the brain during menopause alter a woman's mental landscape. And psychosocial factors affect health. The psychological environment, including stress and support, as well as a woman's knowledge base, plays a critical role in her well-being. A study of Australian women in the menopause transition showed that life satisfaction is predicted by earlier attitudes and is positively associated with exercise and feelings for one's partner—and that it is negatively associated with daily hassles, interpersonal stress, dysphoric symptoms, and current smoking [130].

Brain/Mind Changes

Changes in hormone levels influence both cognitive functions and mood. It appears that hormone changes can affect both major brain functioning (as in Alzheimer's disease) and the "fuzzy thinking" sometimes associated with menopause. The relationship between these hormone changes and brain function has yet to be fully elucidated. It seems likely that adequate levels of estrogen in the female brain are necessary for memory storage and for learning new tasks [131]. The parietal lobes of the cerebral cortex—important for organizational thinking—are affected in early menopause by a changing estrogen concentration and may, along with personal midlife issues, account for the sense of mental fuzz.

Alzheimer's Disease

Alzheimer's disease (AD), while clearly related to estrogen levels, has many more dimensions than the lower levels of estrogen in the parietal lobes that we associate with fuzzy thinking. Legato believes that estrogen replacement therapy lowers the risk of AD by 40% [45]. Henderson et al. found postmenopausal estrogen replacement to be associated with a decreased risk of AD [132], and two studies have confirmed that estrogen use is protective for AD [133, 134]. That there is an association between Alzheimer's and premature menopause is well accepted. Because early menopause can be an autoimmune disorder, as described by Northrup [37], this raises questions about whether estrogen loss is a cause of Alzheimer's or whether the ovarian failure that leads to both menopause and Alzheimer's is related to an immune/inflammation disorder. The inflammatory component of AD (demonstrated by the protective role of nonsteroidal anti-inflammatory drugs [135-138]), along with vascular pathologies and neurotoxic metabolism [137, 139, 140], joins genetics as a cofactor in this complicated disease.

Another aspect of cognitive function is synaptic plasticity. Synaptic remodeling, such as that reported by Naftolin et al. in primates [141] and discussed in the section, "Sex and Stress Hormones," in chapter 2, is clearly associated with estrogen, and is modulated or negated by progesterone and other estrogen antagonists (such as tamoxifen). Research in this area should yield interesting results in the years to come.

The ability of physical activity to provide minor, temporary reduction of symptoms of AD, reported anecdotally, may be related to improved cerebromicrovascular blood flow or other antiaging mechanisms that preserve neurotransmission, including gene expression of integrin-associated proteins. *Integrins* are heterodimeric glycoproteins that undergo changes in distribution, possibly in relation to sex hormones, in the communication network among neurons, organs, and the immune system. There is no direct evidence in this area. Exercise has been shown to have numerous positive effects in persons who are elderly, and one can hope that continuing research in the fitness arena will include the role of exercise in AD.

Mood in Midlife

The impact of exercise on mood in midlife is profound. In two studies on mood and symptom reporting among middle-aged women, Slaven and Lee found that both chronic and acute exercise had a positive effect on mood and reduced the levels of somatic and vasomotor symptoms compared with those in nonexercisers. Menopause status and whether or not the women were taking hormone replacement did not affect these results [142].

Depression may have been more common in women than in men in the 1950s, but by the late 1970s the occurrence of depression was more equal between the sexes [143]. At present, while patterns of depression vary between men and women, the frequency is similar [144]. Changing societal roles, improving research methods, and understandings of sex differences in patterns of depression probably all contribute to a change in the statistical information in this regard. Looking at the causes of depression in midlife women in the early 1990s, Kaufert et al. found that depression in this population appears to be related to major life changes that are associated with stress, rather than to changes in hormone status [10].

Stress

Although the stresses in midlife are major (the difficult teen years of one's children, aging parents, job stresses, and changes in identity), group support strategies, self-efficacy, goals, and positive feelings about themselves allow many women to pass through this period of their lives in a happy frame of mind [145]. In practice we find that although women may report lack of time to participate in organized group exercise, given exercise guidelines and permission to drop in on activities, midlife women are quite capable of devising their own activity programs, a viable stress management strategy.

One unstudied potential for stress is what could be termed the "invisibility factor." Western culture bombards us with images. But the images of midlife women are few and not always easy to identify with. The body changes in menopause. Observing the products and sales pitches aimed at the midlife body, one can see that halting the aging of the female body at all costs is a high priority, as this change signals the loss of fertility (i.e., desirability) and presages the woman's mortality. The loss of fertility that signals aging has long been associated in the Western world with the time a woman becomes invisible in society.

Despite the health concerns, increasing responsibilities, and stresses at work and in society, most women pass through their midlife changes without major disturbances. For many, midlife is a time of awesome surprises, new vistas, questions, comparisons of experience, annoyances, wry humor, laughter, and a humbling before the power of time, but not a depressing, painful, or intolerable experience.

The Need for Support and Education

In 1989, Spiegel et al. published a landmark study showing that breast cancer patients who participated in a supportive weekly group therapy program lived significantly longer than patients who did not attend the support sessions [146]. As noted in chapter 7, women with female labor support have shorter and less complicated births than those without that support. Research tells us that social support has a positive effect on health in relation to CVDs (and that lack of support has a negative influence) [147]. Evidence continues to point us toward the realization that social networking—a hallmark of the female life cycle—is a key component in women's wellness.

By midlife, many women have already developed skills for adjusting or acquiring an appropriate support network. If they have friends of a similar age, these women may be the basis of a support group as well as sources of information. One friend may like to look up medical information and pass it on. Another may uncover a health care provider who is a particularly good communicator; still another may discover a great lecture series. Fitness professionals can be another source of reliable information and support as the population boom moves into menopause.

What else helps women deal with the changes and decisions that midlife entails? Women's own views of their gynecological status [148], their awareness of their personal value system [149], and their exposure to appropriate educational materials [148-150] have been shown to be influential. These factors help give women a sense that the plan of action they have chosen for themselves is appropriate, as well as producing high levels of adherence, whatever the treatment of choice [150]. One of the major questions women have concerns their risk of developing estrogen-dependent cancers (breast, ovarian, and endometrial) if they take hormone replacement. Despite the much greater prevalence of heart disease, cancer seems to frighten women more. Only 8% of women consider CVD a personal health threat [101]. Midlife women are able to understand the complex information that decisions about menopause entail. There is a need for public education that helps women interpret information on ways of achieving a healthy, active lifestyle within their particular domain, time, family, and individual constraints [151].

Clearly support and education are vital for a woman in the process of deciding how to approach this important time of life. Not only do we not have clear-cut answers for every symptom; but with so much individual variation in women's experience of menopause, it is almost impossible to say with certainty what women should do. Each woman should be encouraged to learn as much as she can about the choices she can make.

APPROACHES TO MIDLIFE CHANGES

In seeking advice from experts trained in the chemical model of the body (modern Western medicine), do women cut themselves off from traditional means of dealing with menopause, and particularly from role models of women who have successfully navigated this transition without a high degree of medical intervention? This possibility, suggested by Rousseau [6], brings into question the neutrality of research findings that focus primarily on treating clinical populations with chemicals. What is the actual rate of adherence to chemical treatments in the clinical setting, and how do outcomes compare to those obtained with other methodologies?

Hormone Replacement Therapy

The creation, production, and sales of synthetic or laboratory-enhanced sex hormones, as well as drugs called selective estrogen receptor modulators (SERMs), now constitute a vast industry. Following the development of synthetic estrogen in 1938, the use of estrogen replacement therapy for natural and surgical menopause increased in practice over the next decades, leading to what might be termed the *medicalization of menopause*. In 1975, strong evidence of the increased risk of endometrial (uterine) cancer among users of unopposed conjugated estrogens began to be published [152-154]. Progestogen, a progesterone-like substance, was added to estrogen to combat this effect, and the term *hormone replacement therapy* was born.

The pharmaceutical industry continues to explore the impact of exogenous substances on the health status of midlife women. Drugs that have positive effects on the cardiovasculature and bone density are being refined. The so-called designer estrogens—or SERMs—may eventually include an array of substances that have positive influences on some cancers as well as heart disease and bone health. Table 12.2 reviews the major substances that are currently available, including their purposes and risks.

Estrogen and Cancer

Estrogen is a hormone that stimulates cell division and growth. During pregnancy the presence of estrogen helps create a baby. Excess estrogen is a risk factor for estrogen-dependent cancers. Cancer is a disorder characterized

Table 12.2   Hormone Replacement/Drug Therapies in Menopause

Substance	Description and example brands	Use and benefit	Risks
Conjugated estrogens	From urine of pregnant mares/Premarin	Symptom relief; increases BMD; increases HDL; decreases LDL	Increases risk of endometrial (uterine) cancer, breast cancer, gallbladder disease, deep vein blood clots when unopposed
Modified plant estrone	From plant estrogen/ Estratab, Menest	Similar to conjugated estrogens	Similar to conjugated estrogens
Micronized plant estradiol	From plant estrogren/ Estradiol	Similar to conjugated estrogens	Similar to conjugated estrogens
Estropipate	Synthesized from estrone/Ortho-Est	Similar to conjugated estrogens	
Estradiol patch	Estraderm, FemPatch	Similar to conjugated estrogens, less effect on lipid profile	Similar to conjugated estrogens, skin irritation
Estradiol vaginal ring	Estring	Prevent vaginal dryness	
Medroxyprogesterone acetate	MPA-synthetic progesterone/Provera	Modulate estrogen; reduces risk of uterine cancer; reduces E2's effect on HDL/LDL	PMS symptoms
Norethindrone acetate	Synthetic progesterone/ Micronor, Aygestin	Modulate estrogen; reduces risk of uterine cancer; reduces E2's effect on HDL/LDL	PMS symptoms
Micronized plant progesterone	Prometrium	Modulate estrogen; reduces risk of uterine cancer; reduces E2's effect on HDL/LDL, but less decreased effect on HDL	Fewer side effects than synthetic progest
Micronized plant progesterone, IUD time-released	Progestasert	Reduces risk of uterine cancer	Change IUD annually; risk of perforation
Micronized plant progesterone, vaginal gel	Crinone	Reduces risk of uterine cancer	
Conjugated estrogens with MPA	Prempro, Premphase	Combination provides symptom relief, some effect on lipid levels, reduces risk of estrogen-dependent cancers	Bleeding
Estrone and methyl testosterone	Estratest	Similar to estrogens; may improve libido	May reduce benefits to lipids
Raloxifene	Synthetic selective estrogen-receptor modulator/Evista	Increases bone density (less than estrogen); decreases LDL, but not increase HDL; increases risk of estrogen-dependent cancers	Hot flashes; vaginal dryness
Tamoxifen	Synthetic selective estrogen-receptor modulator/Nolvadex	Prevention/treatment of E-dependent cancers (only U.S. studies show success)	Hot flashes; nausea; bone pain; uterine cancer; blood clots; elevated lipids, triglycerides
Calcitonin	Natural hormone produced by thyroid; synthetically produced/Calcimar, Miacalcin	Reduce calcium resorption to reduce bone loss	Allergies: skin with shots (Calcimar); nasal membranes with nasal spray (Miacalcin)
Alendronate	synth. receptor-site modulator/Fosomax	Increases bone density	Gastrointestinal discomfort; must adhere to strict dosing requirements

From Rousseau [6]; Northrup [37]; *Physician's Desk Reference; Harvard Women's Health Watch.*

in its early stages by *hyperplasia*—increased, abnormal cell production. Lifetime exposure to estrogen is a factor in the development of these cancers, whether the estrogen is endogenous (produced internally) or exogenous (introduced from the outside). As discussed previously, early menarche results in increased lifetime exposure to endogenous estrogen and increased cancer risk. The effect of exogenous estrogen depends on dose and duration, as well as on whether or not it is opposed by progesterone, testosterone, or another chemical that is an estrogen antagonist or modifier. In 1992, a meta-analysis of breast cancer risk from HRT indicated an increased risk of breast cancer even when estrogen is combined with opposing substances [155]. A prospective study of the use of HRT published in 1995 demonstrated that the risk of breast cancer increases as duration of estrogen and progestin use increases, to 1.3 times with 5 years of use and 1.7 times for more than 10 years of use [156]. The authors of a 1998 review study found a causal relationship between HRT and breast cancer based on consistency, dose-response pattern, biologic plausibility, timing and duration of use, strength of association, and coherence [157].

Hormone Replacement Therapy, Cancer, and Diet. The correlation of dietary saturated fat with the higher levels of circulating estrogen implicated in the development of hormone-related cancers [158] has helped to establish the significance of diet, particularly the avoidance of saturated fat and the inclusion of dietary fiber (such as fruits and vegetables), in reducing risk of some cancers. While a nutrient-dense diet is clearly important for maintaining adequate fuels, the importance of diet is enhanced in conjunction with other health-inducing behaviors.

Hormone Replacement Therapy, Cancer, and Exercise. Decreased risk of estrogen-dependent cancers occurs in women who have a life habit of intense exercise, due to reduced exposure to estrogen. Increased risk occurs as a consequence of genes, metabolic factors, weight, race, nutrition, chronic inflammation, and age; these factors are equal in significance to hormonal factors, or even more significant [159]. Estrogen-dependent cancers have etiologies that are not totally understood, although it does appear that estrogen is implicated in a process that stimulates the expression of estrogen receptor sites in uterine and breast tissue [160-162].

A report published in 1997 sheds some light on the mechanisms involved in heavy exercise as a possible preventative for breast cancer. Alterations in catecholestrogen metabolism in response to heavy exercise include changes that may undermine fertility while preventing free radicals and exposure of breast epithelium to endogenous estrogens [163]. One study followed 25,624 women, ages 20 to 54 years at entry into the program, over a mean period of 13.7 years [164]. Results on recreational exercise and breast cancer showed that the greater the leisure-time activity of the participants, the lower the risk of breast cancer. In regular exercisers, the reduction of risk was greater in premenopausal than in postmenopausal women. Risk was lowest in lean women (< 22.8 BMI, or body mass index) who exercised at least 4 hours per week. Risk was also reduced with higher levels of activity at work.

What emerges from research at this point is that having borne and breast-fed children, and living a healthy lifestyle that includes regular exercise and a good diet, are the factors that are most effective in reducing risk of estrogen-dependent cancers [165]. At the same time, genetics (at least two breast cancer-associated genes have been identified) and environmental factors can come into play that are more significant in determining whether a person will develop such cancers. Other issues that are emerging are factors such as the timing of weight gain—particularly in young adulthood—in relation to breast cancer. It appears that the metabolic effect of puberty, pregnancy, or menopause may play a greater role in a woman's predisposition for breast cancer than her weight at the time of cancer onset, with gain at these transitional phases contributing to metabolic dysfunction that creates a link to increased risk [166].

Other Findings on Hormone Replacement Therapy

Other tangential findings in this area include evidence that ingestion of sufficient amounts of alcohol increases estrogen levels threefold in postmenopausal women who are taking estrogen replacement [167] and that hormone replacement may be a risk factor for low back pain [168]. There are interesting findings on hormone replacement and CVD; for example, one study showed that among black women, those at risk for CAD were not more likely to use HRT than those at lower risk and that the predominant medication was unopposed estrogen [169]. Regarding the prevention of stroke, it appears that the role of 17-beta estradiol in this process is to inhibit platelet aggregation by promoting Ca^{2+} reuptake and increasing nitrite/nitrate synthesis [170]. However, a more recent mega analysis has revealed increased risk of stroke may be associated with hormone replacement [171].

Drugs for Bone Strength

The substances known as SERMs that have been designed (hence the popular term "designer estrogens") to affect various receptor sites are an interesting class of chemicals. The chronology of findings regarding hormone replacement has led to an attempt to limit the action of substances to receptors with specific characteristics, thus achieving a positive result and avoiding an allied negative one. Three such drugs are primarily used for increasing bone density when estrogen replacement is clearly contraindicated for physical or psychological reasons: Raloxifen, calcitonin (which also occurs naturally), and alendronate. Their actions are reviewed in table 12.2. Although the efficacy of these substances has been demonstrated for periods as long as two or three years, there are no long-term longitudinal studies to indicate what the results and side effects may be over a decade or more of use.

Diet

Given the evidence covered so far regarding the physiology and psychology of menopause, it should be clear that the nutritional status of a woman plays a critical role in her health status as she proceeds through her middle and later years. Body/mind viability to a large extent depends on the availability of fuels that can be used to accomplish biochemical functions. The brain responds to and produces many molecules that derive from nutritional building blocks. The many structures and organs of the body depend on nutrition-dense calories in order to maintain their complex functions. As the body ages, catabolic processes (e.g., bone resorption, loss of muscle mass) create an increased demand for a body-building diet if one wants to remain physically strong and mentally alert. Chapter 14 provides more detail on this topic.

Exercise

The health benefits of exercise or physical activity extend to women in menopause as they do to all populations. The list of specific benefits for this group includes prevention of falls and fractures through increased balance and strength, limiting of bone loss, cognitive and mood benefits, reduction of CAD risk from obesity and poor lipid profiles, control of BP, some reduction in cancer risk, reduced risk of adult-onset diabetes, and enhanced metabolic function. The program design section of chapter 14 covers the exercise components that are effective, dose effects, and the formatting of midlife fitness programs.

Stress Management

The underlying physiological mechanisms that produce relaxation and a mental state of well-being, and that reduce trait and state anxiety, have been examined in some detail in previous chapters. It is important to note here, within the context of findings on the symptoms of menopause, that the impact of stress on menopause

is as a physiological state that aggravates these symptoms. Hence it is important to tap into the relaxation response as a way to manage stress. Techniques abound for producing the state of relaxation. Talking about it does not work. Achieving the state of relaxation once, using the simplest technique available, is the best way of getting women to do it again. The following chapters on goals, priorities, and program design for midlife women includes information on incorporating stress management into the fitness program for this population.

REFERENCES

1. Locke, M. 1991. Contested meanings of the menopause. *Lancet* 337:1270-1272.
2. Locke, M. 1986. Ambiguities of aging: Japanese experience and perceptions of menopause. *Culture, Medicine and Psychiatry* 10:23-46.
3. Kaufert, P., Gilbert, P., and Hassard, T. 1988. Researching the symptoms of menopause: An exercise in methodology. *Maturitas* 10:117-131.
4. Notman, M.T. 1990. Menopause and adult development. In Flint, Kronenberg, and Utian (eds.), *Annals of the New York Academy of Sciences* 592:149-155.
5. Kaufert, P., and Syrotuik, J. 1981. Symptom reporting at the menopause. *Social Science and Medicine* 15E:173-184.
6. Rousseau, M.E. 1996. Midlife health. In H. Varney Burst (ed.), *Varney's midwifery,* 3rd ed. Boston: Jones & Bartlett, pp. 201-225.
7. Collins, A., and Landgren, B.-M. 1994. Reproductive health, use of estrogen and experience of symptoms in perimenopausal women: A population-based study. *Maturitas* 20(2-3):101-111.
8. Dennerstein, L., Smith, A.M.A., and Morse, C. 1994. Psychological well-being, mid-life and the menopause. *Maturitas* 20(1):1-11.
9. Liao, K.L.-M., Hunter, M., and Weinman, J. 1995. Health-related behaviors and their correlates in a general population sample of 45-year old women. *Psychology & Health* 10(3):171-184.
10. Kaufert, P., Gilbert, P., and Tate, R. 1992. The Manitoba Project: A re-examination of the link between menopause and depression. *Maturitas* 14(2):143-155.
11. Koster, A. 1991. Change of life anticipations, attitudes and experiences among middle-aged Danish women. *Health Care of Women* 12:1-13.
12. Speroff, L., Glass, R.H., and Kase, N.G. 1994. *Clinical gynecologic endocrinology and infertility.* Baltimore: Williams & Wilkins.
13. Smith, K.E., and Judd, H.L. 1994. Menopause and postmenopause. In A.H. DeCherney and M.L. Pernoll (eds.), *Current obstetric and gynecologic diagnosis and treatment,* 8th ed., Norwalk, CT: Appleton & Lange.
14. McKinlay, S.M., and McKinlay, J.B. 1989. The impact of menopause and social factors on health. In C.B. Hammod, F.P. Hazeltine, and I. Schiff (eds.), *Menopause: Evaluation, treatment, and health concerns.* NY: Alan R. Liss, pp. 137-162.
15. Whelan, E.A., Sandler, D.P., McConnaughey, D.R., and Weinberg, C.R. 1990. Menstrual and reproductive characteristics and age at natural menopause. *American Journal of Epidemiology* 131(4):625-628.
16. Brambilla, D.J., and McKinlay, S.M. 1989. A prospective study of factors affecting age at menopause. *Journal of Clinical Epidemiology* 42(11):1031-1039.

17. McKinlay, S.M., Jefferys, M., and Thompson, B. 1972. An investigation of the age at menopause. *Journal of Biosocial Science* 4:161.

18. Frommer, D.J. 1964. Changing age of menopause. *British Medical Journal* 2:349.

19. Morce, C.A., Smith, A., Dennerstein, L., Green, A., Hopper, J., and Burger, H. 1994. The treatment-seeking woman at menopause. *Maturitas* 18(3):161-173.

20. McKinlay, J.B., McKinlay, S.M., and Brambilla, D.J. 1987. Health status and utilization behavior associated with menopause. *American Journal of Epidemiology* 125 (1):110-121.

21. Wilson, R.A. 1966. *Feminine forever.* NY: Evans.

22. Hawkes, K., O'Connell, J.F., and Blurton Jones, N.G. 1997. Hadza women's time allocation, offspring provisioning and the evolution of long postmenopausal life spans. *Current Anthropology* 38(4):551-577.

23. Change, R.F., Plouffe, L., and Schaffer, K. 1994. Physiology of the menopause. In J. Lorrain, L. Plouffe Jr, V. Ravnikar, and L. Speroff (eds.), *Comprehensive management of the menopause.* NY: Springer-Verlag, pp. 3-14.

24. Cauley, J.A., Gutai, J.P., Kuller, L.H., Ledonne, D., and Powell, J.B. 1989. The epidemiology of serum sex hormones in postmenopausal women. *American Journal of Epidemiology* 129:1120-1131.

25. Meldrum, D.R., Davidson, B.J., Tataryn, E.V., and Judd, H.L. 1981. Changes in circulating steroids with aging in postmenopausal women. *Obstetrics and Gynecology* 57:624-628.

26. Hemsell, D.L., Siiteri, P.K., and MacDonald, P.C. 1972. Estrogen derived from plasma androstenedione, presented to the Armed Forces District Meeting of the American College of Obstetricians and Gynecologists, Seattle, October 1972.

27. Sowers, J.R. 1998. Diabetes mellitus and cardiovascular disease in women. *Archives of Internal Medicine* 158(6):617-621.

28. Legato, M. 1997. Gender-specific aspects of obesity. *International Journal of Fertility and Women's Medicine* 42(3):184-197.

29. Strollo, F. 1999. Hormonal changes in humans during spaceflight. *Advances in Space Biology and Medicine* 7:99-129.

30. Ueda, M., and Tokunaga, M. 2000. Effects of exercise experienced in the life stages on climacteric symptoms for females. *Journal of Physiological Anthropology and Applied Human Science* 19(4):181-189.

31. Navarro, A., Lopez-Cepero, J.M., and Sanchez del Pino, M.J. 2001. Skeletal muscle and aging. *Frontiers in Bioscience* 6:D26-D44.

32. Short, K.R., and Nair, K.S. 2000. The effect of age on protein metabolism. *Current Opinion in Clinical Nutrition and Metabolic Care* 3(1):39-44.

33. Moulias, R., Meaume, S., and Raynaud-Simon, A. 1999. Sarcopenia, hypermetabolism, and aging. *Zeitschrift fur Gerontologie Geriatrie* 32(6):25-32.

34. Sehl, M.E., and Yates, F.E. 2001. Kinetics of human aging: I. Rates of senescence between ages 30 and 70 years in healthy people. *The Journals of Gerontology. Series A, Biological Sciences and Medical Sciences* 56(5):B198-B208.

35. Veyrat-Durebex, C., Boghossian, S., and Alliot, J. 1998. Age-related changes in adaptive mechanisms of macronutrient self-selection: Evidence for a sexual dimorphism. *Mechanisms of Ageing and Development* 103(3):223-234.

36. Skerry, T.M. 1999. Identification of novel signaling pathways during functional adaptation of the skeleton to mechanical loading: The role of glutamate as a paracrine signaling agent in the skeleton. *Journal of Bone and Mineral Metabolism* 17(1):66-70.

37. Northrup, C. 1994. *Women's bodies, women's wisdom.* NY: Bantam, p. 444.

38. Kronenberg, F. 1990. Hot flashes: Epidemiology and physiology. *Annals of the New York Academy of Sciences* 592:52-86.

39. McKinlay, S.M., and Jefferys, M. 1974. The menopausal syndrome. *British Journal of Preventive & Social Medicine* 28(2):108.

40. Kandel, E.R., Schwartz, J.H., and Jessell, T.M. 1991. *Principles of neural science,* 3rd ed. Norwalk, CT: Appleton & Lange, pp. 752-753.

41. Liske, E. 1998. Therapeutic efficacy and safety of Cimicifuga racemosa for gynecologic disorders. *Advances in Therapy* 15(1):45-53.

42. Tyler, V.E. 1993. *The honest herbal,* 3rd ed. Binghampton, NY: Haworth Press.

43. Cohen, S. 1998. *Personal communication.* Yale University School of Nursing. New Haven, CT.

44. Robinson, E. 1998. *The effect of black cohosh on menopausal symptomotology.* Unpublished master's thesis. Yale University School of Medicine.

45. Legato, M.J. 1997. *Gender-specific aspects of human biology for the practicing physician.* Armonk, NY: Futura.

46. Rosenberg, M.J., and Phillips, R.S. 1992. Does douching promote ascending infection? *The Journal of Reproductive Medicine* 37:930-938.

47. Gardner, J.W., Schuman, K.L., Slattery, M.L., Sanborn, J.S., Abbott, T.M., and Overall, J.C. 1991. Is vaginal douching related to cervical carcinoma? *American Journal of Epidemiology* 133:368-375.

48. Peake, S., Manderson, L., and Potts, H. 1999. "Part and parcel of being a woman": Female urinary incontinence and constructions of control. *Medical Anthropology Quarterly* 13(3):267-285.

49. Strinic, T. 1999. Disorders of pulmonary ventilation function in patients with genital prolapse postmenopause. *Lijecnicki Vjesnik* 121(3):78-81.

50. Gosselin, L.E., Adams, C., Cotter, T.A., McCormick, R.J., and Thomas, D.P. 1998. Effect of exercise training on passive stiffness in locomotor skeletal muscle: Role of extracellular matrix. *Journal of Applied Physiology* 85(3):1011-1016.

51. Lees, B., Molleson, T., Arnett, T.R., and Stevenson, J.C. 1993. Differences in proximal femur bone density over two centuries. *Lancet* 341:673-675.

52. Wallace, W.A. 1983. The increasing incidence of fractures of the proximal femur: An orthopaedic epidemic. *Lancet* :1413-1414.

53. Avioli, L. 1992. Osteoporosis: A growing national health problem. *Female Patient* 17:84.

54. Bass, S., Pearce, G., Bradney, M., Hendrich, E., Delmas, P.D., Harding, A., and Seeman, E. 1998. Exercise before puberty may confer residual benefits in bone density in adulthood: Studies in active prepubertal and retired female gymnasts. *Journal of Bone and Mineral Research* 13(3):500-507.

55. Armstrong, A.L., and Wallace, W.A. 1994. The epidemiology of hip fractures and methods of prevention. *Acta Orthopaedica Belgica* 60(Suppl 1):85-101.

56. Baran, D.T. 1994. Magnitude and determinants of premenopausal bone loss. *Osteoporosis International* 4(Suppl 1):31-34.

57. Christiansen, C. 1993. Prevention and treatment of osteoporosis: A review of different methods. *Ugeskrift for Laeger* 155(31):2383-2386.

58. Devogelaer, J.P., and Nagant de Deuxchaisnes, C. 1993. Osteoporosis. (Review). *British Journal of Rheumatology* 32(Suppl 4):48-55.

59. Eisman, J.A., Kelly, P.J., Morrison, N.A., Pocock, N.A., Yeoman, R., Birmingham, J., and Sambrook, D.N. 1993. Peak bone mass and osteoporosis prevention. *Osteoporosis International* 3(Suppl 1):56-60.

60. Notelovitz, M. 1993. Osteoporosis: Screening, prevention, and management. *Fertility and Sterility* 59(4):707-725.

61. Seitz, M. 1994. Osteoporosis—prevention and therapy. *Therapeutische Umschau* 51(6):410-417.

62. Suominen, H. 1993. Bone mineral density and long term exercise: An overview of cross-sectional athlete studies. *Sports Medicine* 16(5):316-330.

63. Ravnikar, V.A. 1993. Diet , exercise, and lifestyle in preparation for menopause. *Obstetrics and Gynecology Clinics of North America* 20(2):365-378.

64. Dook, J.F., James, C., Henderson, N.K., and Price, R.I. 1997. Exercise and bone mineral density in mature female athletes. *Medicine and Science in Sports and Exercise* 29(3):291-296.

65. Taafe, D.R., Robinson, T.L., Snow, C.M., and Marcus, R. 1997. High-impact exercise promotes bone gain in well trained female athletes. *Journal of Bone and Mineral Research* 12(2):255-260.

66. Petranick, K., and Berg, K. 1997. The effects of weight training on bone density of premenopausal, postmenopausal and elderly women: A review. *Journal of Strength and Conditioning Research* 11(3):200.

67. Nelson, M.E., Fiatrarone, M.A., Morganti, C.M., Trice, I., Greenberg, R.A., and Evans, W.J. 1994. Effects of high-intensity strength training on multiple risk factors for osteoporotic fractures. *Journal of the American Medical Association* 272(24):1909-1914.

68. Simkin, A., Ayalon, J., and Leichter, I. 1987. Increased trabecular bone density due to bone-loading exercise in postmenopausal osteoporotic women. *Calcified Tissue International* 40:59-63.

69. Shimegi, S., Yanagita, M., Okano, H., Yamada, M., Fukui, H., Fukumura, Y., Ibuki, Y., and Kojima, I. 1994. Physical exercise increases bone mineral density in postmenopausal women. *Endocrine Journal* 41(1):49-56.

70. Tsukahara, N., Toda, A., Goto, J., and Ezawa, I. 1994. Cross-sectional and longitudinal studies on the effect of water exercise in controlling bone loss in Japanese postmenopausal women. *Journal of Nutritional Science and Vitaminology* 40(1):37-47.

71. Ito, M., Nakamura, T., Ikeda, S., Tahara, Y., et al. 2001. Effects of lifetime volleyball exercise on bone mineral densities in lumbar spine, calcaneus and tibia for pre-, peri- and postmenopausal women. *Osteoporosis International* 12(2):104-111.

72. Martin, D., and Notelovitz, M. 1993. Effects of aerobic training on bone mineral density of postmenopausal women. *Journal of Bone and Mineral Research* 8(8):931-936.

73. Miyamura, T., Yamagata, Z., Iijma, S., and Asaka, A. 1994. Study on the association between risk factors for osteoporosis and bone mineral density. *Japanese Journal of Public Health* 41(12):1122-1130.

74. Preisinger E., Alacamliogu, Y., Pils, K., Saradeth, T., and Schneider, B. 1995. Therapeutic exercise in the prevention of bone loss: A controlled trial with women after menopause. *American Journal of Physical Medicine & Rehabilitation* 74(2):120-123.

75. Norris, D.O. 1997. *Vertebrate endocrinology,* 3rd ed. San Diego: Academic Press.

76. Wachman, A., and Bertstein, D.S. 1968. Diet and osteoporosis. *Lancet* 1:958-959.

77. Kleiman, J.G., and Lemann, J. 1987. Acid production. In M.H. Maxwell, C.R. Leeman, and M.D. Narins (eds.), *Clinical disorders of fluid and electrolyte metabolism,* 4th ed. NY: McGraw-Hill, pp. 159-173.

78. Kurtz, I., Maher, T., Hulter, H.N., Schambelan, M., and Sebastian, A. 1983. Effect of diet on plasma acid-base composition in normal subjects. *Kidney International* 24:670-680.

79. Bushinsky, D.A., Sessler, N.E., and Krieger, N.S. 1992. Greater unidirectional calcium efflux from bone during metabolic, compared with respiratory, acidosis. *American Journal of Physiology* 262:F525-F531.

80. Krieger, N.S., Sessler, N.E., and Bushinsky, D.A. 1992. Acidosis inhibits osteoblastic and stimulates osteoclastic activity in vitro. *American Journal of Physiology* 262:F442-F448.

81. Bushinsky, D.A., and Sessler, N.E. 1992. Critical role of bicarbonate in calcium release from bone. *American Journal of Physiology* 263:F510-F515.

82. Sebastian, A., Harris, S.T., Ottaway, J.H., Todd, K.M., and Morris, R.C. 1994. Improved mineral balance and skeletal metabolism in postmenopausal women treated with potassium bicarbonate. *New England Journal of Medicine* 330:1776-1781.

83. Ziegler, R., Scheidt-Nave, C., and Scharla, S. 1995. Pathophysiology of osteoporosis: Unresolved problems and new insights. *Journal of Nutrition* 125(7 Suppl):2033S-2037S.

84. Pansini, F., Bagni, B., et al. 1995. Oophorectomy and spine bone density: Evidence of a higher rate of bone loss in surgical compared with spontaneous menopause. *Menopause* 2(2):109-115.

85. Barrett-Connor, E., and Kritz-Silverstein, D. 1996. Does hyperinsulinemia preserve bone? *Diabetes Care* 19(12):1388-1392.

86. Hla, M.M., Davis, J.W., Ross, P.D., Yates, J., et al. 2000. Relation between body composition and biochemical markers of bone turnover among early postmenopausal women. *Journal of Clinical Densitometry* 3(4):365-371.

87. Eagan, M.S., and Sedlock, D.A. 2001. Kyphosis in active and sedentary postmenopausal women. *Medicine and Science in Sports and Exercise* 33(5):688-695.

88. Larcos, G., and Baillon, L.B. 1998. An evaluation of bone mineral density in Australian women of Asian descent. *Australasian Radiology* 42(4):341-343.

89. Chien, M.Y., Wu, Y.T., Yang, R.S., Lai, J.S., and Hsu, A.T. 2000. Physical activity, physical fitness, and osteopenia in postmenopausal Taiwanese women. *Journal of the Formosan Medical Association* 99(1):11-17.

90. Ino, Y., Mizuno, K., Suzuki, A., Tamakoshi, A., Kikkawa, F., and Tomoda, Y. 1997. Factors influencing an ultrasound-estimated bone mass in postmenopausal women. *Journal of Obstetrics and Gynecology Research* 23(2):295-300.

91. Kulack, C.A., and Bilexikian, J.P. 1998. Osteoporosis: Preventive strategies. *International Journal of Fertility and Women's Medicine* 43(2):56-64.

92. Heikkinen, J., Kyllonen, E., Kurttila-Matero, E., Wilen-Rosenqvist, G., Lankinen, K.S., Rita, H., and Vaananen, H.K. 1997. HRT and exercise: Effects on bone density, muscle strength and lipid metabolism. A placebo controlled 2-year prospective trial on two estrogen-progestin regimens in healthy postmenopausal women. *Maturitas* 26(2):139-149.

93. Goto, S., Shigeta, H., Hyakutake, S., and Yamagata, M. 1996. Comparison between menopause-related changes in bone mineral density of the lumbar spine and the proximal femur in Japanese female athletes: A long-term longitudinal study using dual X-Ray absorptiometry. *Calcified Tissue International* 59(6):461-465.

94. Parra-Cabrera, S., Hernandez-Avila, M., Tamayo-y-Orozoco, J., Lopez-Carrillo, L., and Meneses-Gonzalez, F. 1996. Exercise and reproductive factors as predictors of bone density among osteoporotic women in Mexico City. *Calcified Tissue International* 59(2):89-94.

95. Ueda, A., Yoshimura, N., Morioka, S., Kasamatsu, T., Kinoshita, H., and Hasimoto, T. 1996. A population based study on factors related to bone mineral density in Wakayama Prefecture. *Japanese Journal of Public Health* 43(1):50-61.

96. Cheng, S., Suominen, H., Rantanen, T., Parkatti, T., and Heikkinen, E. 1991. Bone mineral density and physical activity in 50-60 year old women. *Bone and Mineral* 12:123-132.

97. American College of Sports Medicine position stand. 1995. Osteoporosis and exercise. *Medicine and Science in Sports and Exercise* 27(4):i-vii.

98. Geelhoed, E., Harris, A., and Prince, R. 1994. Cost-effectiveness analysis of hormone replacement therapy and lifestyle intervention for hip fracture. *Australian Journal of Public Health* 18(2):153.

99. Philosophe, R., and Seibel, M.M. 1991. Menopause and cardiovascular disease. *NAACOG's Clinical Issues in Perinatal and Women's Health Nursing* 2(4):441.

100. American Heart Association. 1993. *1993 heart and stroke facts.* Dallas: AHA.

101. Giardina, E.G. 1998. Call to action: Cardiovascular disease in women. *Journal of Women's Health* 7(1):37-43.

102. Sharp, P.C., and Konen, J.C. 1997. Women's cardiovascular health (Review). *Primary Care* 24(1):1-14.

103. Wenger, N.K., Speroff, L., and Packard, B. 1993. Cardiovascular health and disease in women. *New England Journal of Medicine* 329:247.

104. Brochier, M.L., and Arwidson, P. 1998. Coronary heart disease risk factors in women. *European Heart Journal* 19(Suppl A):A45-A52.

105. Panico, S., Galasso, R., Celentano, E., Ambrosca, C., Asti, A., Frova, L., Capocaccia, R., and Berrino, F. 1997. Hormone replacement therapy and cardiovascular diseases: Different populations, different risks. *Annali dell Istituto Superiore di Sanita* 33(2):203-206.

106. Davis, C.E., Deev, A.D., Shestov, D.B., Perova, N.V., Plavinskaya, S.I., Abolafia, J.M., Kim, H., and Tyroter, H.A. 1994. Correlates of mortality in Russian and US women: The lipid research clinics program. *American Journal of Epidemiology* 139:369-379.

107. Haddock, B.L., Marshak, H.P., Mason, J.J., and Blix, G. 2000. The effect of hormone replacement therapy and exercise on cardiovascular disease risk factors in postmenopausal women. *Sports Medicine* 29(1):39-49.

108. Shelley, J.M., Green, A., Smith, A.M., Dudley, E., Dennerstein, L., Hopper, J., and Burger, H. 1998. Relationship of endogenous sex hormones to lipids and blood pressure in mid-aged women. *Annals of Epidemiology* 8(1):39-45.

109. Chemnitius, J.M., Winkel, H., Meyer, I., Schirrmacher, K., Armstrong, V.W., Kreuzer, H., and Zech, R. 1998. Age-related decrease of high density lipoproteins (HDL) in women after menopause. Quantification of HDL with genetically determined HDL arylesterase in women with healthy coronary vessels and in women with angiographically verified coronary heart disease. *Mediz Klinik* 93(3):137-145.

110. Finucane, F.F., Madans, J.H., Bush, T.L., Wolf, P.H., and Kleinman, J.C. 1993. Decreased risk of stroke among postmenopausal hormone users. *Archives of Internal Medicine* 153:73-79.

111. Lalonde, G. 1993. Hormone replacement therapy and cardiovascular disease. In J. Lorrain, L. Plouffe Jr, V. Ravnikar, and L. Speroff (eds.), *Comprehensive management of the menopause.* NY: Springer-Verlag.

112. Hong, M.K., Romm, P.A., Reagan, K., Green, C.E., and Rackley, C.E. 1992. Effects of estrogen replacement therapy on serum lipid values and angiographically defined coronary artery disease in postmenopausal women. *American Journal of Cardiology* 69(3):176-178.

113. Stampfer, M.J., Colditz, G.A., Willett, W.C., Manson, J.E., Rosner, B., Speizer, F.E., and Hennekens, C.H. 1991. Postmenopausal estrogen therapy and cardiovascular risk disease: Ten-year follow-up from the Nurses' Health Study. *New England Journal of Medicine* 325:756.

114. McFarland, K.F., Boniface, M.E., Hornung, C.A., Earnhardt, W., and Humphries, J.O. 1989. Risk factors and noncontraceptive estrogen use in women with and without coronary disease. *American Journal of Cardiology* 69:176.

115. Beard, C.M., Kottke, T.E., Annegers, J.F., and Ballard, D.J. 1989. The Rochester Coronary Heart Disease Project: Effect of cigarette smoking, hypertension, diabetes, and steroidal estrogen use on coronary heart disease among 40 to 59 year old women, 1960 through 1982. *Mayo Clinic Proceedings* 64:1471.

116. Gruchow, H.W., Anderson, A.J., Barboriak, J.J., and Sobocinski, K.A. 1988. Postmenopausal use of estrogen and occlusion of coronary arteries. *American Heart Journal* 115:954.

117. Hassager, C., and Christiansen, C. 1988. Blood pressure during estrogen/progestogen substitution therapy in healthy postmenopausal women. *Maturitas* 9:315.

118. Sullivan, J.M., Vander Sqaag, R., Lemp, G.F., Hughes, J.P., et al. 1988. Postmenopausal estrogen use and coronary atherosclerosis. *Annals of Internal Medicine* 198:358.

119. Wren, B.G., and Routledge, A.D. 1983. The effect of type and dose of estrogen on the blood pressure of postmenopausal women. *Maturitas* 5:135.

120. Bain, C., Willett, W., Hennekens, C.H., Rosner, B., Belanger, C., and Speizer, F.E. 1981. Use of postmenopausal hormones and risk of myocardial infarction. *Circulation* 64:42.

121. Ross, R.K., Paganini-Hill, A., Mack, T.M., Arthur, M., and Henderson, B.E. 1981. Menopausal oestrogen therapy and protection from death from ischaemic heart disease. *Lancet* 1:585.

122. Futterman, L.G., and Lember, L. 2001. Lp(a) lipoprotein—an independent risk factor for coronary heart disease after menopause. *American Journal of Critical Care* 10(1):63-67.

123. Bonow, R.O., Bohannon, N., and Hazzard, W. 1996. Risk stratification in coronary artery disease and special populations. *American Journal of Medicine* 101(4A):A17S-A22S.

124. Wingrove, C.S., Walton, C., and Stevenson, J.C. 1998. The effect of menopause on serum uric acid levels in non-obese healthy women. *Metabolism* 47(4) 435-438.

125. Lev, E.I., Pines, A., Drory, Y., Rotmensch, H.H., Tenenbaum, A., and Fisman, E.Z. 1998. Exercise-induced aortic flow parameters in early postmenopausal women and middle-aged men. *Journal of Internal Medicine* 243(4):275-280.

126. Ickovics, J.R., Morrill, A.C., Meilser, A.W., Rodin, J., Bromberger, J.T., and Matthews, K.A. 1996. Employment and coronary risk in women at midlife: A longitudinal analysis. *American Journal of Epidemiology* 143(2):144-150.

127. Naimark, B.J., Read, A.E., Sawatzky, J.A., Boreskie, S., Ducas, J., Drinkwater, D.T., and Oosterveen, S. 1996. Serum ferritin and heart disease: The effect of moderate exercise on stored iron levels in postmenopausal women. *Canadian Journal of Cardiology* 12(12):1253-1257.

128. Stevenson, E.T., Davy, K.P., Jones, P.P., Desouza, C.A., and Seals, D.R. 1997. Blood pressure risk factors in healthy postmenopausal women: Physical activity and hormone replacement. *Journal of Applied Physiology* 82(2):652-660.

129. Green, J.S., Crouse, S.F., Rohack, J.J. 1998. Peak exercise hemodynamics in exercising postmenopausal women taking versus not taking supplemental estrogen. *Medicine and Science in Sports and Exercise* 30(1):158-164.

130. Dennerstein, L., Dudley, E., Guthrie, J., and Barrett-Connor, E. 2000. Life satisfaction, symptoms, and the menopausal transition. *Medscape Women's Health* 54(4):E4.

131. Barinaga, M. 1994. Watching the brain remake itself. *Science* (Dec. 2):1475-1476.

132. Henderson, V.W., Paganini-Hill, A., Emanuel, C.K., Dunn, M.E., and Buckwalter, J.G. 1994. Estrogen replacement therapy in older women: Comparisons between Alzheimer's disease cases and nondemented control subjects. *Archives of Neurology* 51:896-900.

133. Kawas, C., Resnick, S., Morrison, A., Brookmeyer, R., Corrada, M., et al. 1997. A prospective study of estrogen replacement therapy and the risk of developing Alzheimer's Disease: The Baltimore Longitudinal Study of Aging. *Neurology* 48:1517-1521.

134. Paganini-Hill, A., and Henderson, V.W. 1996. Estrogen replacement therapy and the risk of Alzheimer's Disease. *Archives of Internal Medicine* 156:2214-2217.

135. Vane, J.R., and Botting, R.M. 1998. Mechanisms of action in anti-inflammatory drugs. *International Journal of Tissue Reactions* 20(1):3-15.

136. Stewart, W.F., Kawas, C., Corraa, M., and Metter, E.J. 1997. Risk of Alzheimer's disease and duration of NSAID use. *Neurology* 48(3):626-632.

137. de la Torre, J.C. 1997. Cerebromicrovascular pathology in Alzheimer's disease compared to normal aging. *Gerontology* 43(1-2):26-43.

138. Rich, J.B., Rasmusson, D.X., Folstein, M.F., Carson, K.A., Kawas, C., and Brandt, J. 1995. Nonsteroidal anti-inflammatory drugs in Alzheimer's disease. *Neurology* 45(1):51-55.

139. Reiter, R.J., Carneiro, R.C., and Oh, C.S. 1997. Melatonin in relation to cellular antioxidative defense mechanisms. *Hormone and Metabolic Research* 29(8):363-372.

140. Crawford, J.G. 1996. Alzheimer's disease risk factors as related to cerebral blood flow. *Medical Hypotheses* 46(4):367-377.

141. Naftolin, F., Leranth, C., Perez, J., and Garcia-Segura, L.M. 1993. Estrogen induces synaptic plasticity in adult primate neurons. *Neuroendocrinology* 57:935-939.

142. Slaven, L., and Lee, C. 1997. Mood and symptom reporting among middle-aged women: The relationship between menopausal status, hormone replacement therapy, and exercise participation. *Health Psychology* 16(3):203-208.

143. Murphy, J.M. 1986. Trends in depression and anxiety: Men and women. *Acta Psychiatrica Scandinavica* 73:113-127.

144. Kessler, R.C., McGonage, K.A., Swartz, M.S., Blazer, D.G., and Nelson, C.B. 1993. Sex and depression in the National Comorbidity Survey I: Lifetime prevalence, chronicity and recurrence. *Journal of Affective Disorders* 29:85-96.

145. McQuaide, S. 1998. Women at midlife. *Social Work* 43(1):21-31.

146. Spiegel, D., Boom, J.R., Kraemer, H.C., and Gottheil, E. 1989. Effect of psychosocial treatment on survival of patients with metastatic breast cancer. *Lancet* ii:888-891.

147. Shumaker, S.A., and Czajikowski, S.M. (eds.). 1994. *Social support and cardiovascular disease.* NY: Plenum Press.

148. Bastian, L.A., Courchman, G.M., Rimer, B.K., McBride, C.M., Feagames, J.R., and Siegler, I.C. 1997. Perceptions of menopausal stage and patterns of hormone replacement therapy use. *Journal of Women's Health* 6(4):467-475.

149. O'Connor, A.M., Tugwell, P., Wells, G.A., Elmslie, T., Jollie, E., Hollingsworth, G., McPherson, R., Bunn, H., Graham, I., and Drake, E. 1998. A decision aid for women considering hormone therapy after menopause: Decision support framework and evaluation. *Patient Education and Counseling* 33(3):267-279.

150. Rothert, M.L., Holmes-Rovner, M., Rovner, D., Kroll, J., et al. 1997. An educational intervention as decision support for menopausal women. *Research in Nursing & Health* 20(5):377-387.

151. DiPietro, L. 1996. Habitual physical activity among women. In O. Bar-Or, D.R. Lamb, and P.M. Clarkson (eds.), *Perspectives in exercise science and sports medicine. Vol 9: Exercise and the female: A life-span approach.* Carmel, IN: Cooper Publishing Group.

152. Ziel, H., and Finkle, W. 1975. Increased risk of endometrial carcinoma among users of conjugated estrogens. *New England Journal of Medicine* 293:1167-1170.

153. Mack, T., Picke, M., Henderson, B., Pfeffer, R., Gerkins, V., Arthur, M., and Brown, S. 1976. Estrogens and endometrial cancer in the U.S. *New England Journal of Medicine* 294:1262.

154. Weiss, N., Szekely, D., and Austin, F. 1976. Increasing incidence of endometrial cancer in the United States. *New England Journal of Medicine* 294:1259.

155. Cummings, S.R. 1992. Hormone therapy to prevent disease and prolong life in postmenopausal women. *Annals of Internal Medicine* 117(12):1016-1037.

156. Colditz, G.A., Hankinson, S.E., Huner, D.J., Willett, C.E., Manson, J.E., Stampfer, M.J., Hennekens, C., Rosner, B., and Speizer, F.E. 1995. The use of estrogens and progestins and the risk of breast cancer in postmenopausal women. *New England Journal of Medicine* 331(24):1589-1593.

157. Colditz, G.A. 1998. Relationship between estrogen levels, use of hormone replacement therapy and breast cancer. *Journal of the National Cancer Institute* 90(11):814-823.

158. Risch, H.A., Jain, M., Marrett, L.D., and Howe, G.R. 1994. Dietary fat intake and risk of epithelial ovarian cancer. *Journal of the National Cancer Institute* 86(18):1409-1415.

159. Lauritzen, C. 1994. Cancer risk under hormone therapy (review). *Therapeutische Umschau* 51(11):755-766.

160. Chien, C.H., Wang, F.F., and Hamilton, T.C. 1994. Transcriptional activation of c-myc proto-oncogene by estrogen in human ovarian cancer cells. *Molecular and Cellular Endocrinology* 99(1):11-19.

161. Galtier-Dereure, F., Capony, F., Mandelonde, T., and Rochefort, H. 1992. Estradiol stimulates cell growth and secretion of procathepsin D and a 120 kilodalton protein in the human ovarian cancer cell line BG-1. *Journal of Clinical Endocrinology and Metabolism* 75(6):1467-1502.

162. Bernstein, L., Ross, R.K., and Henderson, B.E. 1992. Relationship of hormone use to cancer risk. *Journal of the National Cancer Institute: Monograms* (12):137-147.

163. DeCree, C., Van Kranenberg, G., Guerten, P., Fujimori, Y., and Keizer, H.A. 1997. 4-Hydroxycatecholstrogen metabolism responses to exercise and training: Possible implications for menstrual cycle irregularities and breast cancer. *Fertility and Sterility* 67(3):505-516.

164. Thune, I., Brenn, T., Lund, E., and Gaard, M. 1997. Physical activity and the risk of breast cancer. *New England Journal of Medicine* 336(18):1269-1275.

165. Love, P.R., and Vogel, V.G. 1997. Breast cancer prevention strategies. *Oncology* 11(2):161.

166. Stoll, B.A. 1995. Timing of weight gain in relation to breast cancer risk. *Annals of Oncology* 6(3):245-248.

167. Ginsbery, E.S., Millo, N.K., Mendelson, J.H., Barbieri, R.L., et al. 1996. Effects of alcohol ingestion on estrogens in postmenopausal women. *Journal of the American Medical Association* 276(21):1747-1751.

168. Brynhildsen, J.O., Bjors, E., Skarsgard, C., and Hammar, H.L. 1998. Is hormone replacement therapy a risk factor for low back pain among postmenopausal women? *Spine* 23(7):809-813.

169. Rosenbery, L., Palmer, J.R., Rao, R.S., and Adams-Campbell, L.L. 1998. Correlates of postmenopausal female hormone use among black women in the United States. *Obstetrics and Gynecology* 91(3):454-458.

170. Nakano, Y., Oshima, T., Matsuura, H., Kajiyama, G., and Kambe, M. 1998. Effect of 17Beta estradiol on inhibition of platelet aggregation in vitro is mediated by an increase in NO synthesis. *Arterisclerosis, Thrombosis, and Vascular Biology* 18(6):961-967.

171. Oger, E., and Scarabin, P.Y. 1999. Hormone replacement therapy in menopause and the risk of cerebrovascular accident [French]. *Annales d'Endocrinologie* 60(3):232-241.

CHAPTER 13

GOALS AND PRIORITIES OF MIDLIFE FITNESS PROGRAMS

This chapter deals with setting goals and priorities of fitness programs for women during the midlife period that encompasses menopause. Goals for this population include enhancing the quality of life, promoting health and preventing disease, and improving balance and posture. Priorities include safety, effectiveness, and advanced networking.

SETTING GOALS FOR WOMEN'S MIDLIFE FITNESS

What direction should our goal setting take when we address the population that is close to, in the process of, or finished with menopause? We are no longer primarily concerned with potential, but rather effects of lifestyle. One woman might flow into midlife with lifelong physical activity, having eaten a healthy diet, practiced stress management techniques, had access to appropriate health care, and experienced her perimenopausal period as largely asymptomatic. Another may have a history of a high volume of high-intensity activity, menstrual dysfunction, osteoporosis, and a genetic predisposition to arthritis or stroke. A third woman might have a sedentary history, obesity, type 2 diabetes, and high blood pressure. A fourth might have health-risk behaviors such as

smoking, yet also enviable genes that have kept her disease free in the first 50 years of life.

There are no guarantees in midlife and beyond. If genetics don't endanger a woman, the effects of aging, risky behavior, or psychosomatic or environmental factors may. But the resources she brings with her to midlife and how she chooses to deal with matters at hand will have an impact on how she weathers this transition, and this is our main direction. Goals that we can reasonably expect to attain to some degree from well-designed fitness programs for midlife women include enhancing the quality of life, promoting health and preventing disease, and improving balance, posture, and weight control.

FIRST GOAL: ENHANCING THE QUALITY OF LIFE

The joy of moving must first be established if any of these goals stand a chance. The capabilities of movement to reduce tension and stress, relieve discomfort, contribute to mental well-being, and improve outcomes are life-enhancing capabilities. For women who tap into the power of moving because it is pleasurable, life enhancement is an obvious goal. The human body is built to move in accordance with the laws of gravity, and if it does not do so frequently, there are negative health consequences. It may be that for many years a woman moved her body to meet the demands of family, home, job, or life situation. Or, professional dance, sport, athletic competition, or recreational exercise regimens may have come to dictate how she moves. Midlife presents an opportunity to invoke the pleasure principle of movement (i.e., moving from internal cues because it feels good). Some women make adjustments that allow them to continue running—or walking—marathons. Others take up the tango.

The capacity of physical activity to relieve physical discomfort is exemplified by its beneficial effect on the disorder called *fibromyalgia*. This disorder, a condition in which tendons, ligaments, and muscles are painfully tender and which often involves fatigue and stiffness, primarily affects women. Some of its symptoms are characteristic of autoimmune or inflammatory disorders. Movement seems a critical component in relieving this condition, as maintaining one position for long periods is poorly tolerated by this population [1]. Exercise seems to be the most effective therapy [2], with stretching, strength training, and moderate cardiovascular activities proving helpful [3].

Midlife can be a time when life challenges come from many directions. Falling levels of estrogen and progesterone are associated with changes in muscle recovery, fat deposition, mental function, joint discomfort, sleep disturbances, dry skin, and painful intercourse. While undergoing such a major physical transition, a woman may also be in the midst of stressful emotional events—relating to aging parents, children with problems, marital difficulties, or financial woes. Women whose resources are already stretched and who have chronic or acute illness may not be looking for an exercise program. Yet appropriate physical activities aimed at bringing together groups of women with the same issue—such as mothers and grandmothers of adolescent mothers, or women with breast cancer— can involve needed support, improve physical outcomes, and lay the groundwork for important personal growth.

As women age, the ability of exercise to improve cognitive function and mood [4] is a clue to how movement creates its own reward. Having a clear mind is pleasurable and meaningful. It is also reasonable to expect that moving with a moderate level of exertion in one's midlife and later years produces heightened awareness and the joyful, exalted feelings associated with the production of endogenous beta-endorphins. The joy of movement is the best basis for commitment to physical fitness, for enjoyment is a critical factor in long-term adherence and mental benefits [5].

SECOND GOAL: PROMOTING HEALTH AND PREVENTING DISEASE

Physical fitness has been shown to be an effective strategy for reducing disease and death [6]. Although various other factors are significant in particular cases, physical activity is the one factor that is consistently significantly associated with health. Recreational exercise or daily physical activity for perimenopausal and menopausal women can be a gateway to lifestyle behaviors that help to optimize women's health as they age. In 1991, Gillis and Perry reported a relationship between physical activity and health-promoting behaviors in rural midlife women. The researchers identified participation in physical activity as a predictor of healthy behaviors in this population [7]. In order for a person to sustain an active lifestyle, other health-promoting behaviors are necessary. Movement involves energy output, which appears to be a key component in healthy human function at many levels from biomechanics to molecular transport. Habituation to physical activity can drive fuel acquisition through eating nutritious food, or provide the impetus to get regular sleep and resist activities that drain energy such as smoking.

But practical interventions for the purpose of disease prevention or treatment have focused largely on getting individuals to make massive, multifaceted lifestyle changes at midlife, instead of directing efforts at simply helping people enjoy moving and thereby creating an innate need for sustaining healthy behaviors. For women, success in lifestyle change depends on high levels of support from health care providers and significant social contacts [8]. Change is a slow, incremental process. Moreover, we don't know whether massive interventions really work with adult women [9].

What other evidence do we have that focusing on physical activity might be an effective centerpiece for health promotion and disease prevention for this population? What about the impact of exercise on immune function in postmenopausal women? Women experience higher levels of autoimmune disorders and inflammatory responses following menopause [10], when estrogen falls to very low levels, than do men or premenopausal women. Nieman et al. conducted an interesting study to examine the influence of physical activity on immune function in Caucasian women in their 60s, 70s, and 80s. The control group consisted of 12 highly conditioned women, active in endurance competitions. Thirty-two sedentary women were randomized into two experimental groups, participating in either a calisthenics or a walking program. The researchers found that the highly conditioned group had superior natural killer and T-cell function, but that neither experimental group showed any improvement in these measures following a 12-week program [11]. The incidence of upper respiratory tract infections was lowest in the highly conditioned group and highest in the calisthenics group, with the walking group in an intermediate position [11]. The walking group also showed improved $\dot{V}O_2$max .

Nieman and Pedersen also found that the summation effect of a 12- to 15-week general-population program of near-daily brisk walking reduced the incidence of illness and infections (as measured by sickness days) by half [12]. In addition, the most dramatic preventative effects of an intervention on the stress of intense exercise—which appears necessary for disease protection at the cell level—may be those of carbohydrate ingestion (which has been associated with higher plasma glucose levels, attenuated cortisol and growth hormone response, fewer perturbations in oxidative burst activity, and diminished pro- and anti-inflammatory cytokine response) [12]. Indications are that both long- and short-term physical activity histories have some, albeit small, impact on immune function, and that the effect of diet in regard to a well-functioning immune system may be a critical factor as level of activity increases.

What about other areas of women's health such as bones, heart, and psychosomatic problems like stress? We have already seen a fair amount of evidence that exercise contributes to positive outcomes in these areas. What other information promotes the idea that exercise is a factor in health? In an Australian study by Ward et al., superior quadriceps strength, nonsmoking, and high levels of current physical activity were significantly associated with high bone density at the femoral neck in a cohort of 311 women aged 60 to 91 (mean age 72.2) [13]. Those with little childhood activity were significantly associated with low bone density [13]. Interestingly, although many anthropomorphic, health, and lifestyle measures were included in the study, only physical activity and smoking status were significant and independent predictors of bone density with physical activity predicting greater bone mineral density (BMD) and smoking predicting lower BMD. Gender differences in muscle sympathetic nerve activity that affect cardiovasculature [14, 15] help explain why premenopausal women are protected from cardiovascular diseases but "catch up" following menopause [16]. The effect of physical activity on older adults may well include influence on muscle sympathetic nerve activity changes associated with aging [14], and theoretically explains some of the heart protection that exercise offers older individuals, including women. For women, stress is a major psychosocial factor associated with non-insulin-dependent diabetes mellitus, or type 2 diabetes [17], and coronary heart disease [18]. The ability of vigorous exercise and

stress management techniques to offset the effects of stress has been discussed often in this text.

THIRD GOAL: IMPROVING BALANCE, POSTURE, AND WEIGHT CONTROL

A number of issues related to biomechanics confront midlife women, including osteoporosis, sarcopenia (loss of muscle mass), arthritis, and other inflammatory and autoimmune disorders. But in this portion of the life cycle we have to be efficient. Just as physical activity provides an impetus for other health-inducing behaviors, focusing on balance and posture gives us more than just these two outcomes.

Balance can be a gateway competency. There is a balance exercise to suit every level of skill and experience. We can ask women with limited fitness to sit in a chair and raise one leg, putting the arms out to the side for balance. We can ask our highly fit women to do this on an exercise ball or standing on one leg. Women can walk and freeze, or jog and stop on one leg. They can participate in tai chi or adapted yoga. Balance skills that result from exercise are clearly useful in the older population to help prevent falls, and efforts can begin in midlife to optimize the coordination and strength levels that contribute to balance.

Posture and weight control appeal to our vanity. They are worth working on so that women feel strong and look attractive. To attain healthy posture, women can load bones and muscles, lift weights or move furniture for upper-body strength, then reach up and out for objects on shelves to stretch these muscles. They can do squats (with chairs under the buttocks for safety) to develop hip and thigh strength, and jump or jog to improve BMD. We learned in the last chapter that a high level of body fat is a predictor of kyphosis, one of the major postural deformities seen in older women. Strength and changes in body composition intersect at their impact on BMD. Consequently, body fat is a factor we can also use to track prediction of postural problems.

Acquiring and Developing Balance and Posture Skills

The ability of exercise to reduce the risk of falls and fractures in later years is a significant aspect of the long-term beneficial outcomes associated with physical activity for women. As our knowledge in this area grows, we are finding that not only general aerobic exercise provides this benefit for older women [19]; tai chi and computerized balance training [20] also help to reduce risk of falls and fractures, as well as producing improvements in ankle dorsiflexion, hip extension, and hip flexion strength [21].

The impact of postural sway (i.e., the incipient stabilizing actions of the muscles) on stability and injury prevention is significant [19, 22]. We can reasonably expect some degree of benefit in this area from strength training for postural muscles and from participation in antigravity cardiovascular activities from midlife forward. The techniques mentioned earlier, and also the centering activities described in previous chapters, help a woman sense upright and develop righting skills. These techniques can easily be incorporated into programming for midlife women both as a means of helping prevent falls as women age and as a means of providing improved leverage and force for powerful movement.

In practice, activities promoting centering, proprioceptive skills, and postural strength are among those most appreciated by a diverse sample of midlife women participating in physical activity in a variety of settings [23]. Learning to sense one's central axis while seated and standing, and learning to rise from a chair without using one's arms while maintaining a balanced center of gravity (see figure 13.1), have proven popular with women from varying educational, socioeconomic, and racial

backgrounds [23]. Once the ability to sense balance and carry it into larger movements is acquired, it becomes easier to ensure its presence in daily biomechanical challenges such as lifting or carrying household and work-related objects, or in coordination challenges such as tripping on a rug.

Reducing Body Fat

The level of body fat as a marker for possible bone deformity may not be an independent factor. In older obese females and males, the combination of resistance training and hypocaloric dieting has the effects of augmenting lean body mass, reducing fat mass, and increasing trabecular bone in the lumbar spine [24]; in contrast, the combination of aerobic exercise and hypocaloric diet is associated with loss of both fat and lean mass [24]. This finding, along with the association of chronic exercise with body fat reduction and increases in BMD in postmenopausal women [25], contributes to our understanding. It is the combination of metabolic processes resulting in postmenopausal increases in BMD and muscle mass that affects the association of body fat and bone deformity. For midlife and older women with high body fat, the exercise prescription should include a combina-

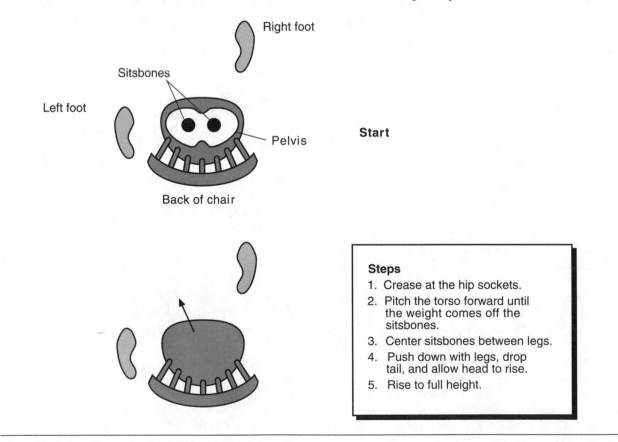

Figure 13.1   Standing up from a chair while centered.

tion of resistance training and calorie restriction for best results.

Ovarian hormones contribute to differences in how energy is mobilized, utilized, and stored, leading to variations in body composition, control of feeding, and tolerance of starvation conditions (fertile women tolerate starvation more readily than men) [26]. Current thinking suggests that falling levels of female hormones shift the energy balance in midlife women, increasing the tendency for women to develop central adiposity (abdominal fat). This places a woman at risk for adverse metabolic consequences because central adiposity is more resistant to aerobic exercise intervention than is fat deposited in the buttocks or thigh [27-29].

Weight Gain in Midlife

The phenomenon of weight gain during the midlife period is controversial. Although weight gain in menopause is commonly remarked on and is sometimes associated with hormone replacement therapy (HRT) in popular thinking, the Massachusetts Women's Health Study analysis of the relationship between menopause transition and weight status did not show a link between menopause transition and weight gain [30]. Other findings from this study included no significant relationship between HRT and weight gain; the relationship between behavioral factors— particularly exercise and alcohol consumption—and weight in this period was stronger [30]. The researchers concluded that the weight increases experienced by midlife women in the United States are not a result of the menopause transition [30].

So, where does reported weight gain come from? One possibility is that once a woman reaches menopause, subsequent weight gain reflects increases in body fat and abdominal fat related to aging. Changes in body composition in this time may reflect the accumulating effects of sarcopenia and insulin resistance, and the increasing need for exertion to stave off these effects. As noted by Astrup, cross-sectional studies indicate that postmenopausal women with high levels of physical activity have less body fat and abdominal fat than those without, and longitudinal studies show that physically active women are less prone than sedentary women to gaining body fat and abdominal fat after menopause [31].

Hormone Replacement Therapy and Weight Gain

What about weight gain and HRT? As already mentioned, despite the common view that hormone replacement is responsible for weight gain in menopause, the evidence does not support this view. Statistical analysis using weighted mean difference for continuous outcomes shows no effect of either unopposed estrogen or the combination of estrogen and progesterone on weight gain and body fat distribution in perimenopausal and postmenopausal women [32]. There is a need for further research to explicate the issues of midlife weight gain, changes in body composition and fat deposition, and the role of exercise in prevention of bone deformities associated with high levels of body fat. In any case, exercise that helps maintain lean body mass appears to be important for maintaining a healthy skeleton in midlife and beyond.

SETTING PRIORITIES

An essential function of programming for this population is to help women experience physical activity as a joyful feeling within themselves. Learning to center, to exert oneself, and to relax puts the knowledge into the body. Being centered while seated or standing leads to moving in a centered way. Women can sense from the inside how weight is borne in the body before stressing the system with movement. They can sense the impact of motion and learn to move the body's energy where it is needed to maintain safety.

Safety is the first priority, for without it, we cannot expect to meet the second priority, effectiveness. The third priority, advanced networking, is a nod to the realization that by the time a woman has survived a half-century, she has mastered the basics of community building. The information she needs from here on is more technical than the information she needed previously and evolves constantly. Her support system may be evolving, too, for friends and family are going through their own life changes.

FIRST PRIORITY: SAFETY

Safety, as always, consists of both physical and psychological aspects. Everything from the character of the space to the appropriateness of the activities affects the physical aspect. Physical safety itself is a factor in psychological safety, along with instructional methodologies, education, and support. Program format and time structure bear on whether activity becomes a safe haven or a source of stress.

Physical Safety

Issues surrounding physical safety can be deterrents to women's participation in physical activity [33]. The physical characteristics of a space, its location (is the neighborhood safe and/or familiar?), cleanliness, attractiveness, and lack of physical hazards affect women's responses. And women are more resistant to cooling as they age [34], so temperature control is important, along with comfort in clothing. A safe place that encourages sociability, that has a forgiving floor, and that has a bathroom nearby is important. Whereas a percentage of women accept a gym or health club atmosphere and some are comfortable in a women's gym, many (especially in the inner city) are more willing to participate at a more familiar location, such as a church or community center where they are already active.

Procedural issues—intake and screening, needs assessments, and prescription adherence in the case of a medical referral—take on added importance as people age. Modifications of movements to increase joint protection or to allow for postural anomalies may be indicated. Assessment of safe intensities, frequencies, and durations is necessary for strength, endurance, and flexibility activities. These won't necessarily follow standard guidelines, either, as the effects of lifestyle and personal tolerances, as well as life's other demands, impinge on the process. For example, a woman who has been sedentary for many years, and who has good genes for endurance, may have a cardiovasculature willing to progress normally to 30 minutes of moderate-intensity walking five days a week. However, her knees may not be able to keep up. Or, a woman who lifts and carries her grandchildren every other week may need a rotating weight-training schedule that takes this into account. Monitoring for unusual back or chest pain, dizziness, or other complaints that could indicate a problem is essential, as is making sure that women understand they should not continue exercising if they feel something is not right.

Psychological Safety

Perhaps for the first time ever, a woman in midlife is facing the reality that her body is aging, and she may be fearful. On the other hand, she may be thrilled that her children have left the nest and she is free to join a masters women's rowing team, lift weights, take her first tap dance class, or return to the ballet technique she loved as a young girl. Eaton and Enns have pointed out that the physiological determinants associated with gender and age are likely to affect the motivation for a person to participate in activities at which she is competent [35]. For a trainer or group instructor, this means not only finding out what movements a woman already does well and reinforcing them, but also telling her about her progress—and not just numbers, but also style and enthusiasm. These aspects require exertion and affect intensity. Triathlon will be a truly equal sport when points are given for style, too!

According to DiPietro, one can say that women have a cyclical relationship with conditioning because of the impact of life events, and there may well be a need for multiple assessments of conditioning status during a woman's lifetime to accurately reflect the impact of physical activity on women's long-term health [36]. It may benefit a midlife woman if a practitioner who is doing assessments recognizes that her body has a story to tell about her life and accomplishments. Finding out about her prior and present physical capacities takes on the function of explicating this story. Such questioning uncovers events that may have profoundly affected her identity or emotional life through their physical impact, such as how many children she has given birth to, which activities she enjoyed in high school, or the nature of injuries she sustained as a college athlete. In this way, assessment serves educational and discovery functions for the practitioner and the woman. Moving away from a linear approach to thinking about fitness, and acknowledging the circular nature of the female life cycle, may help women open up psychologically safe avenues to tap prior accomplishments of their lives as a basis for present-day healthy living. And it may also provide clues to areas that require delicacy or discretion on the part of the instructor or trainer. An instructor who can bring central issues—be they osteoporosis, heart disease, cancer, bladder control, or simply wrinkles—into an open and supportive discussion, provides a safe place for individual concerns to be aired as well.

SECOND PRIORITY: EFFECTIVENESS

If a person makes lifestyle changes that are sufficiently demanding, in terms of time for exercise, to produce measurable increases in strength or $\dot{V}O_2$max, the assumption is that the program is effective. But for a woman with heart disease or bone loss, is this the only case scenario? We want our program to alter this woman's risk factors for a cardiovascular event or further bone loss. For women, though, the prognosis is poor for a lifestyle change involving the time commitment necessary in standard male models of exercise to improve measurable physical performance [8, 9]. Could there be another effective strategy?

Deconstructing Male-Centered Models

As part of the larger mandate to discover exercise determinants and create effective interventions aimed at increasing public participation for all adults, researchers have focused on developing cognitive and behavioral theories and models. While many important contributions [37-50] have added to an evolving picture of the perceived benefits/barriers, motivations, modification factors, learning steps, stages of change, and methods of support, there has been little effect on the level of participation by midlife women. Slowly, though, we are focusing in on understanding the real issues involved in bringing inactive women into the circle: doing things that women want to do in ways that women want to do them, and educating women through a corresponding shift in promotional imagery.

In the early 1990s, researchers in sport and exercise began to publish work on the need for changes in psychosocial models to reflect the presence of women. Messner noted that, fundamentally, the sociology of sport absorbed women without making theoretical changes [51]. As discussed by Henderson, the study of recreational or leisure activities had focused largely on activities appealing to men, dismissing the lower levels of female participation as merely a result of less leisure time due to family obligations [52]. And Lee argued that the existing models were not capable of distinguishing between male and female experience in a way that revealed the true barriers for women (especially midlife and older women) to participation in health-promoting physical activities [53]. As we go back through existing models to uncover where underlying assumptions go awry—and scuttle a lot of the theory base, retaining only ideas, concepts, and words generated by women-centered thinking—we are making some progress in assessing ways to improve the health of women through greater inclusion in physical activity.

For one thing, self-efficacy has been consistently found to be positively associated with physical activity in adults of both sexes, including working women [54]. This has raised questions. Are we asking women what they like to do, and might some of these things be included in the category of physical activity? If we do ask this question, might more women see themselves as at least somewhat physically active (and be counted as such)? And, if more women see themselves as physically active, might they be willing to increase their participation toward greater health promotion? Such thinking has brought gardening, housework, child care, ballroom dancing, ballet, and yoga into the realm of effective physical activity.

Constructing the Social Female Model

To ensure that cardiovascular rehabilitation formats for women meet their needs, Arnold suggests something similar to what we have found effective with postpartum women: provide an opportunity for women to share their experiences of a stressful life event with other women [18]. In the area of osteoporosis, we know that group community exercise programs are effective in reducing fracture risk factors for older women [19, 20]. Gender differences in psychosocial variables and response to lifestyle management programs make it clear that women benefit the most in women's groups [55-57]. Research on older women reinforces the idea that the social model discussed in chapter 1 is an effective women's model of physical activity [58].

With time-commitment and financial barriers, it might make sense to provide community education about a given condition and exercise instructions to improve outcomes, then let women proceed largely on their own; but this strategy needs refinement. One study involving a five-year follow-up showed that although women who had been educated about menopause were more knowledgeable than those who had not, there were no differences in health or mood [59]. In another study, an unvarying home exercise program for an experimental group of women at risk for osteoporosis promoted general agility but resulted in no significant improvements in strength or postural stability over values in the control group at a seven-year follow up [60]. A personal trainer may be a viable solution for the portion of the population that has adequate social support already, has time issues but understands the need for compliance, and can afford to hire such a person. Work with trainers in a gym or club setting may be effective, but there are no data on the outcomes of this approach, and it may be financially out of the reach of many women with health problems.

One portion of the population we have little information about is the self-efficacious group of women who—already aware through public education or their own research efforts that physical activity is important—have independently developed strategies such as walking groups, bicycling or in-line skating groups, or women-only drop-in facilities with brief modular conditioning routines. An example is the walking group shown in figure 13.2, which emerged spontaneously among neighbors. The National Black Women's Health Project's Walking for Wellness program represents a larger effort. Given issues of safety, time pressures in women's lives, and the inability of measurement techniques to account for the effect of activities of daily living on women's overall activity levels [36], these case-by-case strategies, tailored by the participants to meet their own needs and experience, may be the most effective ones we have. Clearly, we need research that helps us clarify the relationship between public education, peer pressure, media imagery, use of the Internet, and other factors that prompt midlife women to devise their own effective strategies.

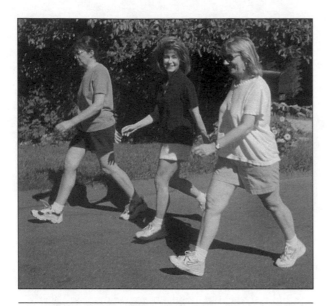

Figure 13.2 Neighborhood walking group. Although little is known about the impact on women's health of spontaneously generated groups of walkers, they may be a highly effective factor. This group, which has been walking together for several years, consists of two women with very long-term commitments to walking and one woman they recruited to join their group. They describe themselves as benefiting physically and spiritually from their near-daily walks.

THIRD PRIORITY: ADVANCED NETWORKING

By midlife, many women already have a community for emotional support. But they may need new information sources for menopause or the symptoms or disorders that accompany a midlife transition. They may need help finding the physicians and midwives with the best track record in a specific area, books or research studies that are worth reading, or Internet sites that have legitimate information. Some women may find themselves in need of financial planning or better survival skills. Others may be looking for support groups around a particular condition, such as breast cancer. Or, they may be looking to get into clinical trials for experimental drugs or other treatments.

As the population of proactive midlife women gets larger and becomes more inclusive of women of color, housewives, and disadvantaged women, the advanced network that is forming is a newly visible and potentially powerful entity. Within it, there are already fitness professionals and researchers. Those designing programs for women in midlife need to remember that these women have been caring for their own and/or their family's health for 20 or 30 years, as well as allocating health dollars. As health care costs rise and health maintenance becomes less accessible to women, this network will need mobi-

lizing so that society does not lose the benefit of its wisdom or shortchange its health status.

Because physical fitness plays a significant role in health, the creation of midlife women's fitness groups represents an important mechanism for bringing greater physical activity into the national health equation. Placing the knowledge and experience to promote physical activity into the hands of women makes it accessible to the entire family. Giving women control of the mode of activity and how progress is assessed could also produce interesting new lines of inquiry. In the next—and final—chapter, designing programs expressly to address the common needs of midlife women is discussed. Bringing such programs into existence can be a first step in improving the market value of an active lifestyle.

REFERENCES

1. Waylonis, G.W., Ronan, P.G., and Gordon, C. 1994. A profile of fibromyalgia in occupational environments. *American Journal of Physical Medicine & Rehabilitation* 73:112-115.
2. Perlmutter, C., and Goldstein, L. 1997. The truth about fibromyalgia. *Prevention* 49:86-91.
3. Roozen, M.M. 1998. Training individuals with fibromyalgia. *Strength and Conditioning Journal* 20(2):64-66.
4. William, P., and Lord, S.R. 1997. Effects of group exercise on cognitive functioning and mood in older women. *Australian and New Zealand Journal of Public Health* 21(1):45-52.
5. Wankel, L.M. 1993. The importance of enjoyment to adherence and psychological benefits from physical activity. *International Journal of Sport Psychology* 24(2):151-169.
6. Blair, S.N., Kohl, H.W., 3rd, Paffenbarger, R.S., Clark, D.G., Cooper, K.H., and Gibbons, L.W. 1989. Physical fitness and all-cause mortality: A prospective study of healthy men and women. *Journal of the American Medical Association* 262:2395-2401.
7. Gillis, A., and Perry, A. 1991. The relationships between physical activity and health-promoting behaviours in mid-life women. *Journal of Advances in Nursing* 16(3):299-310.
8. Mosca, L., McGillen, C., and Rubenfire, M. 1998. Gender differences in barriers to lifestyle change for cardiovascular disease prevention. *Journal of Women's Health* 7(6):711-715.
9. Toobert, D.J., Strycker, L.A., and Glasgow, R.E. 1998. Lifestyle change in women with coronary heart disease: What do we know? *Journal of Women's Health* 7(6):685-699.
10. Tiidus, P.M. 1999. Nutritional implications of gender differences in metabolism: Estrogen and oxygen radicals: Oxidative damage, inflammation, and muscle function. Chapter 11 in M. Tarnopolsky (ed.), *Gender differences in metabolism*. Baton Raton, FL: CRC Press.
11. Nieman, D.C., Henson, D.A., Gusewitch, G., et al. 1993. Physical activity and immune function in elderly women. *Medicine and Science in Sports and Exercise* 25(7):23-31.
12. Nieman, D.C., and Pedersen, B.K. 1999. Exercise and immune function. Recent developments. *Sports Medicine* 27(2):73-80.
13. Ward, J.A., Lord, S.R., Williams, P., Anstey, K., and Zivanovic, E. 1995. Physiologic, health and lifestyle factors associated with femoral neck bone density in older women. *Bone* 16(4 Suppl):373S-378S.
14. Ettinger, S.M., Silber, D.H., Enders, B.G., Gray, K.S., Sutliff, G., Whisler, S.K., McClain, J.M., Smith, M.B., Yang, Q.X., and Sinoway, L.I. 1996. Influences of gender on sympathetic nerve responses to static exercise. *Journal of Applied Physiology* 80:245-251.

15. Ng, A.V., Callister, R., Johnson, D.G., and Seals, D.R. 1993. Age and gender influence muscle sympathetic nerve activity at rest in healthy humans. *Hypertension* 21:498-503.

16. Lerner, D.J., and Kannell, W.B. 1986. Patterns of coronary heart disease morbidity and mortality in the sexes: A 26-year follow-up study of the Framingham population. *American Heart Journal* 111(2):383-390.

17. Bell, R.A., Summerson, J.H., Spangler, J.G., and Konen, J.C. 1998. Body fat, fat distribution, and psychosocial factors among patients with Type 2 diabetes mellitus. *Behavioral Medicine* 24(3):138-143.

18. Arnold, E. 1997. The stress connection: Women and coronary heart disease. *Critical Care Nursing Clinics of North America* 9(4):565-575.

19. Lord, S.R., Ward, J.A., Williams, P., and Zivanovic, E. 1996. The effects of a community exercise program on fracture risk factors in older women. *Osteoporosis International* 6(5):361-367.

20. Wolf, S.L., Barnhart, H.X., Kutner, N.G., McNeely, E., Coogler, C., and Xu, T. 1996. Reducing frailty and falls in older persons: An investigation of Tai Chi and computerized balance training. *Journal of the American Geriatrics Society* 44(5):489-497.

21. Lord, S.R., Wolf, J.A., and Williams, P. 1996. Exercise effect on dynamic stability in older women: A randomized controlled trial. *American Journal of Physical Medicine & Rehabilitation* 77(3):232-236.

22. Sweigard, L. 1974. Skeletal deviations identified in postural alignment. Chapter 17 in *Human movement potential*. NY: UPA.

23. Cowlin, A.F. 1994-99. Unpublished participant evaluations from a diverse population of midlife women in several unrelated settings: Unsolicited comments. New Haven, CT.

24. Singh, M.A. 1998. Combined exercise and dietary intervention to optimize body composition in aging (Review). *Annals of the New York Academy of Sciences* 854:378-393.

25. Douchi, T., Yamamoto, S., Oki, T., Maruta, R., Yamauchi, H and Hagata, Y. 2000. The effects of physical exercise on body fat distribution and bone mineral density in postmenopausal women. *Maturitas* 35(1):25-30.

26. Cortright, R.N. 1999. Sex differences on regulation of energy homeostasis, growth, and body composition during periods of energy imbalance: Animal studies. Chapter 9 in M. Tarnopolsky (ed.), *Gender differences in metabolism*. Baton Raton, FL: CRC Press.

27. Kissebah, A., and Krakower, G. 1994. Regional adiposity and morbidity. *Physiological Reviews* 74:761-811.

28. Bjorntorp, P. 1990. Adipose tissue adaptation to exercise. In C. Bouchard, R.J. Shephard, T. Stephens, and J.R. Sutton (eds.), *Exercise, fitness and health: A consensus of current knowledge*. Champaign, IL: Human Kinetics, pp. 315-323.

29. Despres, J.P., Tremblay, A., and Bouchard, C. 1989. Sex differences in the regulation of body fat mass with exercise training. In Bjorntorp and Rossner (eds.), *Obesity in Europe: Proceedings of the 1st Congress of the European Association for the Study of Obesity*. London: Libbey.

30. Crawford, S.L., Casey, V.A., Avis, N.E., and McKinlay, S.M. 2000. A longitudinal study of weight and the menopause transition: Results from the Massachusetts Women's Health Study. *Menopause* 7(2):96-104.

31. Astrup, A. 1999. Physical activity and weight gain and fat distribution changes with menopause: Current evidence and research issues. *Medicine and Science in Sports and Exercise* 31(11 Suppl):S564-S567.

32. Norman, R.J., Flight, I.H., Rees, M.C. 2000. Oestrogen and progestogen hormone replacement therapy for peri-menopausal and postmenopausal women: Weight and body fat distribution. *Cochrane Database of Systematic Reviews* [computer file] (2):CD001018.

33. King, A.C., Blair, S.N., Bild, D.E., et al. 1992. Determinants of physical activity and intervention in adults. *Medicine and Science in Sports and Exercise* 24(Suppl):S221-S236.

34. Bar-Or, O. 1996. Thermoregulation in females from a life span perspective. In O. Bar-Or, D.R. Lamb, and P.M. Clarkson (eds.), *Perspectives in exercise science and sports medicine*. Vol 9: *Exercise and the female: A life-span approach*. Carmel, IN: Cooper Publishing Group.

35. Eaton, W.O., and Enns, L.R. 1986. Sex differences in human motor activity level. *Psychological Bulletin* 100:19-28.

36. DiPietro, L. 1996. Habitual physical activity among women. In O. Bar-Or, D.R. Lamb, and P.M. Clarkson (eds.), *Perspectives in exercise science and sports medicine*. Vol 9: *Exercise and the female: A life-span approach*. Carmel, IN: Cooper Publishing Group.

37. Skinner, B.F. 1953. *Science and human behavior*. NY: Free Press.

38. Bandura, A. 1977. Self-efficacy: Toward a unifying theory of behavioral change. *Psychological Review* 84:191-215.

39. Brownell, K.D., Stunkard, A.J., and Albaum, J.M. 1980. Evaluation and modification of exercise patterns in the natural environment. *American Journal of Psychiatry* 37:1540-1545.

40. Prochaska, J.O., and DiClemente, C.C. 1984. *The transtheoretical approach: Crossing traditional boundaries of change*. Homewood, IL: Dorsey Press.

41. Bandura, A. 1986. *Social foundations of thought and action: A social-cognitive theory*. Englewood Cliffs, NJ: Prentice-Hall.

42. Brownell, K.D., Marlatt, A.G., Lichtenstein, E., and Wilson, G.T. 1986. Understanding and preventing relapse. *The American Psychologist* 41:765-782.

43. Dishman, R.K., and Steinhardt, M. 1990. Health locus of control predicts free living, but not supervised, physical activity: A test of exercise specific control and outcome-expectancy hypotheses. *Research Quarterly for Exercise and Sport* 61:383-394.

44. Israel, B.A., and Schurman, S.J. 1990. Social support, control and the stress process. In K. Glanz, F.M. Lewis, and B.K. Rimer (eds.), *Health behavior and health education: Theory, research, and practice*. SF: Jossey-Bass.

45. Godin, G., Valois, P., Jobin, J., and Ross, A. 1991. Prediction of intention to exercise of individuals who have suffered from coronary heart disease. *Journal of Clinical Psychology* 47:762-772.

46. Marcus, B.H., Selby, V.C., Niaura, R.S., and Rossi, J.S. 1992. Self-efficacy and the stages of exercise behavior change. *Research Quarterly for Exercise and Sport* 64:447-452.

47. Prochaska, J.O., De Clemente, C.C., and Norcross, J.C. 1992. In search of how people change: Applications to addictive behaviors. *The American Psychologist* 47:1102-1114.

48. Sallis, J.F., Howell, M.F., and Hofstetter, C.R. 1992. Predictors of adoption and maintenance of vigorous physical activity in men and women. *Preventive Medicine* 21:237-251.

49. Glanz, K., and Rimer, B.K. 1995. *Theory at a glance: A guide for health promotion practice*. US Department of Health and Human Services, Public Health Service, NIH, National Cancer Institute, Bethesda, MD.

50. Godin, G., Desharnais, R., Valois, P., and Bradet, R. 1995. Combining behavioral and motivational dimensions to identify and characterize the stages in the process of adherence to exercise. *Psychology and Health* 10:333-344.

51. Messner, M.A. 1990. Men studying masculinity: Some epistemological issues in sport sociology. *Sociology of Sport Journal* 7:136-153.

52. Henderson, K.A. 1990. The meaning of leisure for women: An integrative review of the research. *Journal of Leisure Research* 22:26-38.

53. Lee, C. 1993. Factors related to the adoption of exercise among older women. *Journal of Behavioral Medicine* 16(3):323-334.

54. Marcus, B.H., Pinto, B.M., Simkin, L.R., Audrain, J.E., and Taylor, E.R. 1994. Application of theoretical models to exercise behavior among employed women. *American Journal of Health Promotion* 9:49-55.

55. Brezinka, V., Dusseldorp, E., and Maes, S. 1998. Gender differences in psychosocial profile at entry into cardiac rehabilitation. *Journal of Cardiopulmonary Rehabilitation* 18(6):445-449.

56. Toobert, D.J., Glasgow, R.E., Nettekoven, L.A., and Brown, J.E. 1998. Behavioral and psychosocial effects of intensive lifestyle management for women with coronary heart disease. *Patient Education and Counseling* 35(3):177-188.

57. Castaneda, D.M., Bigatti, S., and Cronan, T.A. 1998. Gender and exercise behavior among women and men with osteoarthritis. *Women & Health* 27(4):33-53.

58. Conn, V.S. 1998. Older women's beliefs about physical activity. *Public Health Nursing* 15(5):370-378.

59. Hunter, M., and O'Dea, I. 1999. An evaluation of a health education intervention for mid-aged women: Five year follow-up of effects upon knowledge, impact of menopause and health. *Patient Education and Counseling* 38(3):249-255.

60. Kerschan, K., Alacamlioglu, Y., Kollmitzer, J., Wober, C., et al. 1998. Functional impact of unvarying exercise program in women after menopause. *American Journal of Physical Medicine & Rehabilitation* 77(4):326-332.

CHAPTER 14

PROGRAM DESIGN FOR MIDLIFE WOMEN

This chapter addresses program design for midlife fitness programs based on the goals and priorities outlined in the previous chapter. It presents suggestions on intake procedures; exercise components, prescription, and format; and program evaluation. Among midlife women, the divergence in programming needs is apparent. Not only are there issues around dose effect, depending on a woman's particular menopause status and health status; but also her exercise history and the domain (sport/exercise, active living, occupational and household/caregiving) in which she is most active produce variables affecting the type and amount of activity in which she participates [1]. The promotion of physical activity in midlife women needs to take into account differences in the demographic and psychosocial correlates of activity domain. This sensitivity extends all the way from the language used in promotional materials and questionnaires to the selection of sites and the creation of activities that reflect competencies.

INTAKE PROCEDURES FOR MIDLIFE EXERCISE

Information gathering for the midlife population includes data collection to establish motivation and needs and/or the reason for medical referral, to make sure that the client understands the nature of exercise, to obtain an exercise history, and to determine prior and current activity domain(s). In addition, screening procedures to assess health, fitness, and nutritional status help the instructor or trainer ensure a safe and effective program for each individual.

When midlife women enter organized fitness programs for the first time, it is critical to collect data efficiently because we need to know many things in order to prepare prescriptions or make modifications for individuals who are not familiar to us. We also need to gather information about women who have been active for some time before becoming menopausal, because, as we have seen, the stage of life profoundly affects how we set goals for women's fitness programs. Midlife is another time of physical change, and sometimes asking familiar clients to assess their life stage causes them to refocus the direction in which they wish to take their physical activities.

With some groups of women there may be good reasons not to introduce a large amount of paperwork at the onset of an activity program. While efforts need to be made to acquire as much information as possible for safety reasons, some groups—especially those with high levels of psychosocial risks (e.g., abuse, depression, poverty) or time constraints—may not tolerate extensive data collection. Moreover, it may not be essential to get lots of information at first, especially with women who are not initially performing vigorous exercise but instead are gaining a sense of kinesthesia or body acceptance or are starting at a very low level of activity. Sometimes demographic and nonmedical information can be collected over the course of a program or near the end, when trust may be greater.

Data Collection

Certain steps are necessary to obtain essential background information about women participating in midlife programs. These include obtaining a physician referral, having the client sign a physical activity contract or liability waiver, determining exercise history and concerns, and filling out a domain of activity questionnaire.

Medical Referral or Approval

Women referred to a menopause group that includes exercise for health-related purposes should provide physician or midwife referral. If a woman is motivated to participate because she perceives potential health benefits, social benefits, or both, it is still a good idea to get a referral or approval from a health care provider as a first step in assuring that regular exercise is appropriate. The form "Health Care Provider's Referral" is an example of a form for this purpose. In any case, a woman's motivation for participation should be noted. As always, the keys to compliance lie within the desire or need.

Activity Contract and Liability Waiver

To ensure that a woman is cognizant of the effects of exercise and of her responsibility in an activity program, it is a good idea to have a contract regarding the interaction between instructor or trainer and the participant. A waiver can be included in the language of the contract, or a separate waiver can be signed. The form "Group or Individual Physical Activity Participation Agreement" is an example of a contract form for group activities or individual programs. In settings where contract forms may be inappropriate (e.g., women's shelters, or knowledgeable women's groups to which an instructor or trainer is invited), one should obtain a waiver in accordance with state regulations.

Exercise History and Concerns

To make sure that activities are appropriate for a given woman, an exercise history and a record of the concerns of an individual woman are essential pieces of information. Sometimes group programs are formulated around specific concerns, goals, or purposes, such as those of women who have been abused, who want to lose weight, or who have had particular cancers. Getting as much information as possible about exercise history and concerns allows an instructor to plan types of activities that will interest various participants. The form "Exercise History and Concerns of Midlife Women" is an example of a general form for this purpose.

Domain of Activity

One last piece of information that can be extremely helpful for creative purposes and for helping women develop self-efficacy relates to the arenas in which a woman has experienced being physically active. The movements that a woman has done over and over again form a rich base from which to expand her movement vocabulary, improve her biomechanics, and help her learn to strengthen her muscles and bones through resistance training. Asking questions about her domains of activity provides a starting point. An example of such a form is "Domain of Activity Questionnaire."

Screening Procedures

An exercise stress test, health and fitness assessments, and determination of nutritional status are screening procedures that are standards of practice in developing an exercise prescription. While not all of these procedures may be practical, financially feasible, or even desirable in some situations, they form the best protection for instructors and facilities in dealing with clients who are at risk for the disorders that can accompany menopause and the midlife period. Sometimes the aim of the program is limited in scope or is to develop a joy of moving; in other cases, the health care provider referral indicates a Class I cardiovascular status, and testing is not possible. In these cases, the program developer or researcher must weigh the benefits and risks of proceeding and determine the safest manner in which to do so. Sometimes a participant must be restricted or turned away from a group activity and referred to a clinical setting.

Criteria for a Stress Test

The leading cause of death in the United States is myocardial infarction, with 63% of the women who die suddenly from acute coronary events having had no prior symptoms of coronary artery disease [2]. While regular aerobic activity promotes heart health, intense activity in persons with heart disease can be fatal. For women over 50 and those with multiple cardiac risk factors, the American College of Sports Medicine recommends an exercise stress test prior to starting a vigorous exercise program [3].

Clients with an intermediate likelihood of coronary artery disease may be referred for myocardial perfusion scintigraphy, a nuclear imaging technique that has been developed to overcome limitations of exercise stress testing. A multicenter study showed that an emergency room protocol using myocardial perfusion nuclear imaging reduced the rate of later diagnosis of myocardial infarction from 1.8% to 0.1% in patients discharged with chest pain [4]. Although this procedure is invasive and still not

Health Care Provider's Referral

Date: _____

Dear Health Care Provider:

Your patient _____ has contacted me to help her develop a program of physical activity appropriate for the condition(s) you have identified. To ensure safety and effectiveness in this endeavor, I request that you fill in the needed information, sign the referral form, and return the form in the envelope provided.

1. I am referring this patient for physical activity due to the following condition(s):

_____

_____

_____

_____

2. It is appropriate for this patient to participate in the following exercise components, as long as they are appropriate to her age and fitness level (check all that apply):

☐ Activities to improve balance and coordination   ☐ Flexibility exercises

☐ Cardiovascular conditioning activities   ☐ Strength or resistance training

☐ Stress management techniques (such as relaxation)

3. Regarding cardiovascular health, I consider this patient (check one):

☐ Class I: Presumably healthy without apparent heart disease.

☐ Class II: Presumably healthy with one or more risk factors for heart disease.

☐ Class III: Patient is not eligible for cardiovascular conditioning.

4. Does this patient have any preexisting medical/orthopedic conditions not described above requiring continued or long-term medical treatment or follow-up? ☐ Yes ☐ No If yes, please describe:

_____

_____

_____

5. Please list any currently prescribed medications: _____

_____

_____

_____

_____   _____

Referring provider's signature   Date

Thank you for your time. Please feel free to contact me at any time should you have questions.

Sincerely,

A.F. Cowlin, 2002, *Women's fitness program development* (Champaign, IL: Human Kinetics).

Group or Individual Physical Activity Participation Agreement

Congratulations on making your choice of a physically active healthy lifestyle! By participating in regular physical activity, you improve your potential for maximum health benefits.

It is important for you to follow program guidelines not only in supervised sessions but unsupervised sessions as well to gain maximum results.

Your activity sessions will be designed to assure safety at all times. However, as with any exercise program, there are risks, including heart stress and the chance of musculoskeletal injuries. In volunteering for this program, you agree to assume responsibility for these risks and waive any possibility for personal damage. You also agree that, to your knowledge, you have no limiting physical conditions or disability that would preclude an exercise program.

A physician's examination is recommended for all participants with any exercise restrictions and for those persons over 40. If you do not wish to receive a physician's examination, you have been informed of its importance and accept full responsibility for your health and well-being. You also understand that no responsibility is assumed by your instructor, _____.

PARTICIPATION and PAYMENT POLICY (if applicable): _____

_____

_____

_____

_____

_____

Having agreed to participate in a program for a specified period of time, and having paid for that period of time, you have the right to make use of the full program now or—if make-up sessions are necessary—any time (within four months) following payment. There are no refunds.

_____

Participant's name (please print)

_____   _____

Participant's signature   Date

A.F. Cowlin, 2002, *Women's fitness program development* (Champaign, IL: Human Kinetics).

Exercise History and Concerns of Midlife Women

ID # (or Name): _____ Date: _____

Birth date: _____

1. Description of how client currently feels: _____

_____

_____

2. Description of typical day: _____

_____

_____

3. Menstrual history: _____

_____

4. Client stresses: _____

_____

5. General goals: _____

_____

_____

_____

Physical Activity Experience

1. How long has it been since last participated? _____

Past activities: _____

_____

_____

2. Current activities/exercise routine: _____

_____

_____

_____

Specific Exercise History or Concerns/Goals

Aerobic fitness: _____

Coordination/balance: _____

Flexibility: _____

Muscular endurance: _____

Muscular strength: _____

Stress management or mind/body work: _____

Weight management: _____

Reasons for Achieving Goals

General health: _____

Injury rehabilitation: _____

Prevention: _____

Sport-specific training: _____

Strength: _____

Other: _____

Problem Areas, Discomforts

Abdominals: _____

Low back strengthening/flexibility: _____

Lower-body strengthening/flexibility: _____

Upper-body strengthening/flexibility: _____

Client Exercise Restrictions

1. Restrictions: _____

_____

_____

_____

2. Were they diagnosed by a physician/midwife? _____

3. Contraindicated exercises: _____

_____

4. Recommended exercises: _____

_____

5. Exercise preferences: _____

_____

Stress Management

Describe if currently practicing: _____

_____

Availability

1. Time(s): _____

2. Day(s):   Sunday   Monday   Tuesday   Wednesday   Thursday   Friday   Saturday

A.F. Cowlin, 2002, *Women's fitness program development* (Champaign, IL: Human Kinetics).

Domain of Activity Questionnaire

1. Did you have children? How many? _____ When? _____ How were the births?

   _____

   _____

2. What did you do when they were toddlers?

   _____

   _____

3. What are your favorite memories of playing with your children? (Or trips, games, events, etc.)

   _____

   _____

4. If you didn't have children, were you around children? What do you remember doing with them?

   _____

   _____

5. Do you provide care for children, elderly parents, or others? Describe these activities. How much time do you spend doing this on a daily basis?

   _____

   _____

6. What are your most favorite and least favorite household tasks?

   _____

   _____

7. How much time do you spend each week on household tasks?

   _____

   _____

8. Do you do the grocery shopping? Do you carry your own bags?

   _____

   _____

9. Do you work? Describe your work activities. Are they light, fairly light, somewhat hard, hard, or very hard physically?

   _____

   _____

10. Do you play sports? Which ones? How many days per week do you play each activity? How long each session?

    _____

    _____

11. Do you participate in recreational exercise? Describe, tell how many days, how long each time, and how hard you work.

    _____

    _____

A.F. Cowlin, 2002, *Women's fitness program development* (Champaign, IL: Human Kinetics).

readily available, it may prove helpful for women with the resources and the relevant risk factors. The technique is also useful for the diagnosis of hyperthyroidism, including Graves disease and postpartum thyroiditis.

Health and Fitness Assessment

A detailed but user-friendly form for gathering information on health status is a vital tool. Reviewing the responses helps provide a basis for including or restricting exercise components. "Health and Well-Being Status" is a form for this purpose, designed with midlife women in mind. Readers are also referred to the health status instruments mentioned in chapter 11, pages 219 and 221.

In addition to determination of cardiovascular fitness, the results of tests of strength, flexibility, balance, and body composition are valuable. Using the procedures for these tests as educational opportunities is one way to engage women and help them feel more comfortable. Teaching women the language of fitness and allowing them to perform some small steps in the testing process, such as taking their own pulse, help them learn skills and develop competence. It can also be useful to look carefully at the exercise history before conducting a fitness assessment. While some women handle traditional fitness equipment and procedures with equanimity, others would rather find out how heavy a bag of groceries they can lift than how much resistance they can push. The form "Fitness Assessment" can be used to maintain a record of intake fitness levels and progress when the program is oriented toward measurable outcomes and is of sufficient duration to log changes.

Nutritional Status

In addition to general health status, a woman in menopause is affected by her nutrition history and current dietary practices. If, for example, she is at risk for osteoporosis, she may need to be encouraged to take in adequate amounts of calcium and vitamin D. Although the health and fitness professional may not be a dietitian, she is likely to be a major avenue of support for healthy eating behaviors. If a woman's diet is inadequate to support vigorous exercise, having the information on paper provides a tangible tool in the better-eating negotiations! Food diaries are useful for this purpose.

If fitness professionals are to be supportive of healthy nutrition, it is also useful for them to know the elements of a balanced, nutrition-dense diet that helps maintain energy production and provide raw chemicals as building blocks for hormones and neurotransmitters, as well as dietary restrictions that may have been imposed on an individual woman. The effects of aging and menopause translate into demands that the diet be a low-acid-producing, low glycemic index, low saturated fat, and high antioxidant and trace mineral diet. Although a fitness professional can feel quite comfortable supplying information about the food sources of many nutritional elements, only someone licensed to prescribe a diet should actually be making nutritional prescriptions.

To acquire a nutrient-dense diet, women can be encouraged to eat whole foods as opposed to highly processed foods. During processing, nutrients are often lost through heat or by stretching the food substance to produce more profit. Eating a potato rather than potato chips is an example of this principle.

Red meat is a high acid, high phosphorous food that can cause calcium resorption. Consequently, other protein sources are often preferable. Fish, such as salmon, which are also high in omega-3 oils, are desirable, as well as skinless fowl. Women can be encouraged to avoid carbonated beverages (high in phosphorous) and excess alcohol or caffeine. Instructors are encouraged to keep abreast of the current recommended daily allowance (RDA) of vitamins and minerals, and also to be aware of other sources of information about research findings that address dose effect [5, 6]. Sources of vitamin C include citrus fruits, strawberries, and tomatoes; vitamin D sources include 15 to 30 minutes in the sun with some exposed skin, or fortified milk or fish. Beta carotene (vitamin A precursor) sources include yellow and orange colored foods, such as carrots and squash; vitamin E sources include nuts, vegetable oils, whole grains, olives, asparagus, and spinach. B vitamins are plentiful in green leafy vegetables and whole grains. Minerals are also available from whole foods. Supplementation is subject to medical supervision.

The impact of soy in the diet of menopausal women has been the source of much interest and some controversy. Early findings on soy—a staple of the diet in many Asian cultures where menopause is considered less obtrusive—were hopeful. Positive and perhaps significant effects on chronic disease, as well as symptoms such as hot flashes and adverse conditions such as bone loss, hypertriglyceridemia or pre-cancerous changes in breast tissue often associated with hormone replacement are associated with the dietary use of soy and soy products [7-15]. However, large prospective studies will be needed to verify many of the effects. It is also difficult to know how the Americanization of the world's diet will affect health research and whether a soy diet in non-Asian races will have the same effect as it does in Asians. Sources of isoflavones or plant-derived estrogen precursors (phytoestrogens) include soybeans (by far the greatest source), cashews, peanuts, almonds, oats, corn, wheat, apples, melons, as well as most fruits and vegetables to a lesser degree [16-18]. A phytonutrient source of progesterone precursors is a standardized preparation of black cohosh.

Health and Well-Being Status

ID# (or Name): _____ Date:_ _____

D.O.B.:_____

Address:_____
          Street   City   State   Zip

Phone (H):_____ (W):_____ E-mail:_____

In case of emergency, whom may I contact?

Name:_____ Relationship:_____

Phone (H):_____ (W):__ _____

Race:_____ Education:_____

Household income: ☐ < 20,000   ☐ 20,000-40,000   ☐ 40,000-60,000   ☐ > 60,000

Please answer all of the questions as completely and accurately as possible. The information is important for safety and helping you achieve your goals.

Section 1: Have You Had? (Check if yes.)

☐ Amenorrhea	☐ Heart attack	☐ Obesity
☐ Asthma	☐ High blood pressure	☐ Osteoarthritis
☐ Bladder or uterus prolapse	☐ High cholesterol	☐ Osteoporosis
☐ Cancer type ___ ___	☐ Hysterectomy	☐ Pregnancy # ____
☐ Cesarean	☐ Incontinence	☐ Rheumatic fever
☐ Chest pains	☐ Injury to spine or seizures	☐ Shortness of breath
☐ Diabetes type _____	☐ Leg injuries (R or L)	☐ Stroke
☐ Edema (ankle swelling in A.M.)	☐ Low blood pressure	☐ Thyroid disease
☐ Fainting	☐ Lung disease	
☐ Fibromyalgia	☐ Lupus	
☐ Recent operations: Type: _____ Date: _____		

What is your menopause status?   ☐ Perimenopausal   ☐ Menopausal   ☐ Postmenopausal

Section 2: Have Any Relatives Had?

☐ Allergies or arthritis	☐ Heart attacks
☐ Alzheimer's	☐ Heart operations
☐ Breast cancer	☐ High blood pressure
☐ Other cancers	☐ High cholesterol
☐ Congenital heart disease	☐ Other major illness
☐ Diabetes type _____	

Please explain checked items: _____

_____

_____

_____

Section 3

	Yes	No
1. Have you had high blood pressure (> 140/90) on more than one occasion?	☐	☐
2. Have you ever been told that your blood cholesterol was high (> 200)?	☐	☐
3. Do you currently smoke? If yes, how much per day and at what age did you start? _____ a day ____ age	☐	☐
4. Do you drink alcohol? How much? _____ How often? _____	☐	☐
5. Have you ever been told that you have diabetes?	☐	☐

6. Has anyone in your immediate family (parents, siblings) had any heart problems or coronary disease before the   ☐   ☐ age of 55? If yes, describe:

_____

_____

7. Do you currently participate in any aerobic activity on a regular basis? If yes, describe: ☐   ☐

_____

_____

8. Are you presently employed? If yes, what is your present occupational position?   ☐   ☐

_____

_____

9. Do you work at home? If yes, ☐ job related ☐ home related: ☐   ☐

_____

Section 4

	Yes	No

1. Have you had back problems, any problems with joints, or been diagnosed with arthritis? If yes, describe: ☐   ☐

_____

_____

2. Do you have any other medical conditions or health problems which may affect your exercise program   ☐   ☐ or safety in any way? If yes, describe:

_____

_____

Mark any medications taken in the last six months:

☐ Blood pressure medicine	☐ Epilepsy medicine
☐ Blood thinner	☐ Heart rhythm medicine
☐ Cholesterol medicine	☐ Hormone replacement, name: _____
☐ Diabetes medicine	☐ Nitroglycerin

Other: _____

Section 5

How were you referred? _____

List in order YOUR personal fitness objectives:

1. _____

2. _____

3. _____

4. _____

A.F. Cowlin, 2002, *Women's fitness program development* (Champaign, IL: Human Kinetics).

Fitness Assessment

ID# (or Name): _____ Date: _____ ☐ Pre ☐ 1 ☐ 2 ☐ 3

Address: _____

           Street   City   State   Zip

Phone (H): _____ (W): _____

Age: _____ Max HR (225 – age): _____ Target HR: _____ – _____

	Pretest	Post #1	Post #2	Post #3
Resting HR	_____	_____	_____	_____
Resting BP	_____	_____	_____	_____
Weight	_____	_____	_____	_____
Body fat %	_____	_____	_____	_____
Triceps	_____	_____	_____	_____
Thighs	_____	_____	_____	_____
Abdominals	_____	_____	_____	_____
Aerobic capacity	_____	_____	_____	_____
Push-ups	_____	_____	_____	_____
Curl-ups	_____	_____	_____	_____
Quadriceps	_____	_____	_____	_____
Flexibility	_____	_____	_____	_____

Comments: _____

_____

_____

_____

_____

_____

_____

_____

_____

_____

_____

_____

_____

_____

_____

_____

_____

_____

A.F. Cowlin, 2002, *Women's fitness program development* (Champaign, IL: Human Kinetics).

Developing Research Questions

In addition to research topics already referred to in this section, as well as the instruments suggested for research purposes in previous sections and especially chapter 11, readers interested in developing research questions may find the following suggestions useful. Demographics can be obtained using instruments from studies concerning body image and sexuality in this population [19, 20]. Also available are established procedures for monitoring and measuring physical activity in women [21-23], assessing issues concerning quality of life and precursors for exercise adherence [24-27], assessing body composition in obese women [28], and assessing various psychosocial issues [29-32].

EXERCISE COMPONENTS, PRESCRIPTION, AND FORMAT FOR WOMEN'S MIDLIFE FITNESS PROGRAMS

The breadth of activity histories, predispositions, effects of lifestyle, and life situations that we encounter in midlife women results in a vast array of effective exercise routines for this population. In contrast to the situation with adolescence (in which we are largely concerned with introducing girls to the myriad possibilities for an active life) or with childbearing (in which despite variations in exercise history and body type, all participants are involved in the same athletic event, i.e., pregnancy, birth, and recovery), with women at midlife we are confronted by huge differences in skill, functional capacity, and will. So that this section can be truly helpful, it focuses on the common fitness needs that face this population, regardless of history or body type. Beyond this, many women are capable of many things. But some will be capable of only the minimum, and reaching these women will produce the greatest gain in public health.

Essential Midlife Exercise Components

Based on the information discussed in this and the previous chapter, these are components and volumes for an ideal activity program aimed specifically at the needs of midlife women:

- Bone-loading resistance and impact training two or three days per week
- Weight-bearing aerobic activity for 20 to 30 minutes, five days per week
- Centering, relaxation, and other stress management techniques as needed

Some women need to take a few minutes to center and clear their minds every day, while others need to do relaxation activities on the weekend to maintain an inner calm. It is easy to incorporate stretching into the strength routine, where it is most effective. An effective midlife program encompasses these components in a mood-enhancing interactive strategy. The following sections cover these components in some detail.

Prescription and Format for Midlife Programs

The routine need not be a linear progression of exercises that continues over a long time, but can change focus, expand, or contract to meet ongoing needs. For example, a woman concerned primarily with general health and mental well-being may belong to a neighborhood walking group, participate in a rotating weightlifting program at the gym or at home, and take a yoga class once a week. Periodically, she may switch her activities. Perhaps she is a spring and summer gardener, so in those seasons she substitutes carrying rocks, moving dirt, and planting flower beds for weightlifting and yoga, and rides her bicycle instead of walking so she can check out more gardens.

Short commitments of time toward specific individualized or group goals may be more effective for another woman. Someone with type 2 diabetes in a less safe neighborhood might go to a special program at her church where eight-week sessions are run in the fall, winter, and spring in a creative social format two or three evenings a week. In between sessions and over the summer, she may take a break or join with others from her group to walk or swim at a local school. Still another woman may attend a lecture on menopause and exercise, then make a plan with her physician or midwife. She might get started by convincing members of her book club to walk while they discuss their reading. Or, she might look at her weekly schedule and figure out that she can pack her grocery bags a little heavier, take the stairs at work, park farther from the train station, play more Frisbee with the dog, and join her husband for a little yard work or walk her grandchildren home from school more often.

More specialized exercise groups for purposes such as breast cancer surgery rehabilitation are needed. In addition to immediate effects due to surgery, chemotherapy, or radiation, the physical and emotional sequellae of this cancer and its treatment include psychological distress, fatigue, weight gain, premature menopause, and changes in body image [33]. All of these can be addressed in an exercise group. Groups for people with diabetes, cardiovascular disease, osteoporosis, or autoimmune disorders are examples of other specialized groups.

Masters sport programs for women are an area in which active midlife and older women are addressing their personal and group needs. Over-50 or over-60 women's basketball leagues are one example. In all these programs, an essential element is the socializing and networking. It is useful to keep in mind that the more visible these programs are, the more they help those on the sideline. Women can be brought into the circle of activity by osmosis.

DESCRIPTION OF EXERCISE COMPONENTS

The following paragraphs describe the essential components already mentioned. In addition to these, strength exercises such as abdominals, Kegels, biceps and triceps curls, and seated hamstring curls form an integral and interesting aspect of a well-rounded midlife fitness program. It is easy to include stretching by following several sets of strength activities with stretches for those muscles; or, if instructors are so inclined, they can choreograph strength and stretch moves.

Bone-Loading Resistance or Impact Training

Age is a major determinant of bone strength, mass, and microarchitecture [34], as well as muscle mass. These factors are also affected by loading, and consequently it is important to do bone loading training throughout the aging years. By the time a woman is perimenopausal she is losing bone and muscle mass. One study indicates that there is a concomitant loss of muscle strength and bone density in women between 45 and 65 irrespective of HRT, and that the loss of lower-body strength is 50% greater than the loss of upper-body strength [35]. Hopefully women have prior experience that drove up their peak BMD in their teens and 20s and helped maintain bone mass in their 30s; but by their 40s it is critical that women are doing activities that load bone, especially the spine, pelvis, and femurs, to help minimize bone and muscle loss.

What about load intensity? One study showed that either high-load (80% 1 repetition maximum [1RM], 8 reps) or high-repetition (40% 1RM, 16 reps) exercise was effective in increasing muscle strength and size in early-postmenopausal women and that neither regimen resulted in significant increases in spine or hip BMD over a six-month period, with calcium supplementation to 1500 milligrams daily [36]. The threshold for an intensity that has an effect on bone may be sensitive to genetics [37] and sex [38].

Bone is also responsive to impact activities. As noted in chapter 12, the highest peak bone mass is attained in young healthy athletes involved in impact sports such as gymnastics and dance. In their five-year follow-up study of jumping in weighted vests, Snow et al. found that the program helped prevent significant loss of femoral neck, trochanter, and total hip BMD in older postmenopausal women [39]. An exciting finding of this particular study was the long-term compliance of participants [39], indicating that a high-intensity impact activity involving coordination skills can be challenging and interesting enough to retain women in their mid to late 60s.

Modifications for Currently Active Midlife Women

Even at the molecular and cellular level, women respond somewhat differently to conditioning than men. Research indicates that estradiol provides protection against muscle damage caused by acute exercise with relatively high oxidative stress, because of its role as an antioxidant and membrane stabilizer [40-54]. Resting creatine kinase, while generally lower for women than for men [55, 56], is higher in premenarcheal girls and postmenopausal women and lowest in pregnant women [57, 58], demonstrating the influence of estrogen status on creatine kinase leakage, one marker of level of exertion in resistance training. Since estrogen protects muscle from postexercise damage, and estrogen status is changing, midlife women may experience the need to adjust the level of exertion or the recovery time to prevent inflammation and soreness. Theoretically, HRT will affect this equation. In the absence of specific findings, each woman should make adjustments based on preventing inflammation and soreness.

Core Stabilization During Resistance Training

Stabilizing the lumbar spine during weight training provides important skeletal protection. Figure 14.1 shows the use of tactile aid by another party to assist in developing kinesthesia in the anterior and posterior regions of the abdomen. Exhaling on the effort is a fundamental concept that is critical. People can learn the sensations of core body stabilization in a number of ways. In addition to tactile aid, methods such as centering techniques, tai chi, dance, calisthenics for the core, and exercise balls are all effective.

Meeting Upper-Body Strength Needs

The loss of estrogen associated with menopause is also related to the high levels of autoimmune and inflammatory disorders in midlife and older women [59], and conditions such as shoulder bursitis and fibromyalgia are not

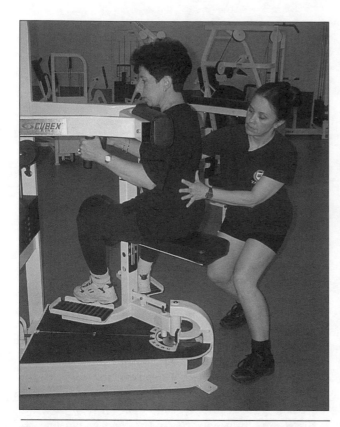

Figure 14.1   Use tactile aid for core stabilization during strength straining.

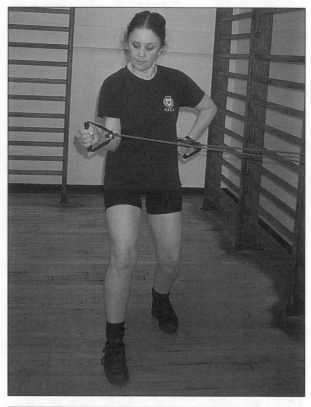

Figure 14.2   Strengthening the external rotator cuff and balancing its strength with that of the internal rotator cuff can be helpful in maintaining the full range of arm motion at the shoulder for midlife and older women.

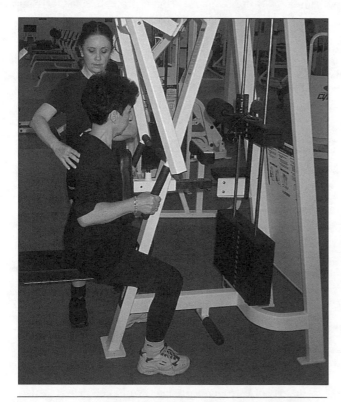

Figure 14.3   Strengthening the upper spine and scapular region helps overcome the propensity for a sunken chest that is sometimes the sequella of pregnancy, nursing, or poor spinal alignment.

uncommon. The shoulders of women are particularly susceptible because of the changes in spinal alignment and stress to the shoulders during the childbearing and nursing years. Internal rotation and a sunken chest posture are common results of uncorrected alignment following childbearing.

To balance the shoulder and protect arm movements above shoulder height, rotator cuff exercises have proven useful. Increasing the strength of external rotators (see figure 14.2) helps counter the effects of internal rotation. Along with balancing the rotator cuff, a good strategy is to strengthen the rhomboids and erector spinae muscles along the upper thoracic region to help overcome ill effects of a sunken chest (see figure 14.3). This is also a good preparation for learning to use the rowing ergometer (see figure 14.4), which involves a greater volume of muscle, thus achieving greater conditioning and laying the groundwork for further upper-body training for those who desire this.

Meeting Lower-Body Strength Needs

An earlier section covered the need to increase muscle strength and load bone in the hip region, as well as the greater loss of strength in the lower body compared to

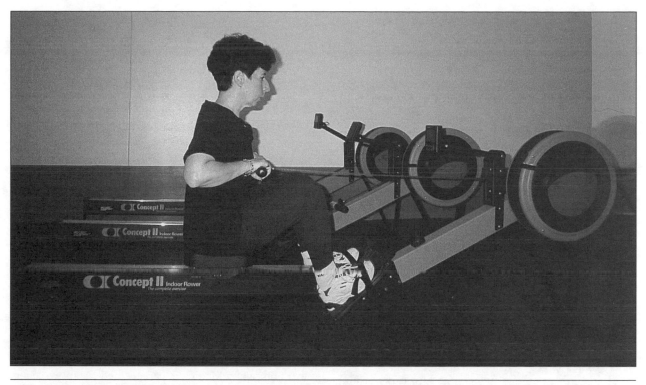

Figure 14.4 Developing strength in the upper back (see figure 14.3) and clean mechanics is advisable before learning to use the rowing ergometer.

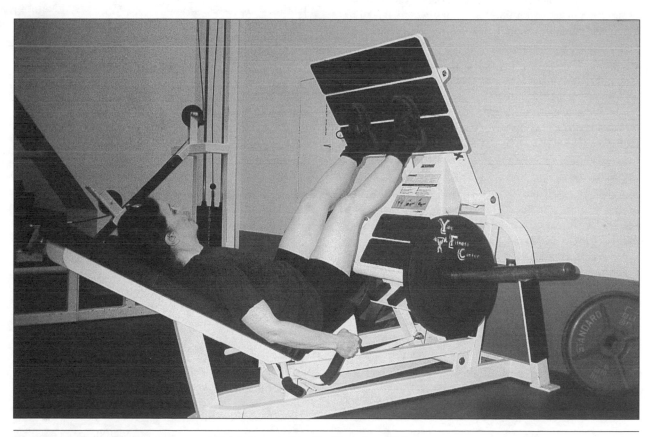

Figure 14.5 Strengthening the legs and hips is important to the prevention of falls.

the upper body in postmenopausal women. We also know that strength in the hips and legs is important in maintaining the maximum balance range and coordinated stability [60]. Among activities that help are standing squats; leg presses (see figure 14.5); standing one-leg balances; and isolated strengthening exercises for the quadriceps, gluteals, hamstrings, and psoas major. Relevé (rising on the balls of the feet) and shifting the weight onto the heels while raising the toes are also helpful.

Weight-Bearing Aerobic or Cardiovascular Conditioning

Rhythmic, repetitive motion that propels one's whole body through space—that's the ticket if you want to feel good and maximize health! Twenty or thirty minutes almost every day is a good thing. The Centers for Disease Control and Prevention and the American College of Sports Medicine recommend accumulations of near-daily moderate-intensity physical activity in the 200-kilocalorie range for health purposes [61]. Why are midlife and older women largely outside the desired range?

As already noted, part of the difficulty is that we do not have a clear idea of how much physical activity women really do. Also, the system of implementing behavior change has become so proliferated that it has lost its strength. Much attention has been given to extending the transtheoretical model of behavior change to exercise adoption [62]. But this construct still approaches the adoption of exercise as something to be added, and it characterizes nonlinear progress as relapse. This leads to a growing list of stage-specific interventions, especially for women, who, as DiPietro has pointed out, may be inclined to cyclical commitments to physical activity [63]. Although the concept of a series of interventions to keep an individual on a linear path may be valid, in practice it is cumbersome.

Let's return to our model of one simple thing that drives further behaviors. The primary "exercise" that is referred to in exercise adoption is the aerobic component. Williams and Lord note that for older women, developing muscle strength best predicts continued participation in structured exercise [64]. First, get them strong. Power strength may well drive the appetite for endurance. If life intervenes and the activity level drops, return to strength. Such an approach has potential for midlife women because the starting point is always the same, it is easy to remember, and there are additional health benefits to increasing strength. Formatting exercises into a circuit with a minute or two of walking, dancing, or jumping rope in between exercises lets women experience the satisfying motor release of cardiovascular activity following the focused effort of strength movements.

Appropriate Activities for Midlife Cardiovascular Conditioning

How hard should midlife women be working and what should they be doing? Most women are doing some activity that involves moving on their feet, so there is always a starting point, even if it is making beds, stacking inventory, or delivering the mail. Take the pulse, assess perceived exertion, calculate METs (metabolic equivalents). The range of capacities is wide.

Intensity. Three major situations come up when one is delineating appropriate intensity levels for midlife women. One is the presence of medication that may alter heart rates. In this case, following medical instructions and relevant guidelines for cardiovascular intensity is absolutely necessary. The second situation is that of the moderately or highly fit woman. She may know her preferred heart rate, and it may be above her age-predicted maximum, although well within an appropriate perceived exertion range. Medical clearance and liability waivers are necessary. The third situation is that of the beginner. For a woman at this level, learning the signs of exertion (breathing changes, heat, alterations in awareness, fatigue), learning how to take her own pulse, and learning how to subjectively assess her own level of exertion are necessary skills. Once her functional capacity has been assessed during the intake process, appropriate intensities can be determined using standards of practice.

Mode. Although walking is the most common example of recreational movement, a wide range of activities will satisfy the need for weight-bearing cardiovascular activity. For a percentage of the population, it is a viable option to walk, jog, or even run outdoors in groups or (for safety reasons) at an indoor track or on a treadmill at a school or community gymnasium. Women who walk for transportation or on the job should count this toward their accumulation of daily activity.

Standard forms of weight-bearing recreational activity, such as step aerobics, appeal to a percentage of women. Aerobics classes designed expressly for the midlife population should be offered for brief periods of time. Commitments for extended periods are difficult for this group to make. In northern climates, winter classes may be full, but summer classes often empty as women take advantage of the warm weather and extended daylight to pursue outdoor activities. In southern climates, moving a class into the pool for a couple of the hottest months makes sense, even though the participant list may vary somewhat. Instructors of general-population classes should be tolerant of these women's waxing and waning attendance. Women may travel or have family demands.

Women from a variety of backgrounds are turning to dance—ballet, salsa, swing, African and Caribbean dance, Asian dance, and others—as programs become more available in many communities. Some of these forms involve impact actions or high-intensity effort at an advanced level. Because they have highly evolved training methods, at the basic level they are relatively safe. Modern dance has an element of individual expression that some women find satisfying. Making beds, stacking inventory, and delivering the mail become abstract aesthetic motions in modern dance!

Competition in Midlife

In some locations, senior women's leagues are being formed, aimed at having fun with friends, providing competitive outlets for those women so inclined, or both. There is a need to track health, injury, and psychosocial consequences of these programs. Their existence brings up interesting questions: Does menopause change the female's nurturing/competitive balance? Do the decreasing levels of female hormones and resulting shift in the balance of female and male hormones affect women's goals, ambitions, or aggressiveness in midlife?

Centering, Relaxation, and Other Stress Management Activities

Previous discussion has included details on centering, relaxation, and stress management. Readers may refer to chapters 8 and 11 for definitions, descriptions, and recommendations regarding the execution of these and other mind/body activities. The sample program presented later in this chapter illustrates how to use these activities within the context of a menopause program.

MOOD-ENHANCING INTERACTIVE STRATEGIES

Fitness professionals need to format and promote activities that are known to improve mood, and need to offer them within a supportive social structure. This text has often referred to the psychological trait of self-efficacy and the social support model of women's activities as critical elements for success in developing a healthy lifestyle. As we search for clues to why different women experience more or less discomfort from the physiologic changes associated with menopause, psychosocial fac-

tors and their association with physical activity are coming to the fore [65-67].

Mood Enhancement

We have previously noted that the combination of vigorous and reflective activities promotes self-confidence, health and well-being, positive mood, and anxiety reduction for women. A study by Long and Haney demonstrated that jogging and progressive relaxation, in eight-week programs, each independently reduced trait anxiety and improved self-efficacy for working women significantly and nondifferentially, with both benefits maintained at an eight-week follow-up [68]. In the Melbourne Women's Midlife Health Project study, researchers found that changes in activity level were positively associated with change in high-density lipoprotein cholesterol and well-being [69], indicating that if less active women increase their activity level they benefit in terms of both their heart health and their sense of well-being. Making small increases in the level of vigorous exercise or relaxation, or maintaining adequate levels if a woman is already involved in these activities, is clearly important to mood enhancement in the midlife period.

Social Interaction

Identifying a supportive social structure for healthy behavior can influence the experience of menopause. We know from previous discussions in this book that interaction with other women having similar needs or goals in a formal program improves outcomes. In a study describing individuals (80% women, 97% white, 67% married, 54% persons with undergraduate or graduate degrees) who were successful at long-term maintenance of substantial weight loss, researchers in the United States found that people who were successful reported regular physical activity, self-monitoring, and coping skills [70] as their methodology. According to other findings from this study, there was a triggering event that precipitated the weight loss, and the individuals often used structured programs to help them develop coping mechanisms [70]. While socially oriented group weight loss programs have come under some criticism for not always being scientifically rigorous, such programs have the best record for enabling this long-term behavior change. Fitness professionals may well gain by borrowing from this model to effect positive physical activity changes for midlife women. One study has demonstrated that reframing the psychosocial context can make physical activity interventions more relevant and thereby more effective for midlife women [71].

SAMPLE MIDLIFE GROUP FITNESS PROGRAM

There is a need for both individualized solutions and structured programs that bring midlife women together for education, support, and group fitness. Many women do well developing their own programs. Once they have the information they need (i.e., that strength, aerobics, and stress management activities are critical), they can figure out how to comply with this routine in ways such as those described earlier. Women also benefit from a social context and a chance to gain new skills, and some women need a great deal of support. Programs can be offered once or twice a week in eight-week sessions, on an as-needed basis in the community or facility. The form "Sample Group Fitness One-Hour Session for Midlife Women" presents an example of a session within such a program.

PROGRAM EVALUATION

Objective participant outcomes for women in midlife can be difficult to determine. If BMD improves, muscle mass increases, type 2 diabetes improves, or body fat goes down, then the activity is working; but these factors have to be monitored. If the program is in a clinical or experimental setting, results are easy to come by. If not, the instructor or personal trainer must develop an appropriate relationship with care providers or researchers, as well as obtaining informed consent and maintaining confidentiality with clients.

Participant satisfaction is easier to determine. As at other stages of women's lives, midlife women are usually willing to tell an instructor or trainer what they like and don't like on an ongoing basis. Because one of the first goals of midlife programs is to help women develop a joy of moving, this needs to be evaluated. Attendance and adherence are clues. If notes on motivation or needs assessment are taken at the start, the evaluation process should also include a before-and-after comparison. Intake forms can be used by the instructor to guide a debriefing discussion at the end of a course (see the form "Exercise History and Concerns of Midlife Women"). Asking clients to rate personal outcomes and elements they found effective on a Likert-type scale is also helpful.

Sample Group Fitness One-Hour Session for Midlife Women

Start seated upright on the sitsbones, in a chair, feet on the floor.

3 minutes: Centering, seated—balance activity, hiss/compress abdominal exercises, associative mental focus.

2 minutes: ROM movements, seated—carve into the space all around you leading with your hands, one at a time, allowing the body to follow; repeat leading with feet.

3 minutes: Leg wake-ups, seated exercises for quadriceps, abductors, adductors—1-2 sets of 8. One leg held up in front—ankle circles, flex/extend leg; sit on one hip—abduct other leg; on sitsbones—squeeze adductors, resisting with hands (NB: exhale on effort).

2 minutes: Standing up from a chair while centered (see figure 13.1)—4 to 8 each, R & L.

3 minutes: Walking, talking, fill and spill (drink water, visit the ladies' room).

20 minutes: Weight-bearing aerobic activities (e.g., aerobic dancing to favorite music; line dancing; modified hip hop; low step aerobics; jog/walk; square dancing; waltzing; polka; etc.) appropriate to level and interest.

20 minutes: Standing strength/stretch for legs—squats, hip extensors, hamstrings, calves. For arms—standing and/or seated—rotator cuff, shoulder retraction, rowing, plus others as needed. Use partners, bands, tubes, hand weights.

Abdominals—from slight wall squat—hiss/compress, then maintaining back of waist on wall, "curl-ups."

7 minutes: Relaxation—start seated on sitsbones, repeat centering; sit back in chair to support back, if needed, but sit on sitsbones; close eyes, breathe deeply and slowly.

Get comfortable, on each exhale let half the tension release until feeling soft/loose.
See in the mind's eye a joyful past event; release the image from the mind. See in the mind's eye a joyful future event; release the image from the mind. When finished, bring mind to surface slowly, be present, smile.

A.F. Cowlin, 2002, *Women's fitness program development* (Champaign, IL: Human Kinetics).

LOOKING AHEAD

The differences between women and men provide the impetus for the question: Do common concepts of physical fitness truly represent the best interests of women? To address this issue, we have looked closely at two things. The first is those times within the female life cycle during which reproductive physiology most profoundly affects women's activity preferences and needs, namely adolescence, pregnancy, the postpartum period, and menopause. The other is the primarily male source of the models for physical fitness. In exploring these areas, we have found that there is still a great deal of ground to cover in order to delineate the effects of biology on women's tolerance for physical activity, to create and uncover forms of activity that benefit girls and women (and perhaps men), and to relocate the venue of activity to a space within people's lives.

At a time when health problems associated with inactivity have become epidemic, efforts to increase physical activity levels in the general public have helped us find several weaknesses in models of fitness based primarily on male-centered values. Despite policies that bring more women into men's activities, doing so has a positive effect on very few women. Hierarchical, aggressive, rules-oriented modalities that were traditionally male have been opened up to females in a social experiment that has benefited some highly aggressive females. But many women are attracted to activities that focus on social network building, helping others, learning new skills, and developing aesthetic sensibilities. Pushing the entire population to go to the gym and work out, to take up running, or to play sports was not the optimal strategy.

The next step was to reach out to "special populations" who were resistant to the male motivation, *You'll live longer.* Despite females' biologically based vulnerability to a variety of sex hormone-related disorders, from osteoporosis and arthritis to lupus and Alzheimer's, women already live longer. This is not a good incentive to become more like a man. Moreover, women are not a special population. Regardless of research arguing that behavior permits individuals to overcome biology, women may not be wise to overthrow their biology and become men. Rather, as the majority, women may find it in their best interest to insist on a large investment in restructuring knowledge and practice to focus more on the health of the earth and the human race, and less on giving a prize to the alpha person or group.

Women are just beginning to be influential on a global scale. This is a major historical change because it affects what we trust in to tell us we are making progress. What we measure, how we measure it, and what we do with the information may well invoke radical changes in how people live. Technology's impact on science—the ability to network large amounts of information to see more profound patterns—speeds the change because this type of networking is sympathetic to female biology and thought.

One of the underlying phenomena giving momentum to this time in human events is the mystery of female reproductive physiology: What does it entail? Who controls it? These are pivotal questions for science and society. Most women spend the majority of life in one stage or another of the cycle of female fertility. There has been little to attract most women to the male models of fitness. As professionals designing women's fitness programs we must ask ourselves questions: What road do we take with the information flowing from scientific discovery? Where do we start? How do we proceed? The creation of new models is a large task, one to which many individuals contribute. Some are motivated by self-preservation, others by growth, and still others by discovery. Imagination and creative problem-solving are helpful to all. The author hopes that for those who work on this project the ideas in this text will be one source of inspiration.

REFERENCES

1. Sternfield, B., Ainsworth, B.E., and Quesenberry, C.P. 1999. Physical activity patterns in a diverse population of women. *Preventive Medicine* 28(3):313-323.
2. American Heart Association. 1997. 97 Update debunks cardiovascular disease myths, press release. Dallas, TX: AHA NR 97-4488.
3. American College of Sports Medicine. 2000. *Guidelines for exercise testing and prescription,* 6th ed. Baltimore: Williams & Wilkins.
4. Janowitz, W.R., Nateman, D.R., and Ziffer, J.A. 1998. Nuclear imaging facilitates patient care at chest pain center. *Diagnostic Imaging* 20(12):13C-14C.
5. Northrup, C. 1994. *Women's bodies, women's wisdom.* NY: Bantam.
6. Balch, J.F., and Balch, P.A. 1997. *Prescription for nutritional healing,* 2nd ed. NY: Avery.
7. Burke, G.L. 1996. The potential use of a dietary soy supplement as a post-menopausal hormone replacement therapy. Second International Symposium on the Role of Soy in Preventing and Treating Chronic Disease. Brussels, 9/19/96.
8. Knight, D.C., and Eden, J.A. 1996. A review of the clinical effect of phytoestrogens. *Obstetrics and Gynecology* 87(5):897-904.
9. Setchell, K.D. 1996. Overview of isoflavone structure, metabolism and pharmacokinetics. Second International Symposium on the Role of Soy in Prevention and Treating Chronic Disease. Brussels, 9/19/96.
10. Anderson, J.W., Johnstone, B.M., and Cook-Newell, M.E. 1995. Meta-analysis of the effects of soy protein intake on serum lipids. *New England Journal of Medicine* 333(5):276-282.
11. Carroll, K.K., and Kurowska, E.M. 1995. Soy consumption and cholesterol reduction (Review). *Journal of Nutrition* 125(3 Suppl):594S-597S.
12. Adlercreutz, C.H., Goldin, B.R., Gorbach, S.L., Hockerstedt, K.A., Watanabe, S., Hamalainen, E.K., Markkanen, M.H.,

Makela, T.H., Wahala, K.T., Adlercruetz, C.H. 1995. Soybean phytoestrogen intake and cancer risk (Review). *Journal of Nutrition* 125(3 Suppl):757S-770S.

13. Messina, M. 1995. Modern applications for an ancient bean: Soybeans and the prevention and treatment of chronic disease (Review). *Journal of Nutrition* 125(3 Suppl):567S-569S.

14. Murikies, A.L., Lombard, C., Strauss, B.J.E., Wilcox, G., Burger, H.G., and Morton, M.S. 1995. Dietary flour supplementation decreases postmenopausal hot flashes: Effect of soy and wheat. *Maturitas* 21(3):189-195.

15. Brandi, M.L. 1992. Flavonoids: Biochemical effects and therapeutic applications. *Bone and Mineral* 19(Suppl):F3-F14.

16. Aldercreutz, H., et al. 1992. Dietary phyto-oestrogens and the menopause in Japan. *Lancet* 339:1233.

17. Elakovich, S.O., and Hampton, J. 1984. Analysis of couvaestrol, a phytoestrogen, in alpha tablets sold for human consumption. *Journal of Agricultural and Food Chemistry* 32:173-175.

18. Clemetson, C.A.B., DeCarol, S.J., Burney, G.A., Patel, T.J., et al. 1978. Estrogens in food: The almond mystery. *International Journal of Obstetrics and Gynecology* 15:515-521.

19. Talor, J.F., Rosen, R.C., and Leiblum, S.R. 1994. Self-report assessment of female sexual function: Psychometric evaluation of the Brief Index of Sexual Functioning for Women. *Archives of Sexual Behavior* 23:627-643.

20. Bellerose, S.B., and Binik, Y.M. 1993. Body image and sexuality in oophorectomized women. *Archives of Sexual Behavior* 22:435-459.

21. Roberts, B.L., and Palmer, R. 1996. Cardiac response of elderly adults to normal activities and aerobic walking. *Clinical Nursing Research* 5:105-115.

22. DiPietro, L., Williamson, D.F., Caspersen, C.J., and Eaker, E. 1993. A survey for assessing physical activity among older adults. *Medicine and Science in Sports and Exercise* 84:14-19.

23. Carter, J.S., Williams, H.G., and Macera, C.A. 1993. Relationships between physical activity habits and functional neuromuscular capacities in healthy older adults. *Journal of Applied Gerontology* 12:283-293.

24. Kaplan, R.M., and Bush, J.W. 1982. Health-related quality of life measurement for evaluation research and policy analyses. *Health Psychology* 1:61.

25. Williams, P., and Lord, S.R. 1995. Predictors of adherence to a structured exercise program for older women. *Psychology and Aging* 10:617-624.

26. Fitzgerald, J.T., Singleton, S.P., Nealve, A.V., Prasad, A.S., and Hess, J.W. 1994. Activity levels, fitness status, exercise knowledge and exercise beliefs among healthy, older African-American and White women. *Journal of Aging and Health* 6:296-313.

27. White, K.P., and Nielson, W.R. 1995. Cognitive behavioral treatment of fibromyalgia syndrome: A follow-up assessment. *Journal of Rheumatology* 22:717-721.

28. Utter, A.C., Nieman, D.C., Ward, A.N., and Butterworth, E.D. 1999. Use of the leg-to-leg bioelectrical impedance method in assessing body-composition change in obese women. *American Journal of Clinical Nutrition* 69(4):603-607.

29. Anderson, B.L., and Cyranowski, J.M. 1994. Women's sexual self-schema. *Journal of Personality and Social Psychology* 67:1079-1100.

30. Wiederman, M.W., and Hurst, S.R. 1997. Physical attractiveness, body image and women's sexual self-schema. *Psychology of Women Quarterly* 21:567-580.

31. McEwen, M. 1993. The Health Motivation Assessment Inventory. *Western Journal of Nursing Research* 15:770-779.

32. Nowack, K.M. 1989. Coping style, cognitive hardiness, and health status. *Journal of Behavioral Medicine* 12:145-158.

33. Pinto, B.M., and Maruyama, N.C. 1999. Exercise in the rehabilitation of breast cancer survivors (Review). *Psycho-Oncology* 8(3):191-206.

34. Mosekilde, L. 2000. Age-related changes in bone mass, structure, and strength—effects of loading (Review). *Zeitschrift fur Rheumatologie* 59(Suppl 1):1-9.

35. Humphries, B., Triplett-McBride, T., Newton, R.U., Marshall, S., et al. 1999. The relationship between dynamic isokinetic and isometric strength and bone mineral density in a population of 45 to 65 year old women. *Journal of Science and Medicine in Sport* 2(4):364-374.

36. Bemben, D.A., Fetters, N.L., Bemben, M.G., Nabavi, N., and Koh, E.T. 2000. Musculoskeletal responses to high- and low-intensity resistance training in early postmenopausal women. *Medicine and Science in Sports and Exercise* 32(11):1949-1957.

37. Woods, D., Onambele, G., Woledge, R., Skelton, D., et al. 2001. Antiotensin-I converting enzyme genotype-dependent benefit from hormone replacement therapy in isometric muscle strength and bone mineral density. *Journal of Clinical Endocrinology and Metabolism* 86(5):2200-2204.

38. Hohsi, A., Watanabe, H., Chiba, M., and Inaba, Y. 1998. Bone density and mechanical properties in femoral bone of swim loaded aged mice. *Biomedical and Environmental Sciences* 11(3):243-250.

39. Snow, C.M., Shaw, J.M., Winters, K.M., and Witske, K.A. 2000. Long-term exercise using weighted vests prevents hip bone loss in postmenopausal women. *The Journals of Gerontology. Series A, Biological Sciences and Medical Sciences* 55(9):M489-M491.

40. Dekkers, J.C., van Doornen, L.J.P., and Kemper, H.C.G. 1996. The role of antioxidant vitamins and enzymes in the prevention of exercise-induced muscle damage. *Sports Medicine* 21:213.

41. Tang, M., Abplanalp, W., Ayers, S., and Subbiah, M.T.R. 1996. Superior and distinct antioxidant effects of selected estrogen metabolites on lipid peroxidation. *Metabolism* 45:411.

42. Bar, P., Radboud, W., Koot, R., and Amelink, G. 1995. Muscle damage revisited: Does tamoxifen protect by membrane stabilization or radical scavenging, rather than via the E2-receptor? *Biochemical Society Transactions* 23:236S.

43. Clarkson, P.M. 1995. Antioxidants and physical performance. *Critical Reviews in Food Science and Nutrition* 35(1-2):131-141.

44. Ji, L.L. 1995. Oxidative stress during exercise: Implication of antioxidant nutrients. *Free Radical Biology & Medicine* 18:1079.

45. Lacourt, M., Leal, A., Liza, M., Martin, C., Martinez, R., and Ruiz-Larrea, M. 1995. Protective effect of estrogens and catechoestrogens against peroxidative membrane damage in vitro. *Lipids* 30:141.

46. Sen, C.K. 1995. Oxidants and antioxidants in exercise. *Journal of Applied Physiology* 79:675.

47. Tiidus, P.M. 1995. Can estrogens diminish exercise induced muscle damage? *Canadian Journal of Applied Physiology* 20:26.

48. Subbiah, M., Kessel, B., Agrawal, M., Rajan, R., Abplanalp, W., and Rymaszewski, Z. 1993. Antioxidant potential of specific estrogens on lipid peroxidation. *Journal of Clinical Endocrinology and Metabolism* 77(4):1095-1097.

49. Huber, L., Scheffler, E., Poll, T., Seigler, R., and Dresel, H. 1990. 17B-estradiol inhibits LDL oxidation and cholesteryl ester formation in cultured macrophages. *Free Radical Research Communications* 8(3):167-173.

50. Niki, E., and Nakano, M. 1990. Estrogens as antioxidants. *Methods in Enzymology* 186:330.

51. Bar, P.R., Amelink, G.J., Oldenburg, B., and Blankenstein, M.A. 1988. Prevention of exercise-induced muscle membrane damage by oestradiol. *Life Sciences* 43:2677.

52. Nakano, M., Sugioka, K., Naito, I., Susmu, T., and Niki, E. 1987. Novel and potent biological antioxidants on membrane phospholipid peroxidation: 2-hydroxy estrone and 2-hydroxy estradiol. *Biochemical and Biophysical Research Communications* 142:919.

53. Sugioka, K., Shimosegawa, Y., and Nakano, M. 1987. Estrogens as natural antioxidants of membrane phospholipid peroxidation. *FEBS Letters* 210:37.

54. Yagi, K., and Komura, S. 1986. Inhibitory effect of female hormones on lipid peroxidation. *Biochemistry International* 13:1051.

55. Harris, E.K., Wong, E.T., and Shaw, Jr, S.T. 1991. Statistical criteria for separate reference intervals: Race and gender groups in creatine kinase. *Clinical Chemistry* 37:1580.

56. Norton, J.P., Clarkson, P.M., Graves, J.E., Litchfield, P., and Kirwan, J. 1985. Serum creatine kinase activity and body composition in males and females. *Human Biology* 57:591.

57. Lane, R.J., and Roses, A.D. 1981. Variation of serum creatine kinase levels with age in normal females: Implications for genetic counseling in Duchenne muscular dystrophy. *Clinica Chimica Acta* 113:75.

58. Bundey, S., Crawley, J.M., and Edward, J. 1979. Serum creatine kinase levels in pubertal, mature, pregnant and post menopausal women. *Journal of Medical Genetics* 16:117.

59. Tiidus, P.M. 1999. Nutritional implications of gender differences in metabolism: Estrogen and oxygen radicals: Oxidative damage, inflammation, and muscle function. Chapter 11 in M. Tarnopolsky (ed.), *Gender differences in metabolism*. Baton Raton, FL: CRC Press.

60. Lord, S.R., Ward, J.A., and Williams, P. 1996. Exercise effect on dynamic stability in older women: A randomized controlled trial. *Archives of Physical Medicine and Rehabilitation* 77(3):232-236.

61. Pate, R.R., Pratt, M., Blair, S.N., et al. 1995. Physical activity and public health: A recommendation from the Centers for Disease Control and Prevention and the American College of Sports Medicine. *Journal of the American Medical Association* 273:402-407.

62. Marcus, B.H., Rakowski, W., and Rossi, J.S. 1992. Assessing motivational readiness and decision making for exercise. *Health Psychology* 11(4):257-261.

63. DiPietro, L. 1996. Habitual physical activity among women. In O. Bar-Or, D.R. Lamb, and P.M. Clarkson (eds.), *Perspectives in exercise science and sports medicine.* Vol 9: *Exercise and the female: A life-span approach.* Carmel, IN: Cooper Publishing Group.

64. Williams, P., and Lord, S.R. 1995. Predictors of adherence to a structured exercise program for older women. *Psychology and Aging* 10(4):617-624.

65. Dennerstein, L. Dudley, E. Guthrie, J., and Barrett-Connor, E. 2000. Life satisfaction, symptoms, and the menopausal transition. *Medscape Women's Health* 54(4):E4.

66. Ueda, M., and Tokunaga, M. 2000. Effects of exercise experienced in the life stages on climacteric symptoms for females. *Journal of Physiological Anthropology and Applied Human Science* 19(4):181-189.

67. Morse, C.A., Dudley, E., Guthrie, J., and Dennerstein, L. 1998. Relationships between premenstrual complaints and perimenopausal experiences. *Journal of Psychosomatic Obstetrics and Gynecology* 19(4):182-191.

68. Long, B.C., and Haney, C.J. 1988. Coping strategies for working women: Aerobic exercise and relaxation interventions. *Behavior Therapy* 19(1):75-83.

69. Guthrie, J.R., Dudley, E.C., Dennerstein, L., and Hopper, J.L. 1997. Changes in physical activity and health outcomes in a population-based cohort of mid-life Australian-born women. *Australian and New Zealand Journal of Public Health* 21(7):682-687.

70. Klem, M.L, Wing, R.R., McGuire, M.T., Seagle, H.M., and Hill, J.O. 1997. A descriptive study of individuals successful at long-term maintenance of substantial weight loss. *American Journal of Clinical Nutrition* 66:239-246.

71. Segar, M.L. 2000. *Fitting in fitness: Midlife women reframe physical activity and remain active.* Paper presented at the 3rd Yale Conference on Women's Health and Fitness, New Haven, CT.

INDEX

ABOUT THE AUTHOR

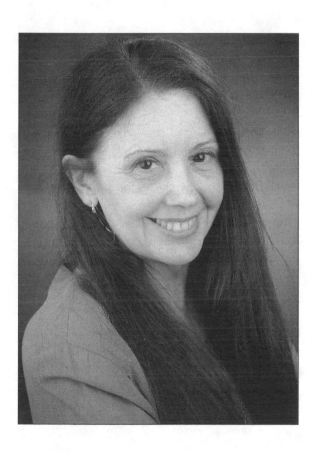

Ann Cowlin is a dance and movement specialist in the Athletic Department at Yale University and assistant clinical professor at the Yale University School of Nursing. A former professional dancer, she has taught both ballet and modern dance at Yale, as well as developed a course for the college seminar program entitled, "Movement and Mind." She danced with the Westchester (NY) Ballet Company, Pasadena Ballet Theater, Mesa Civic Ballet, and The Image Guild integrated arts company. She has performed in works by a number of modern dance choreographers, and appeared on the NBC Today show, as well as other television programs. Ann received her BA in Theater from Occidental College and her MA in Dance from UCLA, taught at Arizona State University, and has pursued interests in kinesiology and the neurology of movement as they relate to women. In 1979, she founded Dancing Thru Pregnancy®, and in 1984 began providing continuing education for professionals working in pre/postnatal health and fitness. She is the author of "Women and Exercise" in *Varney's Midwifery,* is a certified childbirth educator, has spoken at many national conferences on the topic of women and exercise, and has produced women's fitness programs for corporations, health departments, schools, and the U.S. Army.